Interventional Neuroradiology of the Spine

Mario Muto
Editor

Interventional Neuroradiology of the Spine

Clinical Features, Diagnosis and Therapy

Springer

Editor
Mario Muto
Neuroradiology Department
A. Cardarelli Hospital
Naples, Italy

ISBN 978-88-470-2789-3 ISBN 978-88-470-2790-9 (eBook)
DOI 10.1007/978-88-470-2790-9
Springer Milan Heidelberg New York Dordrecht London

Library of Congress Control Number: 2012952595

7 6 5 4 3 2 1 2013 2014 2015
Cover design: Ikona S.r.l., Milan, Italy
Typesetting: Grafiche Porpora S.r.l., Segrate (MI), Italy

Springer-Verlag Italia S.r.l. – Via Decembrio 28 – I-20137 Milan
Springer is a part of Springer Science+Business Media (www.springer.com)

Preface

Interventional neuroradiology is a relatively recently established subdiscipline of neuroscience and radiology that has expanded rapidly and now plays an important role in the diagnosis and treatment of brain and spine pathology of both vascular and non-vascular origin.

Spine pain is a dramatic social problem whose significance has grown even during the short course of the twenty-first century, with annual increases in incidence owing to the increase in average life expectancy, the "silent epidemic" of osteoporosis and the growing number of patients with primary or secondary spine tumors.

Among the many reasons for writing a book in the field of medicine are the desire to share your and your co-authors' experience with the scientific world, the wish to present your point of view on the diagnosis and treatment of particular pathologies and, especially, the importance of transmitting science to those working in other medical disciplines with a view to ensuring that disease is treated in the best possible way.

Bearing this in mind, starting from the basic anatomy and clinical approach, this book presents and describes not only the neuroradiological experience but also the medical, radiotherapy and surgical points of view regarding the optimal treatment of pathologies encountered in daily practice.

I would like to thank all the co-authors for the excellent job that they have done and for their prompt responses to my invitation to contribute to this book, which has ensured publication within a short time.

Naples, November 2012

Mario Muto, MD
Chief, Diagnostic and
Interventional Neuroradiology
A. Cardarelli Hospital, Naples, Italy
President of the Section of Neuroradiology
of the Italian Society of Radiology (SIRM)
Chairman of the Spine Section of the European
Society of Neuroradiology (ESNR)

Contents

Contributors

Cosma Andreula Chief of Radiology Service, Anthea Hospital, Bari, Italy

Giovanni Carlo Anselmetti Interventional Radiology Service, IRCC Candiolo, Italy

Giuseppe Bonaldi Interventional and Diagnostic Neuroradiology, Ospedali Riuniti, Bergamo, Italy

Matteo Bonetti Chief of Radiology Institute, Istituto Clinico Città di Brescia, Brescia, Italy

Paolo Cappabianca Department of Neurological Sciences, University of Naples Federico II, Naples, Italy

Alberto Cauli Rheumatology Unit, AOU Cagliari, Monserrato, Italy

Francesco Causin Neuroradiology Unit, Padua University Hospital, Padua, Italy

Alessandro Cianfoni Radiology Department, Medical University South Carolina, Charleston, SC, USA

Annamaria Colao Department of Molecular and Clinical Endocrinology and Oncology, Federico II University of Naples, Naples, Italy

Arturo Consoli Radiodiagnostic 2-3, Azienda Ospedaliero-Universitaria Careggi, Florence, Italy

Olga Corriero Department of Neurological Sciences, University of Naples Federico II, Naples, Italy

Oreste de Divitiis Department of Neurological Sciences, University of Naples Federico II, Naples, Italy

Pasqualino De Marinis Neurosurgery Unit, A. Cardarelli Hospital, Naples, Italy

Alvaro Antonio Diano Neuroradiology Department, A. Cardarelli Hospital, Naples, Italy

Rossella Di Franco Diagnostic Imaging and Radiotherapy, Second University of Naples, Naples, Italy

Carolina Di Somma IRCCS SDN Foundation, Naples, Italy

Federico D'Orazio Radiology Department, San Salvatore Hospital, L'Aquila, Italy

Massimo Falchini Radiodiagnostic 2-3, Azienda Ospedaliero-Universitaria Careggi, Florence, Italy

Sara Falivene Diagnostic Imaging and Radiotherapy, Second University of Naples, Naples, Italy

Joseph Gabrielli Neuroradiology Unit, Padua University Hospital, Padua, Italy

Massimo Gallucci Neuroradiology Department, San Salvatore Hospital, L'Aquila, Italy

Luigi Genovese Neurosurgery Unit, A. Cardarelli Hospital, Naples, Italy

Gianluigi Guarnieri Neuroradiology Department, A. Cardarelli Hospital, Naples, Italy

Giancarlo Guizzardi Department of Neurological Sciences, Neurosurgical Unit, Azienda Ospedaliero-Universitaria Careggi, Florence, Italy

Roberto Izzo Neuroradiology Department, A. Cardarelli Hospital, Naples, Italy

Marco Leonardi Chief of Neuroradiology Service, Bellaria Hospital, Bologna, Italy

Luigi Manfrè Department of Minimally Invasive Spine Surgery, AOEC "Cannizzaro", Catania, Italy

Stefano Marcia Radiology Department, SS. Trinità Hospital, ASL Cagliari, Cagliari, Italy

Mariangela Marras Radiology Department, AOU Cagliari, Monserrato, Italy

Salvatore Masala Department of Diagnostic and Molecular Imaging, Interventional Radiology and Radiotherapy, University Tor Vergata, Rome, Italy

Ernesto Mazza Radiodiagnostic 2-3, Azienda Ospedaliero-Universitaria Careggi, Florence, Italy

Vitor Mendes Pereira Service Neuro-diagnostique et Neurointerventionnel, Département de l'Imagerie et des Sciences de l'Information Médicale, Hôpitaux Universitaires de Genève, Geneva, Switzerland

Mario Muto Neuroradiology Department, A. Cardarelli Hospital, Naples, Italy

Paolo Muto Radiotherapy Unit, INT IRCCS Fondazione G. Pascale, Naples, Italy

Giovanni Nano Department of Diagnostic and Molecular Imaging, Interventional Radiology and Radiotherapy, University Tor Vergata, Rome, Italy

Pedro Nunnes Neuroradiology Department, Centro Hospitalar do Porto, Porto, Portugal

Emanuele Orrù Neuroradiology Unit, Padua University Hospital, Padua, Italy

Giannantonio Pellicanò Radiodiagnostic 2-3, Azienda Ospedaliero-Universitaria Careggi, Florence, Italy

Vincenzo Ravo Radiotherapy Unit, Cardinale Ascalesi Hospital, Naples, Italy

Jürgen Reul Beta Klinik International Head and Spine Center, Bonn, Germany

Manila Rubino Department of Molecular and Clinical Endocrinology and Oncology, Federico II University of Naples, Naples, Italy

Giovanni Simonetti Department of Diagnostic and Molecular Imaging, Interventional Radiology and Radiotherapy, University Tor Vergata, Rome, Italy

Pia C. Sundgren Diagnostic Radiology, Skåne University Hospital, BFC, Blekinkevägen, Lund, Sweden

Majda M. Thurnher Department of Radiology, University of Vienna, Vienna, Austria

Tommaso Volpi Department of Diagnostic and Molecular Imaging, Interventional Radiology and Radiotherapy, University Tor Vergata, Rome, Italy

Laura Vuolo Department of Molecular and Clinical Endocrinology and Oncology, Federico II University of Naples, Naples, Italy

Biomechanics of the Spine and Etiopathogenesis of Spinal Pain

1

Roberto Izzo and Mario Muto

1.1. Normal Motion in the Spine

The human spine is a multi-joint system controlled by muscles which supports the head and trunk and encloses and protects the spinal cord, the nerve roots and, at the cervical level, the vertebral arteries. Twenty-four highly specialized cervical, dorsal and lumbar motion segments (MS) together provide the significant range of motion (ROM) and load-bearing capacity needed for the physiological activities of daily life. Fused sacral vertebrae form a solid, tilted wedge-shaped base which transmits vertical spinal loads through the pelvic bones and hip joints to the lower extremities.

Within each motion segment MS, the smallest functional spinal unit (FSU) including two adjacent vertebrae with interposing soft tissues, a vertebra can perform, with respect to adjacent ones, three translations along and three rotational movements around each of the x-, y-, z- cartesian axes of space. Various combinations of main and coupled movements can also be carried out, the latter occurring simultaneously along or around an axis different from that of the principal motion [1]. Only limited movements are possible between adjacent vertebrae, but the sum of movements of all MS provides considerable spinal mobility in all major spatial planes. Differences in mobility between regions are due to the effect of the rib cage as well as differences in the shape, orientation and size of the articular and spinous processes.

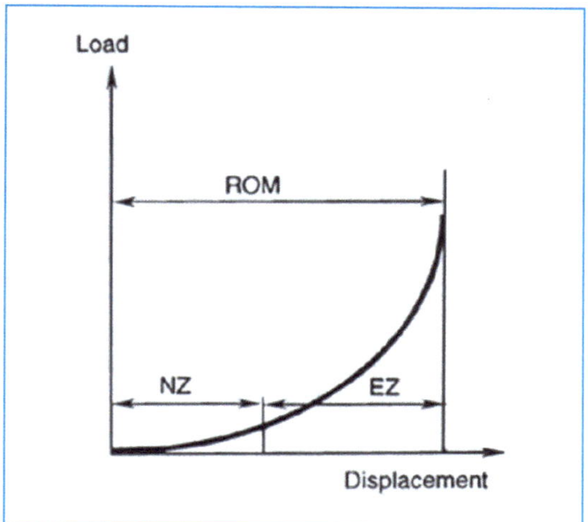

Fig. 1.1 Load/displacement curve of the motion segment. The load/displacement curve of the spine is not linear. The range of motion of the spinal joints includes an initial neutral zone (*NZ*) consisting in relatively large displacements at low load, and an elastic zone (*EZ*) that requires more load per unit of displacement because of the tension of capsules and ligaments

The fundament of the mechanics and motion of the spine is the highly nonlinear load/displacement ratio of the MS. This is because the effort required for movement changes significantly in its various phases [2] (Fig. 1.1). The physiologi-

R. Izzo (✉)
Neuroradiology Department, A. Cardarelli Hospital, Naples, Italy
e-mail: robertoizzo13@virgilio.it

M. Muto (ed.), *Interventional Neuroradiology of the Spine*,
DOI 10.1007/978-88-470-2790-9_1, © Springer-Verlag Italia 2013

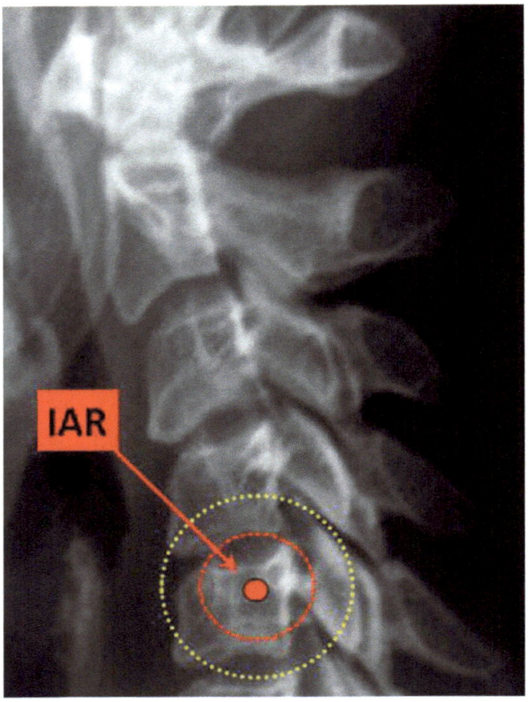

Fig. 1.2 During flexion-extension both vertebral bodies and facets rotate performing two circumference arcs around the same transversal instantaneous axis of rotation whose site changes according to spinal level. In the inferior cervical spine the IAR is located in the superior part of the subjacent vertebral body [3]

cal range of motion (ROM) includes a neutral zone (NZ) and an elastic zone (EZ) [2] (Fig. 1.1). The NZ is the initial part of intervertebral motion on either side of the neutral position, where it meets relatively scarce resistance and the spine exhibits high flexibility owing to the laxity of capsules, ligaments and tendons. The NZ is followed by the EZ, a zone of higher stiffness where the resistance to movement (and the slope of the curve representing it) increase linearly when the ligaments, capsules, fascias and tendons become tense, requiring more load per unit of displacement [2] (Fig. 1.1).

The biphasic nonlinear behaviour of the spinal joints probably meets two opposing needs: (i) to allow for movements near the neutral position to occur with as less muscle effort as possible and (ii) to ensure stability at the ends of joint excursions [2]. Each one of the six degrees of freedom of motion any vertebra can perform with respect to other ones has its own ROM, NZ and EZ [2].

According to Louis, during flexion–extension of the subaxial spine the vertebra moves around a transversal rotation axis placed not in the subjacent disk but in an area within the subjacent vertebral body (VB) [3] (Fig. 1.2). Either the disk and facets perform two circumferential arcs around the same rotation center whose location changes according to the level, being placed two VBs below in the cervical spine and in the superior endplate of the subjacent VB in the dorsal and lumbar spine [3] (Fig. 2.2). The low position of the rotation centers generates a coupled movement of anterolisthesis which varies from a maximum of 2–3 mm at C2-C3 to a minimum of 0.5 mm up to 1.5 mm from D1 to L5 [3].

Kanayama et al. observed that normal cervical and lumbosacral segmental motions occur not simultaneously but stepwise, starting from the upper levels and transmitting in a well-regulated way to the lower segments. In diseased spines, however, motion is initiated at the unstable segments [4]. Axial rotation and lateral bending are always coupled movements because of the oblique orientation of the facet joints and muscles. The coupling of these movements at the cervical level is dramatic [3]. The center of lateral bending will always be between the facets, but the center of axial rotation varies according to the level, being located in the central body for the dorsal spine and in the spinous processes for the lumbar segment [3].

By virtue of its peculiar anatomical and biomechanical features, the craniocervical junction (CCJ) has specific patterns of movement and biomechanics that are completely different from those observed in the subaxial spine. The CCJ is a transitional structure programmed to ensure the maximal mobility of the head in order to guarantee the complete visual and auditive exploration of space [5]. The CCJ, like a cardan joint, allows simultaneous and independent movements of the head around three axes of space to repeat and extend eye movements under the control of visual and vestibular receptors [5].

The occiput-C1–C2 complex is responsible for 40% of all cervical flexion–extension, and for 60% of global rotation [6–8]. Specifically, the

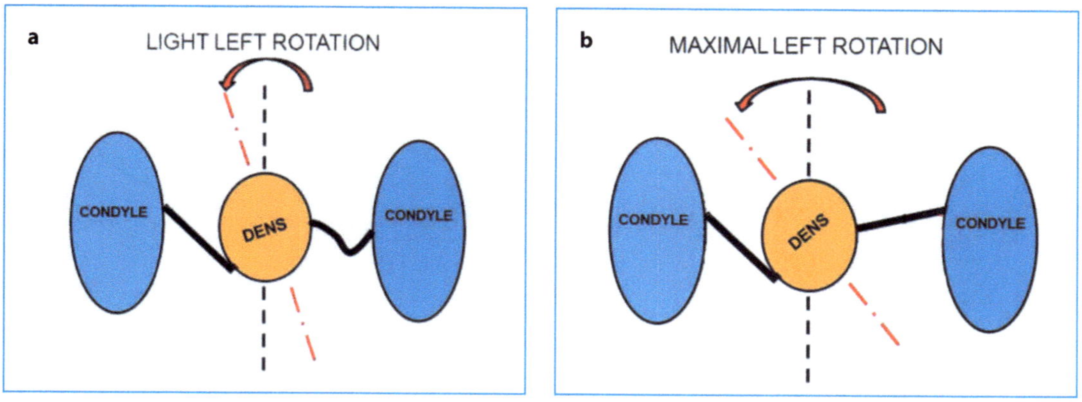

Fig. 1.3 Diagram of the alar ligaments viewed from above. Alar ligaments are the primary restraints of rotation of the head at C1-C2 joint. During axial rotation it comes in tension first the ligament on the side of rotation (**a**), then the contralateral one (**b**). At the end of movement the head is displaced contralaterally

C1-C2 joint (the most mobile individual joint in the entire spine) performs most of the rotation of the head [7, 9]. In the subaxial cervical spine, the frontal inclination of the facets allows much less axial rotation. Panjabi et al. reported a general tendency to decrease with aging for all movements of the cervical spine, except for the axial rotation of the CCJ [7].

The inferior obliquus muscle undertakes the first 30°of head rotation with a relatively fine action through its insertions on the transverse process of C1 and the spinous process of C2. This traction (which is unilateral and not balanced) creates a backwards translation of the atlas ring blocked by the contact with the dens [5]. The movement is therefore continued by the opposing powerful actions of the sternocleidomastoid (SCM) and splenius capitis (SCA) muscles. The superior insertions of these muscles are located far laterally on the mastoids, whereas the inferior attachments are near the median line to obtain the maximal rotation possible despite of the shortening capacity of just one-third of muscular length during contraction [5].

The alar ligaments are the primary restraints of C1-C2 axial rotation [10] (Fig. 1.3). The primary movement of the C0-C1 joint is flexion–extension, during which the occipital condyles rotate and move in posterior and anterior directions, respectively. During flexion–extension, the tectorial membrane and alar ligaments prevent sagittal translation between the basion and the tip of the dens (whose range is ≤1 mm), with a minor stabilising contribution coming from the cup-like facets of C1, whereas the transverse ligament prevents the forward shifting of anterior C1 ring. [11, 12].

1.2 Definition of Stability and Instability of the Spine

Several definitions of spinal stability based on biomechanical and clinical parameters have been postulated, but a specific definition is lacking. White and Panjabi defined the clinical stability of the spine to be "the ability under physiologic loads to limit patterns of displacement to not damage or irritate the spinal cord and nerve roots and to prevent incapacitating deformity or pain caused by structural changes" [12]. Larson defined the stable spine to be symmetrical in movement and configuration (normal or abnormal), with no change with time [13].

Apart from protection of nervous structures, spinal stability is the basic requirement for the: transfer of power forces between the upper and lower limbs; active generation of forces in the trunk; prevention of the early biomechanical deterioration of its own components; reduction of energy expenditure during muscle action [14, 15]. The loss of stability, i.e., instability, is an important often unknown cause of back pain particularly at the lumbar level.

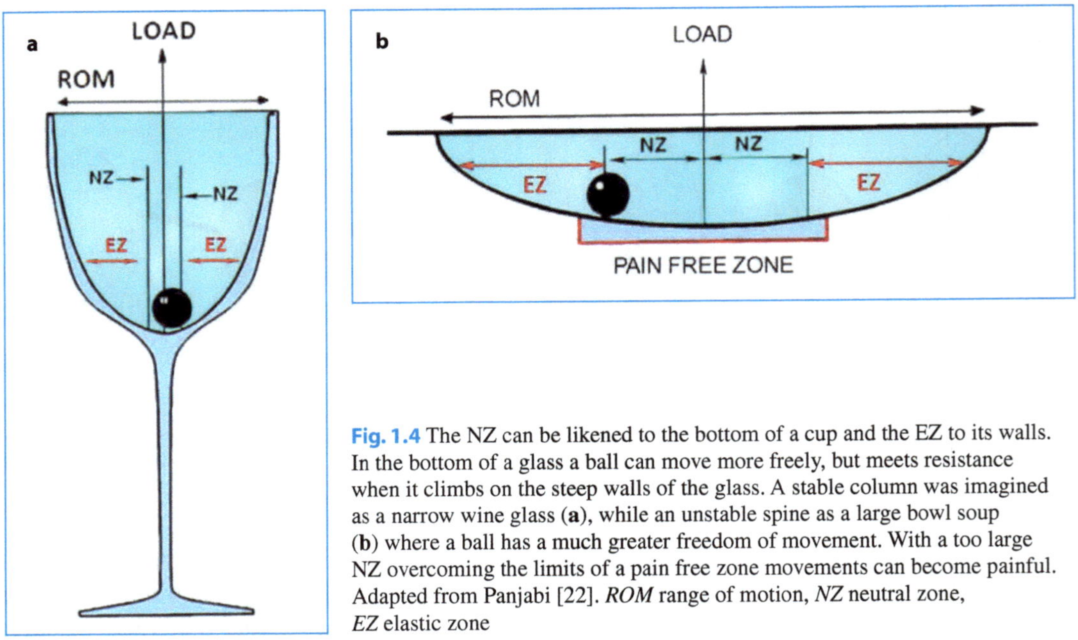

Fig. 1.4 The NZ can be likened to the bottom of a cup and the EZ to its walls. In the bottom of a glass a ball can move more freely, but meets resistance when it climbs on the steep walls of the glass. A stable column was imagined as a narrow wine glass (**a**), while an unstable spine as a large bowl soup (**b**) where a ball has a much greater freedom of movement. With a too large NZ overcoming the limits of a pain free zone movements can become painful. Adapted from Panjabi [22]. *ROM* range of motion, *NZ* neutral zone, *EZ* elastic zone

A widely accepted definition of instability is also lacking. White and Panjabi defined instability as "the loss of the ability of the spine under physiologic loads to maintain its patterns of displacement so there is no initial or additional neurologic deficit, no major deformity, and no incapacitating pain" [16]. Physiological loads are related to normal daily tasks and activities. According to Pope, instability is a loss of stiffness leading to abnormal and increased movement in the MS [17]. Most of the classic definitions of instability refer to a global increase of movements over the "normal limits" associated with back pain and/or root pain [16, 18]. Unfortunately, the definition of "normal or physiological movements" is controversial because the excessive overlap of the patterns of movement between symptomatic and asymptomatic subjects renders it difficult to define standard references and to correlate clinical with imaging findings [19]. Furthermore, with instability, movements can be abnormal in quality (abnormal coupling patterns) and/or in quantity (increased motion) [20]. Finally, because spinal movement is three-dimensional (3D) with coupled movements, dysfunctional motions also tend to occur in more than one direction [21]. This complexity makes clinical and imaging assessment of spinal instability quite challenging.

1.3 Spinal Stabilization

Stability implies an appropriate relationship between NZ and EZ [2, 22]. In reference to the load–displacement curves of the MS, Panjabi compared the NZ to the bottom of a glass in which a ball can move quite freely, and the extremities of the movement, the EZ, to the steeper walls of the cup on whose inclination the ball climbs meeting an increasing resistance [22] (Fig. 1.2a). A stable column was considered to be like a narrow champagne glass, whereas an unstable column like a large soup bowl [22] (Fig. 1.4).

According to a mechanistic hypothesis of spinal pain, in asymptomatic subjects NZ and ROM are normal and contained within the limits of a pain-free zone (PFZ) [22] (Fig. 1.4). In the unstable spine, the NZ increases over the limits of the PFZ [1, 22]. The severe disk collapse and osteophytosis, surgical fusion and muscular training all improve spinal stiffness, reduce the NZ and relieve pain. The size of the NZ has been shown to be the most sensitive parameter for the defini-

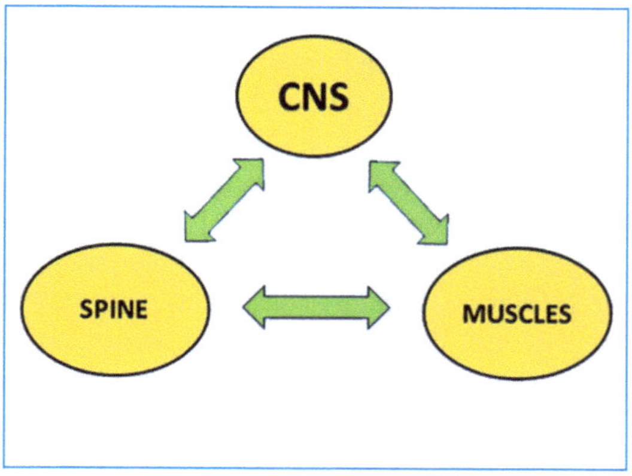

Fig. 1.5 Three subsystems control the stability of the spine: the spinal column, the muscles and the central nervous system. They are strictly related so any acute or chronic damage to a subsystem requires more compensatory work by the other ones. Modified from [77], reproduced with permission

tion of traumatic and degenerative spinal instability: it increases earlier and to a greater extent than ROM and EZ [2, 23, 24]. By observing the behaviour of the NZ in tests on cadaveric specimens and in animals, Panjabi redefined instability as the reduced ability by the stabilizing systems of the spine to maintain the NZs of the FSUs within physiological limits so that deformity, neurological deficit or disabling pain do not occur [2, 25].

The stabilization system comprises three closely related subsystems [25] (Fig. 1.5):

- the column or passive subsystem
- the muscle and tendon or active subsystem
- the unit of central nervous control

In the passive subsystem bones, disks and ligaments have an intrinsic structural role. They mainly control the EZ near the extreme parts of normal movement, where the tension of ligaments tendons, capsules and disk annulus restrain movement [26]. Degeneration or traumatic lesion of bony and soft components of the spine tends to expand the ROM and the NZ. This places a greater demand on the muscles and central nervous systems (CNS) in order to preserve or restrict segmental instability [2, 25]. Disks, ligaments and tendons also behave as "transducers" through mechanoreceptors which send a continuous flow of proprioceptive information about loads, motions and posture from each FSU to the CNS which, in turn, replies *via* an appropriate and coordinated feedback muscular action [22, 25, 27–29]. The muscles and CNS mainly control the NZ of the movement of FSUs, where the intrinsic stiffness and resistance of spinal MS are low [25, 30].

1.3.1 Passive Subsystem

During everyday activities, the spine can support vertical loads of 500–1000 N, over twice the body weight, and, during lifting tasks, up to 5000 N [31] near 50% of final failure load. The passive subsystem is dependent upon the:

- vertebral architecture and bone mineral density (BMD);
- disk–vertebral joints;
- facet joints;
- ligaments;
- physiological spinal curves

1.3.1.1 Vertebral Architecture and the BMD

The load-bearing capacity of the VB is dependent upon its size and shape, the integrity of the trabecular system, and the BMD. The progressive increase in body size downwards in the spine is the only physiological solution to increasing weight loads. The average strength ranges from 2,000 N in the cervical segment up to the 8,000 N in the lumbar spine [32].

The VB mainly consists of spongy trabecular bone having a 3D "honeycomb" structure similar to that of airplane wings that yields the best strength/weight ratio [3]. In the cancellous bone of any VB there are four main trabecular systems having a quite constant orientation [3, 33]:

- A vertical system extending between the endplates which accepts and transmits vertical loads;
- A horizontal system travelling in the posterior arch and joining the transverse processes;
- Two curved oblique systems (superior and inferior) that start from the endplates, cross in the peduncles, and end in the spinous and joint processes, with function of withstanding the horizontal shear stresses.

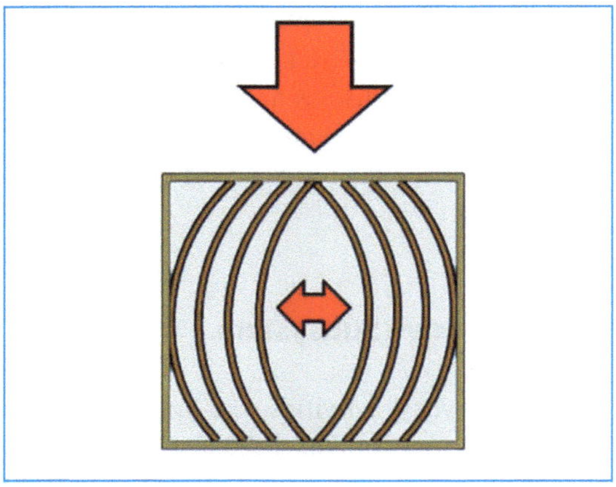

Fig. 1.6 Vertical compressive loads are first accepted by the vertical trabecular columns of the vertebral body. Without the horizontal lamellae which normally favour the radial dispersion of forces, the columns would bow under loads with a consequent loss in resiliency of the vertebral body

Axial loads are initially accepted by vertical "trabecular struts" that would bow if were not restrained by the tension of the horizontal lamellae which favour the horizontal dispersion of the vertical loads and confer resilience to cancellous bone (Fig. 1.6). The endplates, consisting of a thin layer of semiporous subchondral bone and an overlying cartilage layer of similar thickness, prevent extrusion of the disk into the VB, and distribute load evenly to the VB [34].

With respect to spongy bone, the very thin cortical shell (average thickness = 0.4 mm), although highly resistant, has a far lower elasticity and contributes to the overall loadbearing capacity of the VB for less than 15% [35].

The resistance of spongy bone is also heavily dependent upon the BMD. The bone loss in osteoporosis results in a disproportionate exponential reduction of resistance: a bone loss of 25% leads to a reduction of resistance of about 50% [36]. The mechanical resistance of a column decreases by the square of increasing length and by the square of decreasing cross section.

During the early stages of osteoporosis, the resorption of cross-linking trabeculae causes progressive elongation of the vertical columns, with a reduction in the buckling strength. The thinning of the columns themselves in more advanced stages leads to a summation of the two processes.

A strong and continuous correlation between spinal BMD and fracture risk has been established even though a defined threshold value for the BMD under which the vertebral failure occurs has not been established [36]. A vertebra can fatigue after repetitive loading [37]. Vertebral fatigue begins as focal osseous micro-damage that extends until the final failure. The bone resorption observed in osteoporosis is heterogeneous and mainly involves the anterior half of the VBs [38, 39].

In the elderly, because of degenerative disk collapse, forces are no longer evenly distributed on the endplates. Hence, much more load is assumed by the posterior facets when standing erect. This relative stress-shielding effect of the anterior bodies predispose to the local loss and weakening of bone. This is because, according to Wolff's law, bones adapt their mass and architecture in response to the magnitude and direction of forces habitually applied to them [40–42]. If the relative offloading standing posture is followed by spinal flexion, a very high increase in stresses (≤300%) occurs on the weakened anterior bodies [42]. The very high loading disparity could predispose to collapse of the anterior bodies. This explains why this region is frequently the site of osteoporotic fracture, and how forward bending movements often precipitate injury [42]. VB fractures modify the mechanical properties of the injured vertebra as well as the adjacent disks and vertebrae.

1.3.1.2 Disk-vertebral Joints

The disk allows complex motion without the mechanical limitations of the opposing articular surfaces of diarthrodial joints [34].Owing to its peculiar structure, the disk has the tension-resisting properties of a ligament and the compression-resisting properties typical of joint cartilage. The disk behaves as a ligament, allowing and controlling the complex 3D movements of the spine: vertical compression and distraction, flexion–extension, lateral bending, and axial rotation.

The outermost fibers of the annulus are the first controller of the abnormal micro-movements of a normal MS. Experimental diskectomies have been shown to cause a significant increase in movements (especially flexion–extension) [43]. With the nucleus behaving like a pressured cylinder, the disk is also the main "shock-absorber" of mechanical stresses transmitted during motion to the skull and brain. [44]. The nucleus pulposus mainly works in the NZ, bearing low axial loads, whereas the stiffer annulus fibrosus accepts a larger proportion of the highest loads [45].

If the disk is exposed to eccentric loads, the nucleus tends to move toward the region of lower pressure, where the annulus fibers are placed under tension. The biomechanical behavior of a normal, young nucleus is homogeneous and isotropic, equal in all its parts and in all directions. That is, whatever the spatial position of the spine, the load is transmitted evenly on the endplates, thereby avoiding any focal concentration [44, 47]. In contrast, in a degenerated disk, the nucleus loses its normal fluid-like properties and loads asymmetrically, thereby assuming a solid-like behavior [47]. A study of stress profilometry by Adams showed reduction and depressurization of the functional nucleus as well as enlargement of the functional annulus by up to 80%, along with a peak of up to 160% of compressive stresses in the dorsal annulus [48].This irregular distribution and transmission of loads can cause or contribute to acute and chronic pain.

Unlike the nucleus, the fundamental biomechanical property of the annulus is high anisotropy in tension, with a tensile modulus increasing up to 1,000-fold along the alignment of the collagen fibers [46, 49]. In each lamella of the annulus, collagen fibers are aligned strictly with a 30° inclination with respect to the endplate surface. The inclination of the fibers alternates in adjacent lamellae, forming an angle of 120°.

If a normal disk is loaded, the pressurized nucleus transmits loads in all directions, putting the annulus fibers in uniform tension. Bending movements induce maximum tensile and compressive loads on the opposing sides of the outermost annulus layers, along with annulus bulging on the compression side and stretching on the tensile side. During axial rotation, the disk experiences twisting shear stresses with only half of the annulus fibers engaged (those being parallel to the direction of rotation) until delamination eventually occurs. With degenerative depressurization of the nucleus, the annulus fibers are no longer pushed outwards but are instead loaded in compression [48]. The changes in the tensile properties of the annulus that occur with aging and degeneration of the disk are relatively small compared with the morphological changes [34]. Under very high compressive loads, the endplate usually fails first than the disk [50, 51].

The water content and thickness of the disk change continuously during normal daily activities under the opposite influences of hydrostatic and osmotic pressures [52].

Under compressive loads, the high hydrostatic pressure leads to a gradual release of water out of the disk, whose thickness fades until it is counterbalanced by the osmotic pressure exerted by proteoglycans, whose concentration increases progressively [52]. In the recumbent position, the re-prevailing osmotic pressure again recalls water and nutrients back into the disk [53]. In the degenerating disk, the reduced hydrostatic pressure of the nucleus displaces compressive loads on the internal annulus. The internal annulus folds inward and undergoes shearing stresses, predisposing fissures and delamination that can lead to structural fatigue and impaired cellular responses [54]. The fracture of the endplate and the Schmorl herniation drastically reduce the disk pressure, thereby accelerating the degeneration and destruction of the annulus [55].

1.3.1.3 Facet Joints

Facet joints fulfil two basic functions: control of the direction and amplitude of movement; and load sharing. Facet joints resist horizontal forces acting on the spine, and protect the lumbar disks from excessive shear and torsion [56].

According to the three-column model proposed by Louis, the weight of the head and trunk is transmitted first on two columns placed on the same frontal plane (the atlanto-occipital lateral joints) then, from C2 to L5, on three columns arranged like a triangle with an anterior vertex [3]. The anterior column comprises the bodies and disks, the two posterior columns the facet joints. Normally, between the three columns there exists a balanced and modular action for which the posterior facets, according to the posture, accept from 0% up to 33% of the load. However, in the case of hyperlordosis, high and prolonged weight-loading, and disk degeneration, the percentage can increase to 70% [57]. As for the VBs, the increasing size of the facets downwards compensates for the increasing functional demand.

The symmetry of the facet joints is an essential requirement for correct functioning. Each significant asymmetry predisposes to instability and to premature degeneration of the facet joints and disks [58]. Longstanding remodelling and destabilization of the facet joints, along with degenerative changes of the posterior ligaments, lead to degenerative spondylolisthesis, with the sagittal orientation of the facet joints acting as a predisposing factor [59, 60]. Patients showing narrow inferior articular processes and facet joint spaces visible on anteroposterior (AP) radiographs or with narrow facet-joint angles on axial views on magnetic resonance imaging (MRI) and computed tomography (CT) are likely to develop degenerative spondylolisthesis [61].

Facet-joint angles >45° relative to the coronal plane have been found to have a 25-times greater likelihood of developing degenerative slippage [62]. An estimated 15% to 40% of chronic cases of low back pain (LBP) are caused by lumbar facet joints, primarily because of mechanical stresses and deformation of the joint capsule with activation of nociceptors [30].

Pain induced from overpressure originating in the facet joints and/or posterior annulus of the lumbar spine may be relieved by spacing of the interspinous processes [63]. The function of interspinous spacers is to provide a posterior shift of the instantaneous rotation axis (IAR) of MS towards the region of increased stiffness (behind the facet joints), thereby reducing the compressive loads on the facet joints during a standing posture and extension movements.

1.3.1.4 Ligaments

Ligaments act as passive stabilizers of the spine. The stabilizing action of a ligament is dependent not only upon its intrinsic strength, but also on the length of the lever arm through which it acts,

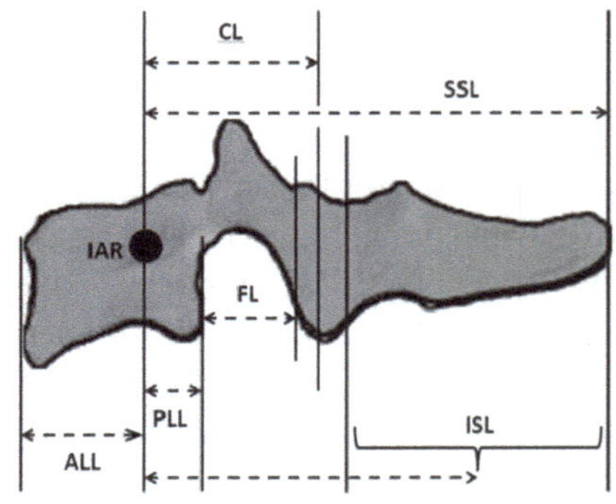

Fig. 1.7 Schematic diagram showing the distance between ligaments insertions and vertebral IAR forming the lever arm through which the ligament acts. The interspinous (*ISL*) and supraspinous (*SSL*) ligaments are located far apart from the IAR and work with a long lever arm. They oppose the spinal flexion more than the flaval (*FL*) and capsular ligaments (*CL*) having a shorter lever arm. The posterior longitudinal ligament (*PLL*), being very close to the spinal IAR and intrinsically less resistant, is twice mechanically disadvantaged. *ALL* anterior longitudinal ligament

corresponding to distance between the bony insertion, point of application of force, and the IAR of the VB, the fulcrum around which the vertebra rotates without moving at any given moment during a movement [64] (Fig.1.7).

A very strong ligament with a short lever arm may contribute to stability less than a weaker ligament working with a longer lever arm that gives it a mechanical advantage. The interspinous ligament (ISL) and supraspinous ligament (SSL) are located far from the IAR and work with a long lever arm. They oppose the spinal flexion more than the flava ligaments (FL), which have a shorter lever arm [65] (Fig. 1.7). The posterior longitudinal ligament (PLL), being very close to the spinal IAR and intrinsically less resistant, is two times mechanically disadvantaged.

An important principle in evaluating the stability of the CCJ is that many ligaments (and bony restraints) control and stabilise the C0-C1 and C1-C2 compartments simultaneously. For example, in the C0-C1 joint, the work of the intrinsic ligaments such as the capsules as well as the anterior and posterior atlanto-occiptal membranes is flanked by "extrinsic" ligaments connecting the occiput and C2, such as the tectorial membrane, the alar ligament and apical ligament [66]. In the CCJ, the alar and transverse ligaments provide much of the stability of the healthy spine. The transverse ligament (the most important component of the cruciate ligament) avoids anterior displacement of the atlas during axial rotation, thereby guaranteeing free pivoting of the dens.

By virtue of a special lattice arrangement of the collagen fibers, the transverse ligament has been shown in biomechanical tests to have a failure strength of 170–700 N (corresponding to about 17–70 kg) [67]. The transverse ligament avoids anterior displacement of the atlas during flexion and axial rotation. An increase >3 mm of the atlantodental space or reduction <13 mm in the distance between the posterior surface of the dens and anterior cortical surface of the posterior ring of C1 can occur only if there is a failure in the transverse ligament (with an intact dens), whose action cannot be supplied by the alar ligaments and tectorial membrane [68].

The alar ligaments control rotation at C1-C2. In the neutral position, the alar ligaments are lax. The rotation first puts in tension the ligament of the same side, then the contralateral one (Fig. 1.3). The failure of the alar ligament (reported to occur at about 200 N [67]) provokes a mean increase in the contralateral rotation of approximately 11–30° which is divided equally between the occipito-atlantal and atlanto-axial joints [69]. The very strong ventral ring of C1 as well as the transverse and alar ligaments guide rotation: an intact dorsal ring of C1 is not necessary for stability.

1.3.1.5 Spinal Curvature

Sagittal curvature represents the evolutionary response to the needs of a standing position and biped walking with little expenditure of energy [70]. Dorsal kyphosis is the only congenital sagittal spinal curvature. Cervical and lumbar lordoses develop with head rising and standing and walking, respectively.

In health and disease, sagittal spine curvature is regulated by pelvic geometry: pelvic incidence, (PI), sacral slope (SS) and pelvic tilt (PT) [70, 71]. The PI is a fixed morphological parameter which remains unchanged for each subject after birth: any change in sagittal balance is obtained through adaptation of other positional parameters [71]. In health and disease, to ensure that the trunk is centred over the femoral heads, an increased SS leads to increased lumbar lordosis and dorsal kyphosis. After lumbar or thoracolumbar wedge fractures, local kyphosis can be compensated by hyperlordosis of the caudal MS and, if necessary, hypokyphosis of the cephalad segment, but always within the limits dictated by pelvic geometry [72]. Sagittal spinal curvatures contribute to spinal stability, increasing ≤17 times the resistance to vertical loads by directing deformations into pre-ordered directions which can be quickly controlled by the fast intervention of muscle contraction [3]. Physiological curvatures can also influence the spinal response to traumatic forces.

In the thoracic spine, owing to kyphosis, the vertebrae are subjected to eccentric loads which concentrate the stresses on the anterior part of the bodies, predisposing to wedge compression fractures [73]. In the lordotic segments, vertical vector forces running near or through the vertebral IARs are more evenly distributed on the endplates. According to the Newton's third law, equal and opposite forces act on the endplates, thereby predisposing to central or burst fractures [73].

1.3.2 Active Subsystem and Central Nervous Control

The active subsystem comprises muscles and tendons which, under control of the nervous system, ensure stability primarily in the NZ (where the resistance to movement is minimal).

Muscle actions are needed to stabilize the spine during standing, lifting and bending. Without muscles, the spine would be highly unstable even under very light loads [25, 30]. Muscles can be divided into superficial (rectus abdominis, sternocleidomastoid) and deep (psoas) flexors as well as superficial (long) and deep (short) extensors. The function of the superficial, multisegmental muscles differs from that of the deep unisegmental muscles [74].

The short muscles (intertrasversous, interspinous, multifidus) are small and located very close to vertebral rotation axes. They act chiefly as "force transducers", sending feedback responses to the CNS about the movement, load and position of the spine [75]. The long superficial muscles are primarily responsible for the genesis of movements. The complexity of the posterior musculature excludes any voluntary control upon single units. The CNS receives extensive inputs from all bones, joints (passive subsystem), muscles and tendons (active subsystem) to regulate and coordinate muscular posture and movement [25, 76]. At the CCJ, the coordinated action of muscles and joints under CNS control probably reaches maximal complexity and sophistication.

In order to obtain a stereoscopic vision and the fusion of the images coming from both halves of the visual scene the light pulses have to be directed on both the maculae [5].

This occur thanks to the coordinated action of the orbital and neck muscles.

The complex coordination between ocular and neck muscles is realized thanks to the fasciculus longitudinalis medialis (FLM), an associative fibers tract that connect the vestibular, oculomotor and XI nerve motor nuclei, and the CCJ which consents simultaneous and independent movements about the three axes of space [5]. If acute or chronic damage occurs to a spinal component and in the mechanoreceptors it contains, abnormal transducer signals are generated and sent to the CNS, causing altered motor responses with impaired temporal and spatial coordination [77]. The altered muscle response, in turn, increases the mechanical stress of spinal bones and joints, and also creates an abnormal feedback response which reaches the CNS. It sets a vicious cycle that leads to the development of inflammation, muscle fatigue, and the stimulation of nociceptors with the onset and maintenance of pain [77] (Fig. 1.8).

Subjects with chronic LBP show impaired neuromuscular control with delayed muscle responses and offset in carrying out voluntary movements as well as a reduced postural control compared with asymptomatic subjects [77–80]. While the transverse abdominis and multifidus muscles stabilize the spine before initiating a movement or accepting a load, in patients suffering from chronic spinal pain such contractions are delayed [78, 81].

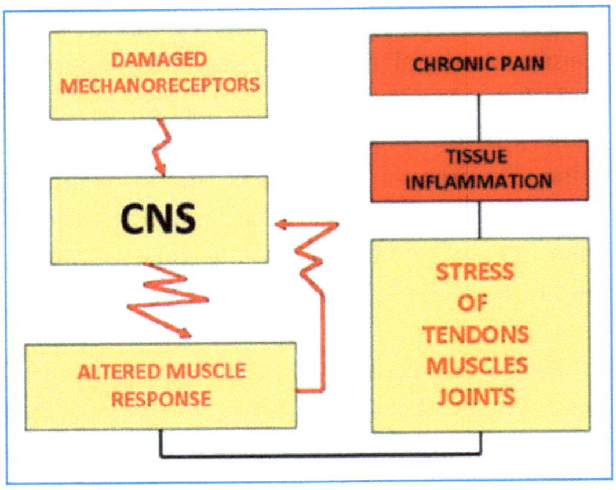

Fig. 1.8 In case damage to ligaments, discs, joint capsules and to mechanoreceptors they contain abnormal transducer signals are generated and sent to the CNS. This causes an altered motor response which, in turn, increases the mechanical stress of bony and joint spinal components and elicits an abnormal feedback response by the FSUs and the muscles themselves. A vicious cycle is so crated that leads with time to the development of inflammation, muscle fatigue, activation of nociceptors. Modified from [77], reproduced with permission

Scheilp suggested that the thoracolumbar fascia (rich of Ruffini and Vater–Pacini corpuscles in all of its three layers), if damaged, could be implicated in the genesis of chronic pain through abnormal stimulation of the CNS [82]. Rehabilitation programs that improve neuromuscular control may also improve functional disability [78].

1.4 Spinal Pain

Spinal pain ,and especially low back pain (LBP), with or without radiculopathy, is extremely common and represents a major cause of disability [83]. The lifetime prevalence of LBP and neck pain in adults is 91% and 66.7%, respectively [84, 85]. In the US, LBP is the leading cause of disability for people aged <45 years and is the second leading cause of disability worldwide [86]. An estimated 1% of the world population are disabled by back pain [84]. The incidence

Table 1.1 Findings that should raise suspicions for more serious causes of low back pain and which should be investigated further

• History of trauma
• Incontinence or retention in the bowel or bladder
• History of cancer
• Unexplained weight loss
• History of intravenous drug use
• Systemic illness or infection
• Low back pain with fever
• Constant progressive pain at night
• Prolonged systemic use of corticosteroids
• Advanced age
• Saddle anesthesia

of LBP is increasing with respect to population growth. This trend represents a major economic burden upon healthcare and welfare systems in western countries. For example, in the USA, it accounts for approximately 70–90% of the total compensation expenditure for workers [87].

LBP can be classified as "acute" (lasting ≤4 weeks), "subacute" (5–12 weeks) and "chronic" (>12 weeks). This distinction has important prognostic implications because, whereas acute forms are considered benign and resolve spontaneously in most cases, chronic pain resolves in <5–10% of cases [88, 89]. Nevertheless, recently the long-held notion that acute non-specific back pain is usually benign, transient and self-limiting [90] has been reconsidered. A 1-year recurrence rate for acute LBP of 20–44% and a lifetime recurrence of ≤72% has been reported [91]. For these reasons, the study of the etiopathogenesis of spinal pain has become very important, deserving special attention to the interaction between the biomechanics and biochemistry of disk degeneration as well as its influence on the other spinal components.

Up to 80% of patients complaining of LBP in the primary care setting present with non-specific LBP [88]. A comprehensive history and physical examination must exclude the small percentage of patients with serious underlying conditions that require further investigation. Findings that should raise suspicion for more serious causes of LBP and which should prompt the clinician to investigate further are shown in Table 1.1 [92]. After excluding serious disease, the next main difficulty is precisely locating the pain source. The complexity of spinal anatomy and its innervation renders such precise localization very difficult.

1.4.1 Neuroanatomy of the Spine

Spinal innervations comprise: somatic sensitive fibers travelling in the spinal nerves; and sympathetic sensitive fibers coming from paravertebral ganglia and chains [93–97]. The nerve supply of the dorsal part of anterior spine is mainly dependent upon somatic sensitive fibers travelling in the sinuvertebral nerve and in a small branch of the primary ventral ramus of the spinal nerve.

The recurrent meningeal or sinuvertebral (Luschka) nerve is formed by union of the gray ramus communicans with a small branch coming from the anterior ramus of the spinal nerve [94, 98, 99] (Fig. 1.9). It immediately re-enters the neural foramen by passing just below the pedicle, runs along the middle of the posterior VB, and finally sends ascending and descending branches in the spinal canal, which anastomose to form a plexus on the dorsal aspect of the posterior longitudinal ligament [94]. The sinuvertebral nerve is a mixed polysegmentary nerve supplying the: external posterolateral annulus; PLL; ventral meninges; anterior epidural vessels; posterior VB and periosteum [96].

Sympathetic trunks and ganglia directly innervate the: anterior longitudinal ligament (ALL); anterior periosteum and VB; perivertebral mus-

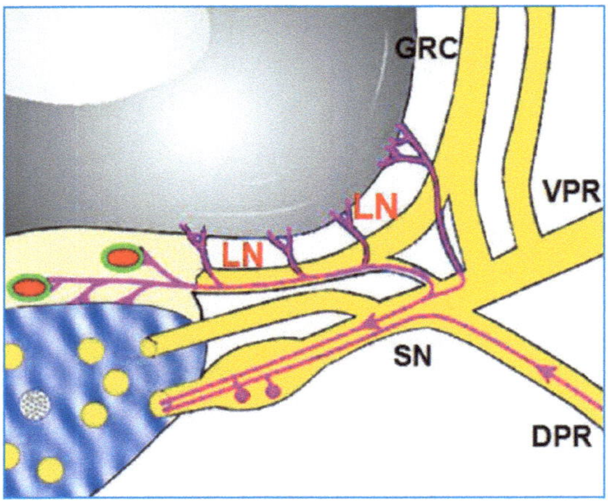

Fig. 1.9 The recurrent meningeal or sinuvertebral (Luschka) nerve is formed by the union of the gray ramus communicans with a little branch coming from the anterior ramus of the spinal nerve. It enters the foramen and divides in anastomizing ascending and descending branches. *SN* spinal nerve, *LN* Luschka nerve, *DPR* dorsal primary ramus, *VPR* ventral primary ramus, *GRC* gray ramus communicans

cle-fascias; most peripheral laminae of the anterolateral disk [93, 98]. From these structures, the fibers passing through the white ramus communicans can directly reach the ventral branch of the spinal nerve and dorsal ganglion (where the cell bodies lie) or enter the sinuvertebral nerve through the gray rami communicantes, distributing in this way directly or indirectly to the whole anterior spine [93, 98, 100].

The autonomic fibers form a nerve plexus along the surface of ALL (paravertebral autonomic neural plexus) containing nociceptive fibers. However, the role of the anterolateral bodies and disks as sources of LBP remains controversial [93, 98, 100]. *Via* the somatosensory fibers reaching directly the spinal cord in a regular way and at every level, any injury in the anterior spine can provoke a well-circumscribed and localized somatic pain [101]. While the somatic fibers account for the well-localized pain, the autonomic afferents are considered responsible for the referred pain [101].

Either radicular and referred pain are "false mental representations of sensory events"being experienced at sites other than the real source. While radicular pain is well-discriminated and distributes in a quite constant cutaneous dermatome, referred pain is diffuse, deep, not well discriminated, and perceived in the somatome area [101, 102]. A somatome area includes all tissues originating embryologically from the same somite, sharing common neural circuitry and common pathway of referral.

Several anatomic factors contribute to the "loose" localization of referred sympathetic sensory inputs: absence of an anatomic midline between sympathetic chains; irregular vertical segmentation of the autonomic plexus; and the ascending diversion of impulses [103]. Because of the absence of white communicantes rami below the L2 level, any sympathetic afferent from the L3–S1 level must ascend in the sympathetic chain at least up to the L2 level before reaching the CNS [103]. In this way, sympathetic pain impulses from the lumbosacral region are referred to somatomes corresponding to level of L2 or above, and the areas of referred pain from all lumbar levels concentrate and superimpose within the superficial somatomes of the upper lumbar nerves [101, 104].

Referred pain can also involve visceral tissues because of the convergence of visceral and somatic sensory afferents on the same fiber tracts of the CNS, and/or the presence of viscerosomatic neurons with bifurcating sympathetic axons distributing in visceral and somatic tissues [105–107]. In both cases of impulse convergence, the CNS may not be able to discriminate the real origin of a painful signal.

Apart from the perception of painful stimuli, the autonomic nervous system can also mediate automatic reflexes and subconscious functions which also may be spatially misregistered. Referred centrifugal autonomic dysfunctions can include vasomotor, pilomotor, and sudomotor activities or muscle spasms [108]. In the cervical spine, intrathecal anastomoses between nerve rootlets contribute to the variability of the patterns of referred pain. In the dorsal spine, referred pain is much more common than radicular pain. Thoracic disk herniations rarely cause radicular pain. Many cases of actual referred pain are misdiagnosed as radicular pain [109].

1.4.2 Pathophysiology of Spinal Pain

Pain is a complex perception influenced by previous experience and by the context in which the noxious stimulus occurs [110]. Any injury involving the disks, ligaments and bones of the spine elicits pain through tissue inflammation and production of a cascade of mediators such as prostaglandins (PGs), bradykinin, serotonin, histamine, excitatory amino acids, nitric oxide (NO), nerve growth factor (NGF) and hydrogen ions, all of which directly activate afferents and/or sensitize nociceptors [111, 112]. Peripheral nociceptors can be specific (thermal, mechanical, chemical) or polymodal, also referred to as "wide dynamic range neurons" (WDRNs) because they can respond to all stimuli.

Fibers transmitting painful stimuli include C-type, unmyelinated (responsible of long-lasting pain), A-delta, myelinated (accounting for fast, sharp pain) and A-gamma, the smallest myelinated fibers. A-beta fibers are normally proprioceptive, but can eventually undergo phenotypic changes and produce nociceptive neurotransmitters.

Acute pain is of recent origin, is related to a specific injury or disease, does not last long and provokes limited and temporary disability [113]. In acute pain, the signals reaching the dorsal horns of the spinal cord have the same intensity as those travelling in neo–paleo–spinothalamic tracts and a descending countersignal coming from supraspinal centers fades and eventually extinguishes arriving painful inputs (eudynia) [113, 114].

1.4.2.1 Central Pain Sensitization

The setting in of complex processes of peripheral and central sensitization may influence the evolution of acute pain and its conversion to chronic pain, i.e., the transformation of a symptom into a disease.

Hypersensitivity or sensitization consists in a decrease in the threshold of neuron activation, increased response to over-threshold stimuli and even spontaneous neuronal activity [110]. While acute pain extinguishes along with the underlying cause, chronic pain is much more difficult to treat. In the case of persistent or chronic pain, altered electrophysiological and biochemical responses mount, having little chance of responding to conventional therapies or fading spontaneously [113].

The continuous stimulation from peripheral nociceptors can lead the spinal cord to reach a "hyper-excitable" state with a "wind-up" response which expands receptive field areas through the properties of the WDRNs: neurons that do not normally transmit pain begin to do so [115, 116]. Simultaneously, others neurons fire with increased frequency and even spontaneously [113], resulting in hyperalgesia and allodynia.

The wind-up response has a biochemical basis involving the action of neurotransmitters. The unrelenting stimulation of the neurons in the dorsal horn promotes excessive release of substance P (SP) and glutamate from the presynaptic nerve endings of the peripheral primary-order neurons. The long-term depolarization of postsynaptic membranes of nociceptive-specific and WDRNs removes the block normally exerted by magnesium ions upon N-methyl-D-aspartate (NMDA) receptors [117].

The binding of glutamate to NMDA receptors and the hyper-activation of the receptors promotes cellular influx of calcium which, in turn, activates nitric oxide synthase (NOS), which then produces NO. NO diffuses across synapses and stimulates the presynaptic release of increasing amounts of SP and glutamate, creating and perpetuating a vicious cycle [117]. Simultaneously, activation of NMDA receptors induces the production and membrane placement of new receptors. Intracellular calcium also promotes the breakdown of prostanoids to arachidonic acid, resulting in CNS inflammation [118]. Just as in acute pain, the brain sends descending signals that modulate afferents but they are rendered ineffective by the wind-up response and by closed and reverberating neuronal circuits. Gamma-aminobutyric acid (GABA), the second most ubiquitous neurotransmitter in the CNS acting in health as a "brake" upon the CNS [113], loses its efficacy in front of excessive release of glutamate in central and peripheral nervous systems (PNS).

In health, several cerebral regions are connected to neo–paleo–spinothalamic tracts, but many more circuits and centers are recruited in chronic pain states. The wind-up response in fact also occurs at supraspinal levels in second-, third- and fourth-order neurons. Although a constant input is needed to initiate the wind-up response, very little (if any) input is needed to maintain it, creating a nightmare scenario of positive feedback with minimal (or absent) peripheral stimuli [113].

Neuroplastic mutations occur peripherally in dorsal ganglia and in the CNS, thereby transforming the symptom into a disease: maldynia [119]. The final result is a diffuse, unrelenting stimulation of brain centers leading to a significant sensitive and emotional response. In chronic pain states along with neuroplasticity and the wind-up response it may also develop neuroimmune and neuroinflammatory changes which contribute to the maintenance and amplification of pain [120]. In response to injury, glial cells and neurons are activated and produce pro-inflammatory cytokines (e.g., interleukin (IL)-1, IL-6, tumor necrosis factor (TNF)-a), which in turn increase the activation of the neurons themselves [121, 122]. Cytokines also promote the migration and infiltration of leukocytes from the periphery into the CNS, with further induction of pain mediators (glutamate, NO, PGs) [123]. In light of this possible evolution, it is very important to treat the symptom and its causes, start the therapy as soon as possible and, if the pain does not resolve, employ more aggressive treatment to prevent the pain from becoming chronic [113].

Interestingly, at the cerebral level, very similar biochemical reactions and events also occur in chronic affective disorders, depression, anxiety, panic and post-traumatic stress [124]. The influence of the CNS on chronic spinal pain has led several authors to reclassify it as a bio–psycho–social syndrome. It can now be seen as the final stage of a complex process that starts acutely due to an anatomical or biological event and then is transformed by psychosocial risk factors into a chronic illness [125, 126].

Psychosocial and economic problems (e.g., unemployment) as well as a history of back pain and unsuccessful treatments contribute to predict which patients will develop chronic pain [126–128]. Knowledge of the central influences on pain is fundamental to prevent conversion of acute spinal pain into chronic disease. While our efforts are focused upon the PNS, the success or failure of therapies are dependent upon how we treat the problem also at the central level [113].

1.4.3 Diskogenic Pain

The estimated prevalence of non-specific chronic LBP in adults varies from 15% to 80% [88, 129]. Only in a limited number of cases is the lumbar pain due to disk herniation. A major cause of non-specific lumbar pain is considered the disk disruption (with or without endplate degeneration), being responsible for diskogenic pain [130].

The type of disk lesion acting as the pain generator remains undefined and debated: disk degeneration, annular tears or endplate changes [131–133]. Moreover, clinically diskogenic pain tends to have a somatotropic rather than a dermatomal distribution pattern, which renders precise localization of the painful level difficult [96].

Within healthy disks, free nerve endings are present only in the outermost few millimeters or 2–3 external lamellae of the annulus, where tensile stresses overcome compressive loads. Nerve endings and capillaries coud not withstand high hydrostatic pressures within the inner annulus and the nucleus of healthy disks, but they can grow in the degenerated disks favored from the depressurization of the nucleus pulposus [87, 134, 135].

In extremely degenerated disks, nervous fibers expressing SP and having nociceptive endings (independent of vessels) can penetrate the nucleus [134, 135]. Freemont et al. analyzed specimens of degenerated lumbar disks deemed to be painful at provocative diskography and normal control disks using immunohistochemical methods. They found nociceptive endings expressing SP only in the nucleus pulposus of disks that were painful, suggesting their important role in the pathogenesis of chronic lumbar pain [134]. On the other hand, healthy nociceptors of the external annulus may be stimulated to undergo abnormal compression, stretching and movements secondary to instability or if peripheral tears expose them to effects of chemical mediators coming from the nucleus.

Distinguishing between the ageing and degeneration of disks is difficult and quite arbitrary. According to Adams et al., disk ageing is primarily associated with biochemical modifications that occur with time in each individual, whereas disk degeneration involves structural disruption and functional impairment beyond the limits of normal aging [136].

With respect to imaging, CT has too-limited contrast resolution for detecting the early signs of disk degeneration, being very sensitive only to detecting a vacuum and calcifications.

MRI consent to evaluate the morphological and biochemical status of the disk, and can equal diskography for showing the internal structure of a disk [137–139].

Pfirrmann et al. distinguished five degrees of progressive disk degeneration on MRI ranging from grade 1 (normal homogeneous hyperintense signal of the nucleus and internal annulus) up to grade 5 (diffuse hypointense signal and collapsed disk) [140]. Despite its high sensitivity, MRI has low specificity and accuracy for the detection of the cause and origin of pain because (i) abnormal findings in disks and endplates are often present in asymptomatic subjects; and (ii) abnormalities are often multiple and of no useful for identifying the origins of the symptoms [141, 142].

The clinical relevance of the abnormalities detected by MRI in subjects complaining of spinal pain has been questioned by several studies showing the frequency of similar findings in asymptomatic individuals. Jensen et al. carried out MRI studies of the lumbar spine in 98 asymptomatic subjects. They noted that 52% of individuals had a bulge in the disk in at least at one level, 27% had a disk protrusion, 1% had a disk extrusion, and only 36% had normal disks at all levels [143]. Kleinstuck et al. found disks to be completely normal in only 11% of asymptomatic individuals [144]. Boden et al. evaluated 67 individuals who had never suffered LBP and found 20% of patients aged <60 years had a herniated nucleus pulposus, and 1 patient with spinal stenosis. In patients aged >60 years, 37% had a herniated disk and 21% had spinal stenosis [145]. Moreover, in a follow-up study of asymptomatic subjects with no history of back pain, abnormal MRI findings, present in 31% of cases, were not predictive of future development or duration of LBP [146]. Imaging studies have only a complementary role to the clinical picture. Clinical correlation is always required to determine the significance of abnormal findings observed on MRI, and therapy cannot rely solely upon imaging abnormalities [146].

Degenerated disks with structural disruption in the annulus or endplate and a decompressed nucleus show high stress concentrations in the annulus (i.e., posterior to the nucleus) [87]. Such stress concentrations and irregular distribution of loads can give rise to pain even if the stresses are not severe enough to cause damage and if imaging studies do not reveal spinal disease to which symptoms can be attributed [87].

1.4.3.1 Peripheral Pain Sensitization

Mechanical phenomena regarding the disc or the nerve roots alone cannot adequately explain the clinics of pain:

- clinical improvement after anti-inflammatory drugs occur without change in pathologic state of the disc.
- very degenerated discs are often not painful

Pain perception is also dependent upon the inflammatory properties of degenerating disks as well as the biochemical mechanisms of pain sensitization.

In health, peripheral nociceptors have a high threshold of activation, and do not respond to physiological joint motion, pressure, stretching or muscular contraction. Inflammatory sensitization reduces the threshold for activation of diskal mechanoreceptors so that disk loading within the physiological range may cause pain. In degenerating disks, in response to abnormal loads or nutritional problems, chondrocytes:

- proliferate;
- replace proteoglycans with abnormal types of collagen;
- upregulate metalloproteinases (MMPs) which degrade the nucleus and annulus matrix;
- promote macrophage infiltration.

- macrophages in turn produce multiple inflammatory mediators: bradykinin, IL-I, NO, TNF-a, phospolipase A2 and NGF [147, 148].

Inflammatory mediators can directly activate nociceptors (bradykinin, serotonin, excitatory amino acids), sensitize them by lowering the thresholds for firing and, by increasing the firing rates and finally recruiting new receptors, broadening the area of perception (PGs, noradrenaline, NGF, serotonin, NO) [149].

Inflammatory sensitization of diskal nociceptors may also arise from nerve fibrils accompanying the ingrowth of granulation tissue into the annular tears or if radial tears reach the external annulus and nociceptors normally present within it. Vascularized granulation tissue and fluid collections within annular tears can be detected on MRI as high-intensity zones (HIZs). These appear as hyperintense compared with the nucleus and are completely included into the fibers of the annulus [150]. The granulation tissue seems to be a healing reaction to the annular injury, and the local inflammation it produces can stimulate the nociceptors generating pain from the fissures [151]. Disks that are simply aging will not be painful because they do not have tears nor granulation tissue along with nerve fibrils [151].

A comparative study between the presence of HIZs on MRI, diskography and post-diskography CT revealed high correlation to exact reproduction of pain with a sensitivity of 82% and specificity of 89% [150]. Similarly, 87% of HIZ disks assessed by Schellhas et al. were concordantly painful at diskography, all containing grade 3–5 annular tears using the modified Dallas diskogram scale [152, 153]. Conversely, Ricketson and Weishaupt did not demonstrate a significant correlation between HIZs on MRI and positive provocative diskography [154, 155].

The degeneration and disruption of disks are very often flanked by endplate changes. Modic et al. described three stages of endplates and subchondral bone modifications accompanying disk degeneration [156]. Several studies have suggested a role for endplate changes in LBP. Braithwaite et al. found good correlation between Modic changes on MRI and diskographic findings with a specificity of endplate abnormalities as markers of painful disks of 96.8%, and a positive predictive value (PPV) of 91.3% [157]. The clinical relevance of endplate changes seems to be confirmed by the low prevalence of Modic changes in asymptomatic subjects: Chung et al. found just 11 type-I lesions in 590 lumbar endplates in asymptomatic individuals [158]. Furthermore, the frequency of type-I changes was shown to increase significantly in the follow-up of subjects with chronic non-specific lumbar pain [159]. Modic type-I changes are common in painful instability and can be converted to more stable type-II and -III changes after fusion surgery, but can persist or reappear in cases of pseudoarthrosis or failed surgery [160] (Fig. 1.10). Weishaupt et al. described four degrees of Modic

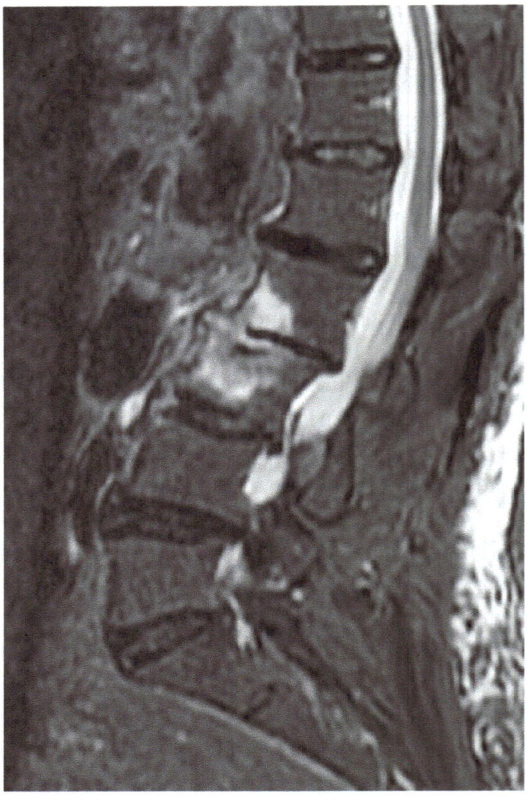

Fig. 1.10 50 year-old male with severe chronic LBP. MR sagittal FSE STIR MRI (TR/TE/TI=300/50/150ms) showing retrolisthesis of L2 secondary to disc collapse. Typical extended Modic type-I changes in the endplates of L2-L3 along with focal hyperintensity in anterior disc due to aseptic discitis is observed

changes ranging from grade I (normal) to grade IV (involving >50% of VH height). They stated that Modic type-I and -II changes of moderate-to-severe degree (degrees III–IV) were valuable indicators of symptomatic disk disease with a PPV of about 100% [161].

Finally, intradiskal nociceptors out from any inflammatory reaction can also be sensitized by the activity of sympathetic nerve efferents. Diskal sensitive endings are very close to sympathetic postganglionic efferent fibers which probably play neuroregulatory functions. The nervous arrangement of the disk (similar to that of enteric structures) suggests that diskal pain may be a form of visceral pain, which is unique in the muscoloskeletal system [162, 163].

1.4.4 Radicular Pain

Radicular pain is generally due to disorders of the nerve root proximal to or at level of the dorsal root ganglion (DRG) [164]. The pathophysiology of radicular pain is incompletely understood. Radicular pain is caused by disk herniation and canal stenosis. Two mechanisms are involved in the genesis of the radicular pain:

- mechanical (i.e., by direct compression of the nerve or DRG, or indirect compression on perineural vessels);
- inflammatory (i.e., by autoimmune cellular responses mounted if the disk is no longer segregated by the annulus and instead is recognized as "non-self" by the immune system) and biochemical (though the action of mediators expressed by disk itself, such as phospholipase-A2, PGE2, IL-6 and MMPs) [165–167].

In a model of lumbar radiculopathy, a positive correlation was found between pain behaviour, levels of messenger ribonucleic acid (mRNA) to produce cytokines and the magnitude of root compression [168]. Consistent with these observations is the graded microglial activation that occurs in the spinal cord in response to various degrees of deformation of the lumbar nerve roots [169]. Inflammatory cells and inflammatory mediators are, in general, more abundant in non-contained herniations than in contained herniations and in degenerative disks, whereas they are absent in healthy disks [170, 171].

The detection by imaging of an extruded or migrated disk herniation with root compression in a patient suffering from acute radiculopathy may represent a plausible cause of pain. However, in front of a prevalence of disc herniations in 20-28% of asymptomatic subjects, a detected herniation may not be the real cause of pain neither can predict its appearance with time [172].

Conversely, a bulging or protruding disk without root compression can generate pain by delivering inflammatory mediators upon the nerve root. For these reasons, as in the case of non-specific LBP, any excessive confidence on imaging signs without concordant clinical findings may lead to incorrect or contraindicated treatments. Also the role of imaging in predicting outcome is controversial. In general, the larger the disk herniation, the more it tends to regress.

The site of herniation is also important; in one study, 56% of the subligamentous, 79% of the transligamentous, and 100% of the sequestered herniations decreased in size with time [173].

Granulation tissue, neovascolarization and macrophage infiltration favour the spontaneous resorption of the herniated tissue [174, 175] (Fig. 1.11). The reactive neovascularisation and consequent degree of contrast enhancement in MRI or CT are proportional to the tendency of spontaneous resorption [176, 177].

Even though extruded disks show greater improvement in patients with acute LBP or sciatica, the type, size, and location of herniation at presentation as well as the changes in the size and type of herniation over time at MRI do not correlate with outcome. MRI does not even appear to be valuable for the prediction of outcome and for planning conservative care [178]. Moreover, in the absence of signs and symptoms suggestive of tumors or infection, early imaging does not elicit findings that would alter the care of patients with LBP or sciatica [178]. In patients with radiculopathy, imaging is recommended only for patients with persistent or worsening symptoms after 4–6 weeks of conservative care who are believed to be candidates for surgery or

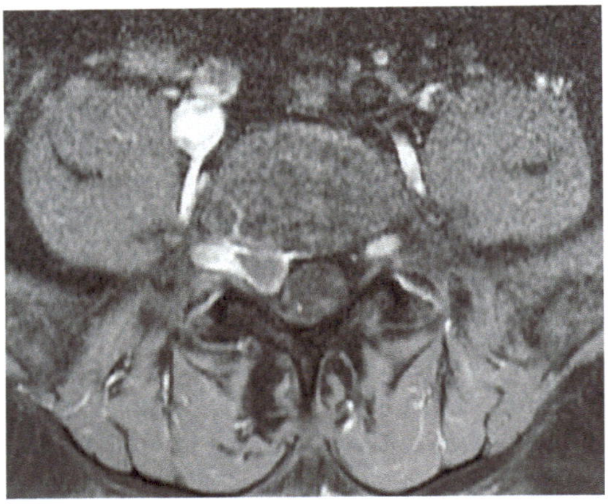

Fig. 1.11 35 years-old male complaining of right L5 acute radicular pain. MR FSE fat-sat axial T1 (TR/TE 450/35ms) image after gadolinium administration showing a cranially migrated posterolateral herniation from the L5-S1 disc encircled by a thick ring of vascularized reactive granulation tissue. This finding is considered predictive of future resorption of the fragment

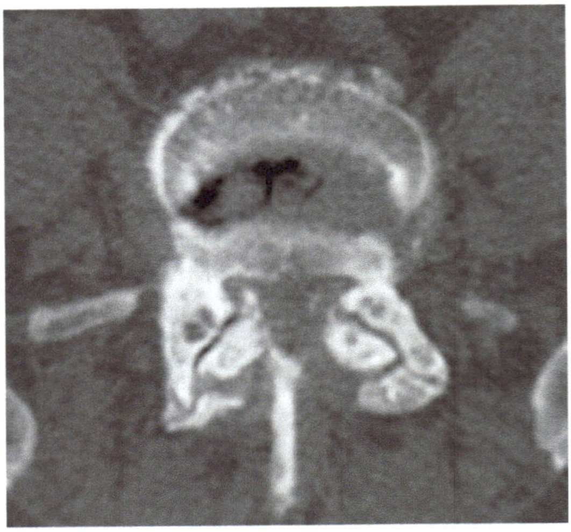

Fig. 1.12 Axial CT scan showing advanced degenerative changes of L5-S1 facet joints with marked hypertrophy and curved osteophytes, geodic cysts, sclerosis along with and joint spaces narrowing (wrap around bumper osteophytes). Bone sclerosis and joint space collapse are better demonstrated by CT than MR

in whom diagnostic uncertainty remains [178]. Pathophysiological studies have been undertaken primarily on lumbar disks because of the higher incidence of lumbar disease. However, it seems reasonable to conclude that parallels may exist for cervical radicular pain.

An unknown source of axial pain that has not been identified definitively by imaging and clinical evaluation in patients with persistent pain may require an interventional approach by diagnostic and therapeutic procedures such as tranforaminal epidural corticosteroids/infiltration of O_2–O_3 mixtures, provocative diskography, and post-diskography CT before more definitive surgical stabilization [179, 180].

1.4.5 Facet Syndrome

Mooney and Robertson as well as McCall et al. elicited axial lumbar pain and referred pain to the extremities by injecting saline solution in synovial spaces and into the capsules of the zygapophysial joints of asymptomatic volunteers [181, 182].

Owing to the rich innervation of capsules, synovial membranes and subchondral bone facet joints are important direct sources of acute and chronic pain. Degeneration of the facet joints is also a frequent cause of radicular pain due to the compression of nerve roots in the lateral recesses and in the foramina secondary to hypertrophic and ostephytic remodeling subluxation, joint effusion with capsular tension, and synovial cysts (Fig. 1.12). The facet joints receive double innervation (somatic and autonomic) and facet pain can be local or distantly referred with significant superimposition among different levels [183, 184].

Arthrosis and arthritis of the facet joints are as many frequent as in patients with as those without lumbar pain even though the most evolved lesions tend to be more often symptomatic. In studies with controlled diagnostic blocks, the origin of pain from the facet joints in subjects with chronic lumbar pain was observed in 15-52% of subjects [183–185].

The primary dorsal ramus of the spinal nerve divides into three branches: lateral (supplying the iliocostalis lumborum muscle and the skin), intermediate (supplying the longissimus muscle and facet joints) and medial (supplying the multifidus muscle, interspinous ligaments and muscles, the facet joints, supraspinous and flava ligament). Each medial branch supplies the apophyseal joints at its own level and the one below. In this way, each joint receives a double sensory afferent.

With respect to imaging, CT is more sensitive and accurate than MRI for depicting thinning of the joint space and bone sclerosis [186]. Pathria et al. and Weishaupt et al. proposed a four-point scale of progressive osteoarthritis ranging from 0 (normal) up to 3 (marked hypertrophy and/or osteophyitosis, erosion and subchondral cysts) [186, 187]. MRI is better than CT for detecting joint effusion and cysts, synovitis, facet edema, periapophyseal edema, and tissue reactions. The optimal depiction of disease of the neural arc involves short TI-inversion recovery (STIR) or T2 fat-suppressed and eventually T1 fat-s with contrast administration MRI sequences [188].

1.5 Conclusions

LBP is second only to upper respiratory diseases as the cause of medical consultations in primary setting care [189]. The complex anatomy and function of the spine render diagnostic assessment of spinal pain very difficult. The first difficulty is excluding the small percentage of subjects having underlying evolving pathologies such as tumours or infections/inflammatory diseases, which account for about 1% of cases of LBP [190]. The diagnosis of idiopathic or nonspecific LBP is inferred after a screening process excluding a series of alarm signs (Table 1.1) [191]. Nearly 80% of cases of LBP are idiopathic or non-specific.

The second step is identification of the exact source of pain. The complex neuroanatomy of the spine and the referral of pain to sites distant from the real location of injury with a somatotropic pattern,make precise localization of the pain level difficult [96].

Only in a limited number of cases is the lumbar pain due to disk herniation. A major cause of non-specific lumbar pain is diskal disruption with or without endplate degeneration, which leads to diskogenic pain [185]. Pain reproduction in provocative diskography is associated primarily with annular tears or disk disruption, and not with age-related biochemical changes manifesting on MRI as a "dark disk." [131–133].

Irrespective of the origin of acute pain, with time, the setting in of complex processes of peripheral and central sensitization may influence the evolution of acute pain into chronic pain, i.e., the transformation of a symptom into a disease. Even though acute pain starts as a consequence of an anatomical and physical derangement, under the influence of the CNS it evolves over time in persistent pain that features as a bio–psycho–social problem in which dysfunction and disability lose any relation to the initial disease [125, 126].

The knowledge of the central influences on pain is the fundament to prevent the conversion of acute spinal pain in a chronic disease and to better control the latter.

While our therapeutic strategies remain focused upon PNS changes the success or failure of patient management also depends upon contemporary treatment of CNS changes [113].

References

1. Panjabi MM (1994) Lumbar spine instability: a biomechanical challenge. Curr Orthop 8:100–105
2. Panjabi MM (1992) The stabilizing system of the spine. Part II. Neutral zone and instability hypothesis. J Spinal Disord 5:390–397
3. Louis R (1989) Chirurgia del rachide. Piccin, Padova
4. Kanayama M, Abumi K, Kaneda K et al (1996) Phase lag of the intersegmental motion in flexion-extension of the lumbar and lumbosacral spine. An in vivo study. Spine 21:1416–1422
5. Rabischong P (1989) Anatomie Functionelle du rachis et de la moelle. In: Manelfe C (ed) Imagerie du Rachis et de la Moelle. Vigot, Paris, p 109–123
6. Panjabi M, Dvorak J, Duranceau J et al (1988) Three dimensional movements of the upper cervical spine. Spine 13:726–730
7. Panjabi MM, Dvorak J, Sandler A et al (1998) Cervical spine kinematics and clinical instability. In: Clark CR (ed) The cervical spine. Lippincot-Raven, Philadelphia
8. Penning L, Wilmink JT (1987) Rotation of the cervical spine. A CT study in normal subjects. Spine 12: 732–738
9. Diano AA (2003) Biomeccanica ed Anatomia della Colonna Vertebrale. Idelson-Gnocchi, Napoli

10. Werne S (1957) Studies in spontaneous atlas dislocation. Acta Orthop Scand 1957 (Suppl. 23).
11. Wiesel SW, Rothman RH (1979) Occipito-atlantal hypermobility. Spine 4:187–191
12. White AA, Panjabi MM (1990) Clinical biomechanics of the spine, second ed. JB Lippincott, Philadelphia
13. Larson SJ (1993) Vertebral injury and instability. In: Holtzman RMN (ed) Spinal instability. Springer, New York
14. Haher TR, O'Brien M, Kauffman D et al (1993) Biomechanics of the spine in sports. Clin Sports Med 12:449–464
15. Guillot M, Fournier J, Vanneuville G, et al (1988) Mechanics of the characteristic geometry of the human spine undergoing vertical pressure. Rev Rhum Mal Osteoartic 55:351–359
16. White AA 3rd, Panjabi MM (1978)The basic kinematics of the human spine. Spine 3:12–20
17. Pope MH, Panjabi M (1985) Biomechanical definitions of spinal instability. Spine 10:255–256
18. Kirkaldy-Willis WH (1985) Presidential symposium on instability of the lumbar spine. Introduction. Spine 10: 254–291
19. Panjabi MM, Krag MH, White AA 3rd et al (1977) Effects of preload on load displacement curves of the lumbar spine. Orthop Clin North Am 8:181–192
20. Dupuis PR, Yong-Hing K, Cassidy JD et al (1985) Radiological diagnosis of degenerative lumbar spinal instability. Spine 10:262–276
21. O'Sullivan PB (1997) The efficacy of specific stabilizing exercise in the management of chronic low back pain with radiological diagnosis of lumbar segmental instability. PhD thesis, Curtin University of Technology, Western Australia
22. Panjabi MM (2003) Clinical spinal instability and low back pain. J Electromyogr Kinesiol 13:371–379
23. Kifune M, Panjabi MM, Arand M et al (1995) Fracture pattern and instability of thoracolumbar injuries. Eur Spine J 4: 98–103
24. Oxland TR, Panjabi MM (1992) The onset and progression spinal injury: a demonstration of neutral zone sensitivity. J Biomech 25:1165–1172
25. Panjabi MM (1992) The stabilizing system of the spine. Part I. Function, dysfunction, adaptation and enhancement. J Spinal Disord 5:383–389
26. Haher TR, O'Brien M, Dryer JW et al (1994) The role of the lumbar facet joints in spinal stability: identification of a alternative paths of loading. Spine 19:2667–2270
27. Indahl A, Kaigle AM, Reikeras O et al (1997) Interaction between the porcine lumbar intervertebral disc, zygoapophyseal joint and paraspinal muscles. Spine 22: 2834–2840
28. Kojima Y, Maeda T, Arai R et al (1990). Nerve supply to the posterior longitudinal ligament and the intervertebral disc of the rat vertebral column as studied by acetylcholinesterase histochemistry. I. Distribution in the lumbar region. J Anat 169:237–224
29. McLain RF (1994) Mechanoreceptor endings in human cervical facet joints. Spine 19:495–501
30. Sharma M, Langrana NA, Rodriguez J (1995) Role of ligaments and facets in the lumbar spine instability. Spine 20:887–900
31. Wilke HJ, Neef P, Caimi M et al (1999) New in vivo measurements of pressure in the intervertebral disc in daily life. Spine 24:755–762
32. Bell GH, Dunbar O, Beck JS et al (1967) Variation in strength of vertebrae with age and their relation to osteoporosis. Calcif Tissue Res 1:75–86
33. Melanotte PL, Volpe A (1987) Il microsubstrato anatomico dell'imaging macroscopico del rachide. In: L'imaging Diagnostico del Rachide. Libreria Cortina, Verona
34. Ferguson SJ, Steffen T (2003) Biomechanics of the aging spine. Eur Spine J 12 (Suppl. 2): S97–S103
35. Silva MJ, Keaveny TM, Hayes WC (1997) Load sharing between the shell and centrum in the lumbar vertebral body. Spine 22:140–150
36. Myers ER, Wilson SE (1997) Biomechanics of osteoporosis and vertebral fracture. Spine 22(24S): 25S–31S
37. Hansson TH, Keller TS, Spengler DM (1987) Mechanical behaviour of the human lumbar spine. II. Fatigue strength during dynamic compressive loading J Orthop Res 5:479–487
38. Simpson EK, Parkinson IH, Manthey B et al (2001) Intervertebral disc disorganization is related to trabecular bone architecture in the lumbar spine. J Bone Miner Res 16:681–687
39. Oda K, Shibayama Y, Abe M, et al (1998) Morphogenesis of vertebral deformities in involutional osteoporosis: age-related, three-dimensional trabecular structure. Spine 23:1050–1055
40. Goodship AE, Lanyon LE, McFie H (1979) Functional adaptation of bone to increasedstress: an experimental study. J Bone Joint Surg Am 61:539–546
41. Rubin CT, Lanyon LE (1984) Regulation of bone formation by applied dynamic loads. J Bone Joint Surg Am 66:397–402
42. Pollintine P, Dolan P, Tobias JH et al (2004) Intervertebral disc degeneration can lead to "stress-shielding" of the anterior vertebral body. A cause of osteoporotic vertebral fracture? Spine 29:774–782
43. Schulte K, Clark CR, Goel VK (1989) Kinematics of the cervical spine following discectomy and stabilization. Spine 14:1116–1121
44. Broberg KB (1983) On the mechanical behavior of intervertebral discs. Spine 8: 151–165
45. Johannessen W, Cloyd JM, Connell GD et al (2006) Trans-endplate nucleotomy increases deformation and creep response in axial loading. Ann Biomech Eng 34: 687–696
46. Elliot DM, Yerramalli CS, Auerbach JD (2008) Biomechanics of the intervertebral disc. In: Slipman CW (ed) Interventional spine. Saunders, Philadelphia p 827–838
47. Horst M, Brinckmann P (1981) Measurement of the distribution of axial stress on the endplate of the vertebral body. Spine 6:217–232
48. Adams MA, McNally DS, Dolan P (1996) 'Stress'

distributions inside intervertebral discs. The effects of age and degeneration. J Bone Joint Surg Br 78:965–972
49. Elliott DM, Setton LA (2000) A linear material model for fiber-induced anisotropy of the annulus fibrosus. J Biomech Eng 122:173-179
50. Brinckmann P, Biggermann M, Hilweg D (1988) Fatigue fracture of human lumbar vertebrae. Clin Biomech 3S: S1–S23
51. Perey O (1957) Fracture of the vertebral endplate in the lumbar spine: an experimental biomechanical investigation. Acta Orthopaed Scand Suppl 25:1–101
52. Adams MA, McMillan DW, Gree TP et al (1996) Sustained loading generates stress concentration in lumbar intervertebral discs. Spine 21:434–438
53. Johannessen W, Vresilovic EJ, Wright AC et al (2004) Intervertebral disc mechanics are restored following cyclic loading and unloaded recovery. Ann Biomedl Eng 32:70–76
54. Kulak RF, Belytschko TB, Schultz AB (1976) Nonlinear behavior of the human intervertebral disc under axial load. J Biomechanics 9:377–386
55. Iatridis JC, Gwynn I (2004) Mechanisms for mechanical damage in the intervertebral disc anulus fibrosus. J Biomech 37:1165–1175
56. Adams MA, Bogduk N, Burton K et al (2002) The biomechanics of back pain. Churchill Livingstone, Edinburgh
57. Dunlop RB, Adams MA, Hutton WC (1984) Disc space narrowing and the lumbar facet joints. J Bone Joint Surg (Br) 66:706–710
58. Noren R, Trafimow J, Andersson JB et al (1991) The role of facet joint tropism and facet angle in disc de generation. Spine 16:530–532
59. Grobler LJ, Robertson PA, Novotny JE et al (1993) Etiology of spondylolisthesis. Assessment of the role played by lumbar facet joint morphology. Spine 18:80–91
60. Varlotta GP, Lefkowitz TR, Schweitzer M et al (2011) The lumbar facet joint: a review of current knowledge: part 1: anatomy, biomechanics, and grading. Skeletal Radiol 40:13–23
61. Kim NH, Lee JW (1995) The relationship between isthmic and degenerative spondylolisthesis and the configuration of the lamina and facet joints. Eur Spine J 4:139–144
62. Boden SD, Riew DK, Yamaguchi K et al (1996) Orientation of the lumbar facet joints: association with degenerative disc disease. J Bone Jt Surg Am 78-A:403–411
63. Wiseman CM, Lindsey DP, Fredrick AD et al (2005) The effect of an interspinous process implant on facet loading during extension. Spine 30:903–907
64. Panjiabi MM, Greenstein G, Duranceau J et al (1991) Three-dimensional quantitative morphology of lumbar spinal ligaments. J Spine Disord 4:54–72
65. Chazal J, Tanguy A, Bourges M et al (1985) Biomechanical properties of spinal ligaments and a histological study of the supraspinal ligament in traction. J Biomech 18:167–176
66. Hecker P (1923) Appareil ligamenteux occipito-atloido-axoidien: etude d'anatomie compare. Arch Anat Hist Embryol 2:57–95
67. Dvorak J, Schneider E, Saldinger P et al (1988) Biomechanics of the cranio-cervical region: the alar and transverse ligaments. J Orthop Res 6:452–461
68. Fielding JW, Cochran GB, Lawsing JF et al (1974) Tears of the transverse ligament of the atlas. A clinical biomechanical study. J Bone Joint Surg (Am) 56: 1683–1691
69. Dvorak J, Hayek J, Zehnder R (1987) CT-functional diagnostics of the rotatory instability of the upper cervical spine: part 2. An evaluation on healthy adults and patients with suspected instability. Spine 12:726–731
70. Morvan G, Wybier M, Mathieu P et al (2008) Plain radiographs of the spine: static and relationships between spine and pelvis. J Radiol 89:654–663
71. Vialle R, Levassor N, Rillardon L et al (2005) Radiographic analysis of the sagittal alignement and balance of the spine in asymptomatic subjects. J Bone Joint Surg 87-A:260–267
72. Koller H, Acosta F, Hempfing H et al (2008) Long-term investigation of nonsurgical treatment for thoracolumbar and lumbar burst fractures: an outcome analysis in sight of spinopelvic balance. Eur Spine J 17:1073–1095
73. Benzel EC (2003) Biomechanics of the spine. Thieme-Verlag, Stuttgart
74. Crisco JI, Panjabi MM (1991) The intersegmental and multisegmental muscles of the lumbar spine: a biomechanical model comparing lateral stabilizing potential. Spine 16:793–799
75. Bogduk N (1997) Clinical anatomy of the lumbar spine and sacrum, 3rd ed. Churchill Livingstone p 67–69
76. Hodges PW, Richardson A (1996) Inefficient muscular stabilization associated with low back pain. Spine 21: 2640–2650
77. Panjabi MM (2006) A hypothesis of chronic back pain: ligament subfailure injuries lead to muscle control dysfunction. Eur Spine J 15:668–676
78. Luoto S, Hurri H, Alaranta H (1995) Reaction times in patients with chronic low-back pain. Eur J Phys Med Rehabil 5:47–50
79. Radebold A, Cholewicki J, Panjabi MM et al (2000) Muscle response pattern to sudden trunk loading in healthy individuals and in patients with chronic low back pain. Spine 25:947–954
80. Taimela S, Osterman K, Alaranta H et al (1993) Long psychomotor reaction time in patients with chronic low-back pain: preliminary report. Arch Phys Med Rehabil 74:1161–1164
81. Hodges PW, Richardson CA (1997) Contraction of the abdominal muscles associated with movement of the lower limb. Phys Ther 77:132–142
82. Schleip R, Vleeming A, Lehmann-Horn F (2007) Letter to the Editor concerning "A hypothesis of chronic back pain: ligament subfailure injuries lead to muscle control dysfunction" (M. Panjabi) Eur Spine J 16:1733–1735

83. Deyo RA, Cherkin D, Conrad D, et al (1991) Cost, controversy, crisis: low back pain and the health of the public. Annu Rev Public Health 12:141–156
84. Kang DJ, Hanks S (2008) Inflammatory basis of spinal pain In: Slipman CW, Derby R, Simeone FA et al (eds) Interventional spine: an algorithmic approach. Saunders Elsevier, Philadelphia, p 17–27
85. Cote P, Cassidy JD, Carroll L (1998) The Saskatchewan health and back pain survey. The prevalence of neck pain and related disability in Saskatchewan adults. Spine; 23:1689–1698
86. Frank JW, Kerr Ms, Brooker AS et al (1996) Disability resulting from occupational low back pain: I. What do we know about primary prevention? A review of the scientific evidence on prevention before disability begins. Spine 21:2908–2917
87. Adams MA. Biomechanics of back pain (2004) Acupuncture Med 22:178–188
88. Nachemson A, Jonsson E (2000) Neck and back pain. The scientific evidence of causes, diagnosis and treatment. Lippincott, Williams and Wilkins, New York
89. Dunn KM, Croft PR (2004) Epidemiology of natural history of low back pain. Eur Med Phys 40:9–13
90. Anderson RE, Drayer BP, Braffman B et al (2000) Acute low back pain–radiculopathy. American College of Radiology (ACR) Appropriateness Criteria. Radiology 215(Suppl):479–485
91. Andersson GBJ (1999) Epidemiological features of chronic low-back pain. Lancet 354:581–585
92. Sizer PS, Brismée JM, Coock C (2007) Medical screening for red flags in the diagnosis and management of musculoskeletal spine pain. Pain Practice 7:53–71
93. Stillwell DL (1956) The nerve supply of the vertebral column and its associated structures in the monkey. Anat Rec 125:139–169
94. Pedersen HE, Blunck CFJ, Gardner E (1956) The anatomy of lumbosacral posterior rami and meningeal branches of spinal nerves (sinu-vertebral nerves). With an experimental study of their functions. J Bone Joint Surg [Am] 38-A:377–391
95. Malinsky J (1959) The ontogenic development of nerve terminations in the intervertebral disc of man. Acta Anat 38:96–113
96. Hirsch C, Ingelmark B-E, Miller M (1963) The anatomical basis for low back pain: studies on the presence of sensory nerve endings in ligamentous, capsular and intervertebral disc structures in the human lumbar spine. Acta Orthop Scand 33:1–17
97. Jackson HC HC, Winkelman RK, Bickel WH (1966) Nerve endings in the human lumbar spinal column and related structures. J Bone Joint Surg [Am] 48-A:1272–1281
98. Bogduk N. Nerves of the lumbar spine (1997) In: Bogduk N (ed) Clinical anatomy of the lumbar spine and sacrum. Churchill Livingstone, London, 127–144
99. Groen GJ, Baljet B, Drukker J (1990) Nerves and nerve plexuses of the human vertebral column. Am J Anat 188:282–296
100. Edgar MA, Ghadially JA. (1976) Innervation of the lumbar spine. Clin Orthop 15:35–41
101. Jinkins JR, Whittemore AR, Bradley WG (1989) The anatomic basis of vertebrogenic pain and the autonomic syndrome associated with lumbar disk extrusion. Am J Roentgenol 152:1277–1289
102. de Palma AF, Rothman RH (1970) Clinical manifestations of lumbar disc syndrome. In: The intervertebral disc. Saunders, Philadelphia, p 203–248
103. Gray H. (1985) Anatomy of the human body. Lea & Febiger, Philadelphia, p 1251–1254 and 1264–1265
104. Hockaday JM, Whitty CWM (1967) Patterns of referred pain in the normal subject. Brain 90:482–496
105. Cervero F (1985) Visceral nociception: peripheral and central aspects of visceral nociceptive systems. Philos Trans R Soc Lond B 308:325–337
106. Wyke B (1987) The neurology of low back pain. In: Jayson MIV (ed) The lumbar spine and back pain. Churchill-Livingstone, New York, p 56–99
107. Bahr R, Blumberg H, Janig W (1981) Do dichotomizing afferent fibers exist which supply visceral organs as well as somatic structures? A contribution to the problem of referred pain. Neurosci Lett 24:25–28
108. Ruch TC (1982) Pathophysiology of pain. In: Ruch TC, Patton HD (eds) Physiology and biophysics. Saunders, Philadelphia, p 508–531
109. Bogduk N (2002) Innervation and pain patterns of the thoracic spine. In: Grant R (ed) Physical therapy of the cervical and thoracic spine, 3rd ed. Churchill Livingstone, New York, p 73–81
110. Rothman SM, Hubbard RD, Leer KE et al (2008) Transduction, transmission and perception of pain. In: Slipman CW, Derby R, Simeone FA et al (eds) Interventional spine: an algorithmic approach. Saunders Elsevier, Philadelphia, p 29–37
111. Dray A, Perkins M (1993) Bradykinin and inflammatory pain. Trends Neurosci 16:99–104
112. Dubner R, Hargreaves KM (1989) The neurobiology of pain and its modulation. Clin J Pain S2:S1–S6
113. Moskowitz MH (2008) Central influences on pain. In: Slipman CW, Derby R, Simeone FA et al (eds) Interventional spine. An algorithmic approach. Saunders Elsevier, Philadelphia, p 39–52
114. Yaksh T (2001) Anatomy of the pain-processing system. In: Waldman S (ed) International pain management. Saunders, Philadelphia, p 11–20
115. Woolf CJ (1983) Evidence for a central component of post-injury pain hypersensitivity. Nature 306:686–688
116. Costigan M, Woolf CJ (2000) Pain: molecular mechanisms. J Pain 1 (3 Suppl.):35–44
117. Coderre C (1999) Excitatory amino acid antagonists: potential analgesics for persistent pain. In: Sawynok, Cowan (eds) Novel aspects of pain management. Wiley Liss, New York, p157–178
118. Yaksh T (2001) Pharmacology of the pain-processing system. In: Waldman S (ed) International pain management. Saunders, Philadelphia, p 21–34

119. Ray AL (2002) Pain perception in the older patient. Geriatrics 57:22–26
120. de Leo JA, Yezierski RP (2001) The role of neuroinflammation and neuroimmune activation in persistent pain. Pain 91:1–6
121. Watkins L, Maier S, Goehler L (1995) Immune activation: the role of pro-inflammatory cytokines in inflammation, illness responses and pathological pain states. Pain 63:289–302
122. Colburn R, Rickman A, de Leo J (1999) The effect of site and type of nerve injury on spinal glial activation and neuropathic pain behavior. Exper Neurol 157:289–304
123. Rutkowski MD, Winkelstein BA, Hickey WF et al (2002) Lumbar nerve root injury induces CNS neuroimmune activation and neuroinflammation in the rat: relationship to painful radiculopathy. Spine 27:1604–1613
124. Mathew SG, Coplan JD, Schoepp DD et al (2001) Glutamate-hypothalamic-pituitary-adrenal axis interactions: implications for mood and anxiety disorders. CNS Spectrums 6:555–564
125. Negrini S, Bonaiuti D, Monticone M et al (2008) Medical causes of low back pain. In: Slipman CW Slipman CW, Derby R, Simeone F, Mayer TG (eds) Interventional spine. Saunders, Philadelphia, p 803–811
126. Waddell G (1987) Volvo Award in Clinical Sciences. A new clinical model for the treatment of low-back pain. Spine 12:632–644
127. Waddel G (1996) Low back pain: a twentieth century health care enigma. Spine 21: 2820–2825
128. Rush AJ, Polatin P, Gatchel RJ (2000) Depression and chronic pain. Establishing priorities in treatment. Spine 25:2566–2571
129. Jacobs JM, Hammerman-Rozenberg R, Cohen A et al (2006) Chronic back pain among the elderly: prevalence, associations, and predictors. Spine 31:E203–E207
130. Schwarzer AC, Aprill CN, Derby R et al (1995) The prevalence and clinical features of internal disc disruption in patients with chronic low back pain. Spine 20:1878–1883
131. Moneta GB, Videman T, Kaivanto K et al (1994) Reported pain during lumbar discography as a function of anular ruptures and disc degeneration. A reanalysis of 833 discograms. Spine 19:1968–1974
132. Videman T, Battie MC, Gibbons LE, et al (2003) Associations between back pain history and lumbar MRI findings. Spine 28:582–588
133. Modic MT, Masaryk TJ, Ross JS et al (1988) Imaging of degenerative disk disease. Radiology 168:177–186
134. Freemont AJ, Peacock TE, Goupille P et al (1997) Nerve ingrowth into diseased intervertebral disc in chronic back pain. Lancet 350:178–181
135. Hurry H, Karppinen J (2004) Discogenic pain. Pain 112:225–228
136. Adams MA, McNally DS, Dolan P (1996) 'Stress' distributions inside intervertebral discs. The effects of age and degeneration. J Bone Joint Surg Br 78:965–972
137. Yu SW, Sether LA, Ho PS et al (1988) Tears of the annulus fibrosus: correlation between MR and pathologic findings in cadavers. Am J Neuroradiol 9:367–370
138. Sether LA, Yu S, Haughton VM et al (1990) Intervertebral disk: normal age-related changes in MR signal intensity. Radiology 177:385–388
139. Modic MT Herfkens RJ (1990) Intervertebral disk: normal age-related changes in MR signal intensity. Radiology 177:332–334
140. Pfirrmann CWA, Metzdorf A, Zanetti M et al (2001) Magnetic resonance Classification of lumbar intervertebral disc degeneration. Spine 26:1873–1878
141. Powell MC, Wilson M, Szypryt P et al (1986) Prevalence of lumbar disc degeneration observed by magnetic resonance in symptomless women. Lancet 2: 1366–1367
142. Savage RA, Whitehouse GH, Roberts N (1997) The relationship between the magnetic resonance imaging appearance of the lumbar spine and low back pain, age and occupation in males. Eur Spine J 6:106–114
143. Jensen MC, Brant-Zawadzki MN, Obuchowski N et al (1994) Magnetic resonance imaging of the lumbar spine in people without back pain. N Engl J Med 331:69–73
144. Kleinstuck F Dvorak J Mannion AF (2006) Are "structural abnormalities" on magnetic resonance imaging a contraindication to the successful conservative treatment of chronic nonspecific low back pain? Spine 31:2250–2257
145. Boden SD, Davis DO, Dina TS et al (1990) Abnormal magnetic-resonance scans of the lumbar spine in asymptomatic subjects: a prospective investigation. J Bone Joint Surg Am 72:403–408
146. Borenstein DG, O'Mara Jr JW, Boden SD et al (2001) The value of magnetic resonance imaging of the lumbar spine to predict low back pain in asymptomatic subjects: a seven year follow-up study. J Bone Joint Surg (Am) 83:1306–1311
147. Gronblad M, Virr J, Ronkko S et al (1996) A controlled biochemical and immunohistochemical study of human synovial-type (group II) phospholipase a_2 and inflammatory cells in macroscopically normal, degenerated, and herniated human lumbar disc tissues. Spine 21:2531–2538
148. Haro H, Shinomiya K, Komori H et al (1996) Upregulated expression of chemokines in herniated nucleus pulposus resorption. Spine 21:1647–1652
149. Kawakami M, Weinstein JN (1986) Associated neurogenic and nonneurogenic pain mediators that probably are activated and responsible for nocicedptive input. In: Weinstein J, Gordon S (eds) Low back pain: a scientific and clinical overview American Academy of Orthopaedic Surgeons, Rosemont, p 265–273
150. Aprill C, Bogduk N (1992) High-intensity zone: a diagnostic sign of painful lumbar disc on magnetic

resonance imaging . Br J Radiol 65 (773):361–369
151. Peng B, Hou S, Wu W et al (2006) The pathogenesis and clinical significance of a high-intensity zone (HIZ) of lumbar intervertebral disc on MR imaging in the patient with discogenic low back pain Eur Spine J 15:583–587
152. Schellas KP, Pollei SR, Gundry CL et al (1996) Lumbar disc high-intensity zone: correlation of magnetic resonance imaging and discography. Spine 21:79–86
153. Sachs BL, Vanharanta H, Spivey MA et al (1987) Dallas discogram description: a new classification of CT/discography in low-back disorders. Spine 12: 287–298
154. Ricketson R, Simmons JW, Hauser BO (1996) The prolapsed intervertebral disc: the high-intensity zone with discography correlation. Spine 21:2758–2762
155. Weishaupt D, Zanetti M, Hodler J et al (1998) MR imaging of the lumbar spine: prevalence of intervertebral disk extrusion and sequestration, nerve root compression, endplate abnormalities, and osteoarthritis of the facet joints in asymptomatic volunteers. Radiology 209:661–666
156. Modic MT, Steinberg PM, Ross JS et al (1988) Degenerative disk disease : assessment of changes in vertebral body marrow with MR imaging. Radiology 166:193–199
157. Braithwaite I, White J, Saifuddin A et al (1998) Vertebral end-plate (Modic) changes on lumbar spine MRI: correlation with pain reproduction at discography. Eur Spine J 7:363–368
158. Chung CB, Vande Berg BC, Tavernier T et al (2004) End plate marrow changes in the asymptomatic lumbosacral spine: frequency, distribution and correlation with age and degenerative changes. Skeletal Radiol 33:399–404
159. Albert HB, Manniche C (2007) Modic changes following lumbar disc herniation. Eur Spine J 16:977–982
160. Parizel PM (2003) Pattern recognition of degenerative disorders in the lumbar spine. Guidelines to MR image interpretation. JBR-BTR 86:222–226
161. Weishaupt D, Zanetti M, Hodler J et al (2001) Painful lumbar disk derangement: relevance ofendplate abnormalities at MR imaging. Radiology 218:420–427
162. Gillette RG, Kramis RC, Roberts WJ (1994) Sympathetic activation of rat spinal neurons response to noxious stimulation of deep tissues in the low back. Pain 56:31–42
163. Simmonds M, Kumar S (1992) The bases of low back pain: review article. Neuro-orthopaedics 13:1–14
164. Ahn SH (2008) Adjuvant analgesics for radicular pain. In: Slipman CW, Derby R, Simeone F, Mayer TG (eds) Interventional spine. Saunders, Philadelphia, p 129–136
165. Saal JS Franson RC, Dobrow R et al (1990) High levels of inflammatory phospholipase A2 activity in lumbar disc herniations. Spine 15:674–678
166. Saal JS (1995) The role of inflammation in lumbar pain. Spine 20:1821–1827
167. Ozaktay AC, Kallakuri S, Cavanaugh JM (1998) Phospholipase A2 sensitivity of the dorsal root and dorsal root ganglion. Spine 23:1297–1306
168. Winkelstein B, Rutkowski M, Weinstein J et al (2001) Quantification of neural tissue injury in a rat radiculopathy model: comparison of local deformation, behavioural outcomes, and spinal cytokines mRNA for two surgeons. J Neurosci Meth 111:49–57
169. Hashizume H, de Leo J, Colburn R et al (2000) Spinal glial activation and cytokine expression following lumbar root injury in the rat. Spine 25:1206–1217
170. Nygaard O, Mellgren SI, Osterud B (1997) The inflammatory properties of contained and noncontained lumbar disc herniations. Spine 22:2484–2488
171. Komori H, Okawa A, Haro H et al (1998) Contrast-enhanced magnetic resonance imaging in conservative management of lumbar disc herniation. Spine 23:67–73
172. Wiesel SW, Tsourmas N, Feffer HL et al (1984) A study of computer-assisted tomography. The incidence of positive CAT scans in an asymptomatic group of patients. Spine 9:549–551
173. Ahn SH, Ahn WM, Byun WM (2000). Effect of the translegamentous extension of human disc herniations in their regression and the clinical outcome of sciatica. Spine 25:475–480
174. Haro H, Shinomiya K, Komori H et al (1996) Upregulated expression of chemokines in herniated nucleus pulposus resorption. Spine 21:1647–1652
175. Haro H, Kato T, Komori H et al (2002) Vascular endothelial growth factor (VEGF)-induced angiogenesis in herniated disc resorption. J Orthop Res 20:409–415
176. Spendiani A, Puglielli E, de Amicis R et al (2004) Spontaneous resolution of lumbar disck herniation: predictive signs for prognostic evaluation. Neuroradiology 46:916–922
177. Komori H, Okawa A, Haro H et al (1998) Contrast-enhanced magnetic resonance imaging in conservative management of lumbar disc herniation. Spine 23: 67–73
178. Modic MT, Obuchowski NA, Ross JS et al (2005) Acute low back pain and radiculopathy. Radiology 237:597–604
179. Lipetz JS (2008) Lumbar axial pain. An algorithmic methodology. In: Slipman CW, Derby R, Simeone F, Mayer TG (eds) Interventional Spine. Saunders, Philadelphia, p 975–989
180. Fritz J, Niemeyer T, Clasen S et al (2007) Management of chronic low back pain: rationales, principles, and targets of imaging-guided spinal injections. Radiographics 27:1751–1771
181. Mooney V, Robertson J (1976) Facet joint syndrome. Clin Othop 115:149–156
182. McCall IW, Park WM, O'Brien JP (1979) Induced pain referral from posterior lumbar elements in normal subjects. Spine 4:441–446

183. Bogduk N (1997) International Spinal Injection Society guidelines for the performance of spinal injection procedures: part 1: zygapophysial joint blocks. Clin J Pain 13:285–286
184. Manchikanti L Singh V, Vidyasagar P et al (2001) Evaluation of the relative contributions of various structures in chronic low back pain. Pain Physician 4:308–316
185. Schwarzer AC, Aprill CN, Derby R et al (1994) Clinical features of patients with pain stemming fom the lumbar zygoapophyseal joints. Is the lumbar facet syndrome a clinical entity? Spine 19:1132–1137
186. Weishaupt D, Zanetti M, Boos N et al (1999) MR imaging and CT in osteoarthritis of the lumbar facet joints. Skeletal Radiol 28:215–219
187. Pathria M, Sartoris DJ, Resnick D (1987) Osteoarthritis of the facet joints: accuracy of oblique radiographic assessment. Radiology 164:227–230
188. D'Aprile P, Tarantino A, Jinkins R et al (2007) The value of fat saturation sequences and contrast medium administration in MRI of degenerative disease of the posterior/perispinal elements of the lumbosacral spine. Eur Radiol 17:523–531
189. Deyo Ra, Phillips WR (1996) Low back pain. A primary care challenge. Spine 21:2826–2832
190. Slipman CW, Patel RK, Botwin KP et al (2003) Epidemiology of spine tumors presenting in musculoskeletal physiatrists. Arch Phys Med Rehabil 84:492–495
191. Koes BW, van Tulder MW, Ostelo R et al (2001) Clinical guidelines for the management of low back pain in primary care: an international comparison. Spine 26:2504–2513

Diagnostic Approaches to Spinal Disease Related to Spinal Intervention

2

Pia C. Sundgren and Majda M. Thurnher

2.1 Introduction

Radiology has an important role in the work-up of potentially treatable lesions in the spine. Computed tomography (CT) and magnetic resonance imaging (MRI) of the spine are the methods of choice for the detection and differentiation of vertebral body (VB) lesions and for demonstration of such degenerative changes in the spine that can be treated with spinal intervention. A common part of the post-interventional procedure is a radiological examination. Several interventional procedures can also be undertaken under fluoroscopic guidance. Here we review the available radiological and magnetic resonance tomographic methods and describe the typical imaging findings in some of the most common conditions that can be treated with non-surgical spinal intervention.

2.2 Imaging Methods

2.2.1 Plain Radiographs

Conventional radiographs of the spine have a very limited role in the work-up of subjects with back pain and in those who are potential subjects for intervention. However, plain radiographs can be used to evaluate the bony structures of the spine in combination with CT or MRI before spinal intervention. In addition, some interventional spine procedures require fluoroscopic guidance (Fig. 2.1).

2.2.2 CT

CT is the examination of choice for assessment of the bony structures of the spine, whereas assessment of the soft-tissue structures of the spine is often limited. The choice of imaging parameters determines the image quality and the radiation dose. High settings for the voltage and current, thin collimation, and low pitch result in the best image quality but also in a high radiation dose to the patient. In recent years, there has been a growing focus on the significant increase in radiation exposure to patients and populations due to the increase in the use of CT worldwide. In the light of these concerns, CT manufacturers have made improvements to CT scanners and developed dose-modulation methods and new reconstruction techniques that decrease the radiation dose to the patient without sacrificing image quality. Rapidly increasing numbers of "low-dose protocols" are being developed and used not only in CT spinal imaging but in all fields of radiology to reduce the overall radiation exposure to patients. Overall, the image quality and

Pia C. Sundgren (✉)
Diagnostic Radiology, Skåne University Hospital, BFC,
Blekinkevägen, Lund, Sweden
e-mail: Pia.Sundgren@med.lu.se

M. Muto (ed.), *Interventional Neuroradiology of the Spine*,
DOI 10.1007/978-88-470-2790-9_2, © Springer-Verlag Italia 2013

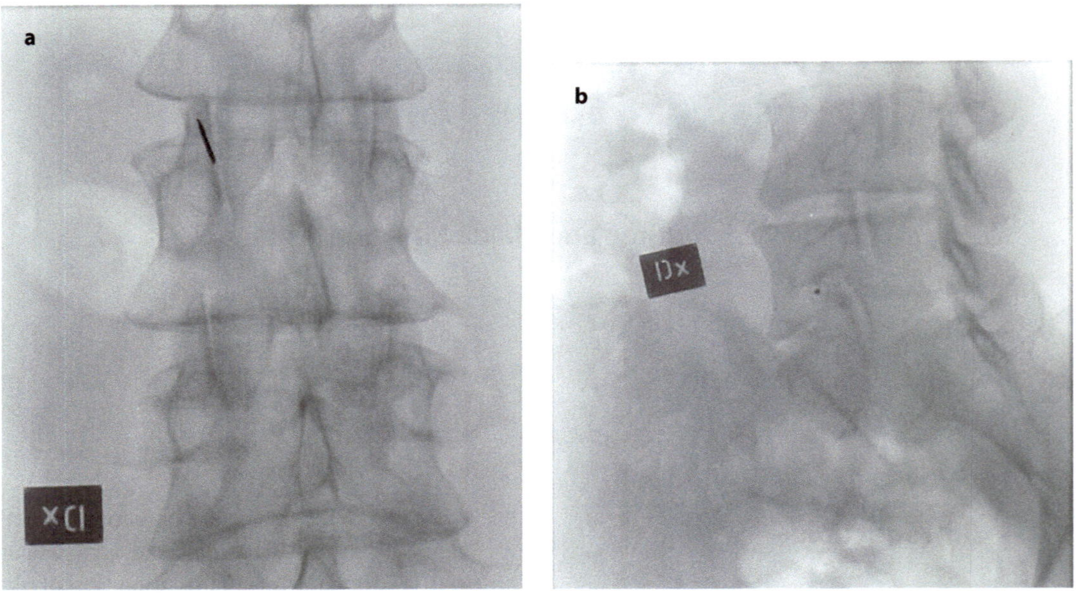

Fig. 2.1 Flouroscopic slightly oblique anteroposterior view (**a**) and lateral view (**b**) of the lumbar spine demonstrating the needle in the right L4–L5 facet joint (images courtesy of Dr R Siemund, Skåne University Hospital, Lund University, Lund, Sweden)

diagnostic performance are dependent upon the choice of imaging parameters and also on post-processing such as reconstruction algorithms and reformatting parameters. For patients who might be subject to intervention, the imaging protocol might vary slightly depending on the type of CT scanner available. In general, thin slices with reconstruction in soft tissue and bone algorithms should be conducted followed by three-dimensional (3D) reformatting in sagittal, coronal, and axial planes [1]. Additional post-processing methods such as volume rendering can be done if necessary. In selected cases, the use of contrast medium can be helpful, especially for the evaluation of paravertebral soft tissue and of the content in the spinal canal (e.g., for differentiating scar tissue from recurrent disk herniation).

2.2.3 Myelography and Myelo-CT

Myelography used to be the only diagnostic method that provided information about soft-tissue structures in the spinal canal. Di Chiro and Schellinger [2] published the first report on myelo-CT in 1976, and it soon became a standard procedure. With the introduction of MRI, the need for myelography decreased. However, myelography remains a valuable method for assessing nerve-root compression in the lateral recess and neural foramina [3]; for assessing stenosis in the spinal canal; and allows for dynamic imaging sequences (including positional changes of the patient) and thereby provides valuable diagnostic information beyond the limits of conventional MRI. Myelo-CT is useful for evaluation of the postoperative spine, with fewer artifacts related to surgical hardware than MRI. Furthermore, myelography or myelo-CT is the only method to evaluate patients in which MRI is not possible for safety reasons (e.g., pacemaker, metallic objects) (Fig. 2.2), if there is a risk of imaging degradation due to metallic implants (Figs 2.3 and 2.4), claustrophobic patients, or those with kyphoscoliosis. A recent study also showed that myelography combined with myelo-CT is more reliable and reproducible than MRI when deciding the level upon which decompressive lumbar surgery should be carried out [4]. Other studies have shown that MRI tends to underestimate the

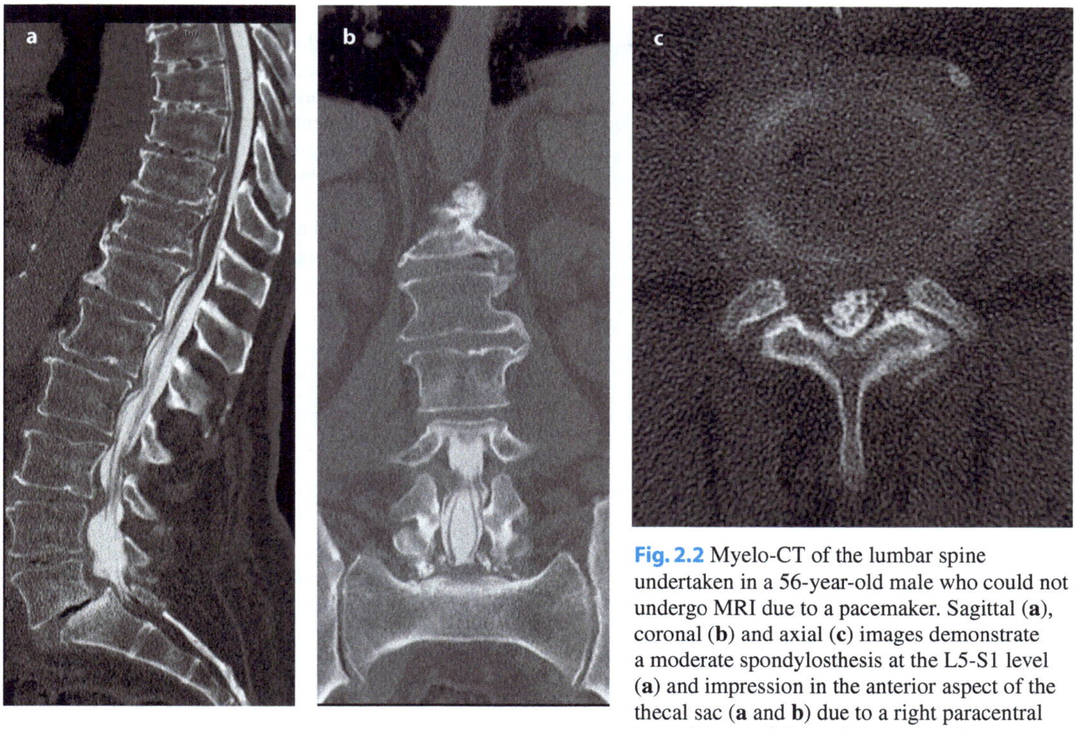

Fig. 2.2 Myelo-CT of the lumbar spine undertaken in a 56-year-old male who could not undergo MRI due to a pacemaker. Sagittal (**a**), coronal (**b**) and axial (**c**) images demonstrate a moderate spondylosthesis at the L5-S1 level (**a**) and impression in the anterior aspect of the thecal sac (**a** and **b**) due to a right paracentral broard-based disk herniation impinging on the right L4 nerve root (**c**)

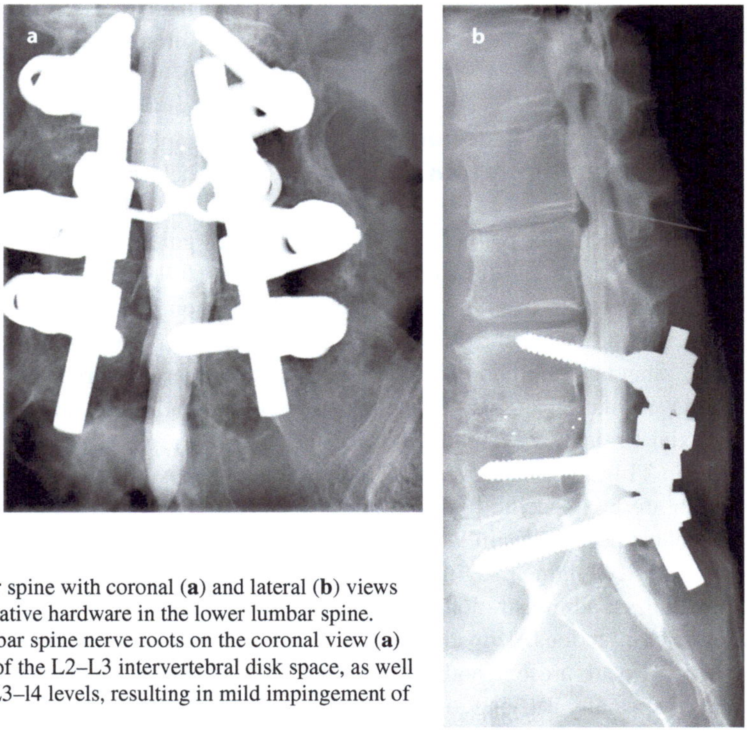

Fig. 2.3 Myelography of the lumbar spine with coronal (**a**) and lateral (**b**) views in a 54-year-old male with postoperative hardware in the lower lumbar spine. A good view is obtained of the lumbar spine nerve roots on the coronal view (**a**) and the needle in place at the level of the L2–L3 intervertebral disk space, as well as bulging disks at the L2–L3 and L3–l4 levels, resulting in mild impingement of the thecal sac

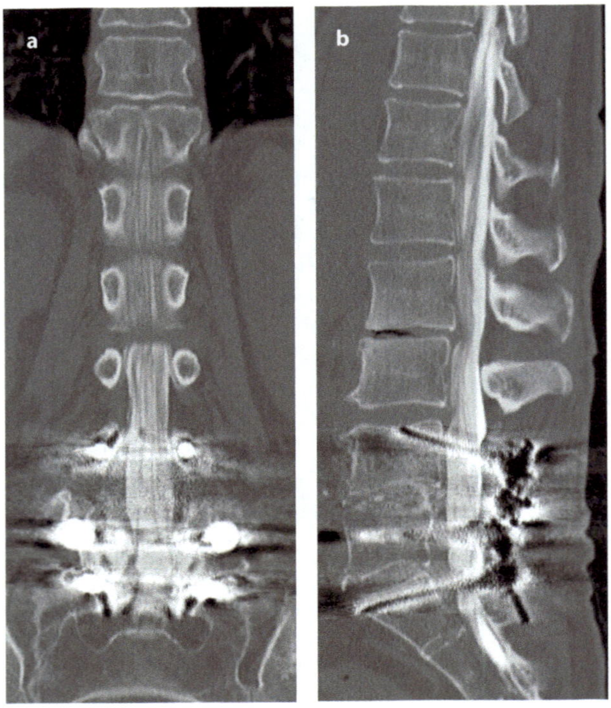

Fig. 2.4 Myelo-CT of the lumbar spine with coronal (**a**) and sagittal (**b**) views in the patient described in Fig. 2.3 demonstrate that, despite metal artifacts from the hardware, good assessment of the lumbar nerve roots (**a**) is possible. Sagittal image (**b**) demonstrates a degenerated bulging disk with vacuum phenomena and mild impingement of the thecal sac at the level of the L2–L3 intervertebral disk space and a bulging disk at the L3–L4 level

width of the spinal canal and the foramina, thereby making spinal stenosis appear more severe on MRI than seen on myelography and myelo-CT [5, 6].

2.2.4 Magnetic Resonance Tomography (MRT)

Currently, MRI is the method of choice for evaluation of the spine and the content of the spinal canal. It is used to examine intervertebral disks, ligaments, the spinal cord and paravertebral soft tissue. Standard morphological MRI sequences for the evaluation of the spine include sagittal and axial T1- and T2-weighted images, and sagittal short TI inversion recovery (STIR) sequences (which are less specific but even more sensitive to signal abnormalities in VBs than T2-weighted images). T1-weighted sagittal and axial images after contrast administration are needed if spinal tumors or infectious, demyelinating or inflammatory disease are present, and in postoperative patients (especially if trying to distinguish between recurrent disk herniation and scar tissue).

New imaging methods such as diffusion-weighted imaging and perfusion-weighted imaging have been suggested to be helpful for the differentiation between benign and pathological VB compression fractures [7–10]. Other MRI imaging methods such as magnetic resonance angiography (MRA) of the spine have been shown to be helpful for assessment of the spinal vasculature and vascular malformations, and particularly as guides for further endovascular assessment and follow-up [11]. The reliability of MRI findings on the lumbar spine varies. In a recent study of 111 lumbar MRI examinations, good inter-observer agreement for rating disk degeneration, and moderate agreement for rating spondylolisthesis, "Modic changes", facet arthropathy, and posterior annular hyperintense zone were shown [12]. The same study demonstrated good intra-observer agreement for rating disk degeneration, spondylolisthesis, Modic changes, facet arthropathy and the posterior annular hyperintense zone but only moderate intra-observer agreement for rating the extent of Modic changes [12]. Other studies demonstrated good intra-observer agreement for the assessment of spinal stenosis but only moderate agreement for assessing foraminal stenosis and nerve-root impingement [13]. The same research team also looked at the reliability for assessing disk herniation on lumbar MRI in 60 patients. They found substantial agreement with respect to disk morphology, moderate agreement for compression of the thecal sac, and moderate agreement for grading nerve-root impingement [14]. They also concluded that quantitative measurements of the spinal canal and thecal-sac area showed good reliability, whereas measurement of disk-fragment area showed more modest reliability [14].

2.3 Degenerative Disk Disease (DDD) and Disk Herniation

Plain radiographs, CT, and MRI of the spine can demonstrate: reduced height of the intervertebral space; osteophytes; sclerosis; Schmorl's nodes; alterations in endplate shape; as well as calcifications and narrowing of the spinal canal and the neural foramina. However, MRI is the best method for the evaluation of DDD because it provides the primary diagnosis as well as grading disk degeneration. Routine morphological sagittal and axial T1-weighted and T2-weighted MRI of the spine as well as post-contrast enhanced T1-weighted MRI are the "gold standard" for evaluation of degenerated disks and disk herniation if the patient has previously undergone surgery for disk herniation. However, studies have shown that MRI has limitations for detection of the early signs of degeneration [15]. Recent studies suggest that axial T2* mapping is effective for detecting the early stages of DDD and has potential diagnostic benefits [16].

Several grading systems used for the classification of DDD focus on the loss of signal intensity on sagittal T2-weighted images [17]. A classification scheme for disk degeneration based on the signal intensity of the disk, differentiation of the annulus and nucleus, and the height of the disk space that demonstrated sufficient intra- and inter-observer agreement has been described by Pfirrmann et al. [18]. Degenerative changes in intervertebral disks demonstrate the development of low T2 signal intensity within the disk with failure to differentiate annulus fibrosis from nucleus pulposis. As disk degeneration progresses, the "vacuum disk phenomenon" can occur, and is manifested as a signal void on T1-and T2-weighted images. A calcified disk typically presents with absent or low signal on MRI but the calcified disk can be hyperintense on T1-weighted images depending on the amount of calcium particulates [19]. Complete or partial tears or fissures of the annulus are due to avulsions in the fibers of the annulus fibrosus and can involve the fibers themselves or their insertions on the adjacent endplates. They can be seen as hyperintense T2 signals just beneath the annulus fibrosus (which normally presents with a low T2 signal).

Three main types of degenerative changes in vertebral endplates and bone marrow have been described [20, 21]. Type-I changes of the endplates and bone marrow demonstrate hyperintensity on T2 images with low signals on T1-weighted images; contrast enhancement after contrast administration may occur. These changes are thought to represent the more acute changes of DDD. Type-II changes present with increases on T1-weighted images and isointense to hyperintense on T2-weighted images.

Type-III changes represent dense woven bone and absence of bone marrow, and are hypointense on T1- and T2-weighted images [21]. Type-III changes correlate with the sclerotic changes seen on spinal radiographs.

Recent studies have demonstrated that DWI might be useful for the differentiation of abnormalities in degenerative and infectious endplates becaue DWI demonstrates the hyperintensity of vertebral bone marrow in patients with spinal infections, but not in subjects with degenerative changes [22].

2.3.1 Disk Herniation

The disk-space margins consist of the superior and inferior bordering vertebral endplates and, peripherally, the vertebral ring apophyses (not including osteophytes) [23]. A disk herniation is defined as extension of disk material beyond the

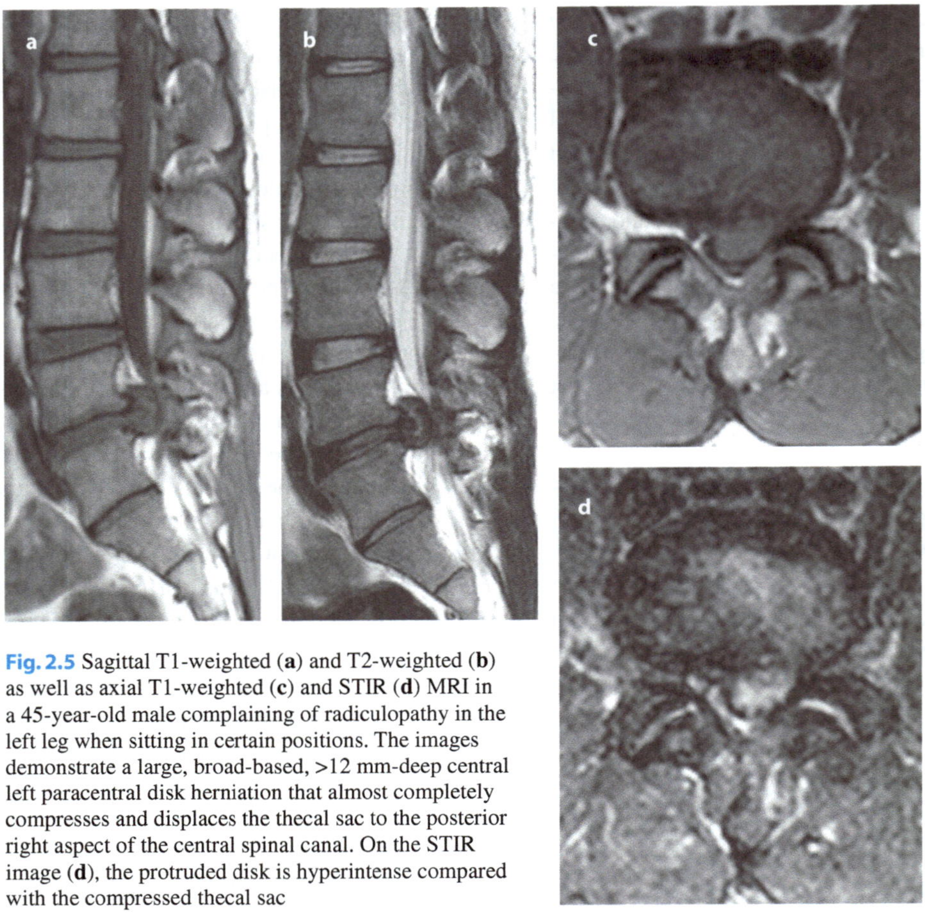

Fig. 2.5 Sagittal T1-weighted (**a**) and T2-weighted (**b**) as well as axial T1-weighted (**c**) and STIR (**d**) MRI in a 45-year-old male complaining of radiculopathy in the left leg when sitting in certain positions. The images demonstrate a large, broad-based, >12 mm-deep central left paracentral disk herniation that almost completely compresses and displaces the thecal sac to the posterior right aspect of the central spinal canal. On the STIR image (**d**), the protruded disk is hyperintense compared with the compressed thecal sac

margins of the disk space. A disk herniation can be considered to be "localized" if <50% of the total circumference of the disk is involved or it can be considered to be "generalized" if >50% is involved [23]. If the disk material extends circumferentially from 50% to 100% beyond the edges of the ring apophyses, it is termed a "bulging" disk. Localized disk herniation is subdivided into "focal" (<25% of the disk diameter) or broad-based (25–50% of the disk diameter) [23] (Figure 5). Disk herniation can be further subdivided in "protruded" or "extruded" disks. A disk protrusion occurs if the base of the herniation is broader than the displaced disk material in any plane. A disk extrusion is present if the base is narrower (in the axial or sagittal plane) than the displaced disk material. If the herniated disk is separated from its origin it is called a "sequestration", and is often termed a "free disk fragment". Posterior and posterolateral ("medial" in previously used terminology) disk herniations are more common than far lateral or extraforaminal disk herniations. Extraforaminal disk herniation is defined as a disk herniation lateral to the foramen without a foraminal component. MRI is the method of choice to evaluate disk herniation regardless of location; a recent study demonstrated that MRI for evaluation of disk morphology has a sensitivity ranging from 60% to 100% and a specificity of 43% to 97% [24]. Usually, central and lateral disk herniations ("medial" in previously used terminology) can be detected readily. However, foraminal and extraforaminal disk herniations with or without foraminal extension are more difficult to detect, and are often overlooked due to the lack of accurate evaluation of foraminal and extraforaminal areas on routine axial and sagittal images. Typical MRI findings that might suggest a far lateral herniation with or without foraminal extension include: focal eccentricity of the disk contour; change in nerve-

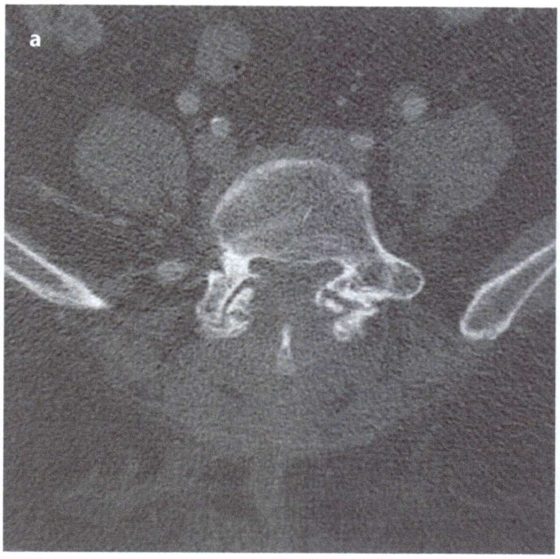

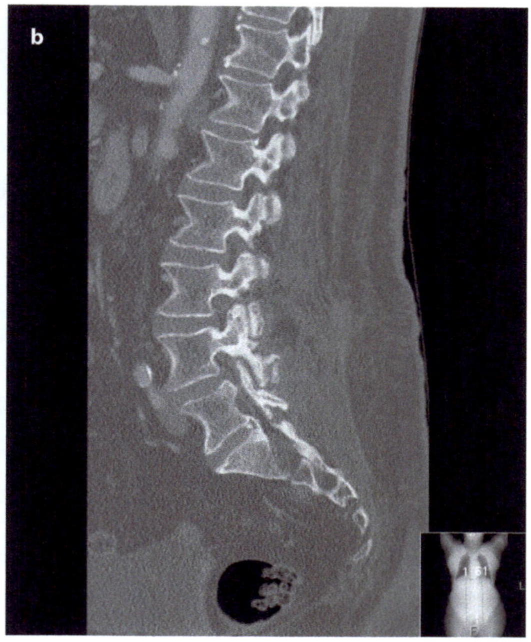

Fig. 2.6 Axial (**a**) and sagittal (**b**) CT with bone algorithms demonstrating typical "wraparound bumper" osteophytes on the right side (**a**) and facet joint arthritis (**a** and **b**)

root thickness due to direct compression by the herniated disk material, compressive nerve-root swelling or nerve-root displacement; and loss of the epidural fat surrounding the nerve root [25]. Recently, other sequences such as obligue coronal view [26], 3D high-spatial resolution diffusion-weighted magnetic resonance (MR) neurography [27], and radiculography through 3D MR rendering using conventional spin-echo sequences and 3D coronal fast-field echo sequences with selective water excitation [28] have been suggested as additional methods to better evaluate far lateral or extraforaminal disk herniation. A recent study using oblique turbo spin-echo T2-weighted sequences showed that this method could provide clear visualization of the dorsal root ganglion and lumbar nerve root in foraminal and extraforaminal areas [26].

2.4 Degenerative Changes and Facet Joint Disease

Lumbar facet joint degeneration is a multifactorial process that occurs independently of the preceding degenerative changes of the intervertebral disk [29–31].

It has been suggested that, in patients presenting with lumbar facet-mediated pain, standard radiographs (including anteroposterior, lateral, and oblique views) should be the initial assessment. In general, the curved configuration and sagittal orientation of the lumbar facet joints limits the utility of frontal and lateral views, but the lateral view gives useful information about possible pars interarticularis defects, as well as showing angulation of facet joints [32]. CT of the spine with reformatted images in sagittal and axial planes with bone algorithms is an excellent way to: demonstrate degenerative changes of the facet joints; show central canal stenosis; grade lateral recess narrowing and neural foraminal narrowing secondary to facet osteoarthritis with associated "wraparound bumper" osteophyte formations along the capsular attachments of the facet joint (Fig. 2.6). Similar findings of hypertrophy of facet joints as well as increased fluid in the facet joint can be seen with MRI (Fig. 2.7). A standard MRI-based classification system for osteoarthritis of lumbar facet joints has been developed by Fujiwara et al. [33]. They also demonstrated that, compared with CT, MRI tends to underestimate the severity of osteoarthritis of the facet joints.

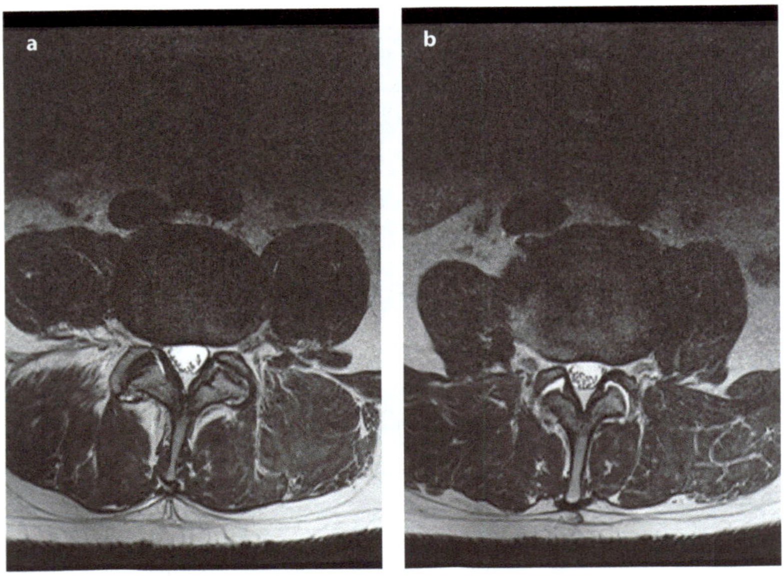

Fig. 2.7 Axial T2-weighted image at the level of the L4–L5 intervertebral disk space (**a**) demonstrating a hypertrophic facet joint with wrap-around osteophytes and hypertrophic ligmanenta flava bilaterally. This results in slight narrowing of the central spinal canal and lateral recesses. Axial T2-weighted image at the level of the L3–L4 intervertebral disk space showing increased fluid in the facet joint bilaterally (**b**)

Synovial cysts associated with arthritis of facet joints and degenerative spondylolisthesis have been noted as potential causes of lower back pain, unilateral radicular pain, neurogenic claudication, and cauda equina syndrome. These cysts are common intraspinal extradural masses located posterolateral to the thecal sac. They are most commonly seen in the L4–L5 region, followed by the L5–S1, L3–4, and L2–3 segments [34]. Lumbar synovial cysts are more commonly seen in patients in their seventh decade of life and have a slight female predominance [35]. The characteristics of the MRI signals of this population are dependent upon hemorrhagic debris or calcification within the cysts but commonly demonstrate hyperintense centers with hypointense rims on T2-weighted images and hypo/isointense areas on T1-weighted images. CT-arthrography has been suggested as an additional test to document communication with a native facet joint before resection or spinal intervention [35].

"Spondylolisthesis" is the term used for anterior or posterior displacement of the VB in relation to an immediately inferior VB. Degenerative spondylolisthesis most often occurs at the L4–L5 level where there is a more vertical orientation of the facet joints. This leads to displacement anterior to the superior VB and to cranio-caudal facet subluxation [23].

Loss of disk height with misalignment of the articular processes, increased segmental axial mobility, degenerative changes (including facet hypertrophy with osteophyte formation, ligamenta flava hypertrophy, fluid with facet joints, synovial facet joint cysts, degenerative spondylolisthesis) may cause narrowing of the spinal canal (especially of the lateral recesses and the neural foramina) [36] (Figs 2.6 and 2.7). Stenosis of the spinal canal or formen may result in compression of the intraspinal or foraminal segments of the nerve roots, and is associated with symptoms that are usually aggravated by the spinal posture [36]. Narrowing of the entire spinal canal is associated with compression of the thecal sac and cauda equina. According to Emch and Modic, the degree of canal narrowing is best classified in the axial plane, and described as "mild" (less than one-third narrowing of the diameter of the spinal canal), "moderate" (one-third to two- thirds) or "severe" (greater than two-thirds) [23]; an identical classification can be applied for grading the degree of neural foraminal stenosis [37].

2.5 Non-traumatic Compression Fractures of the VB

Non-traumatic compression fractures of the VB are common in the elderly population. The most common cause of non-traumatic VB fractures is

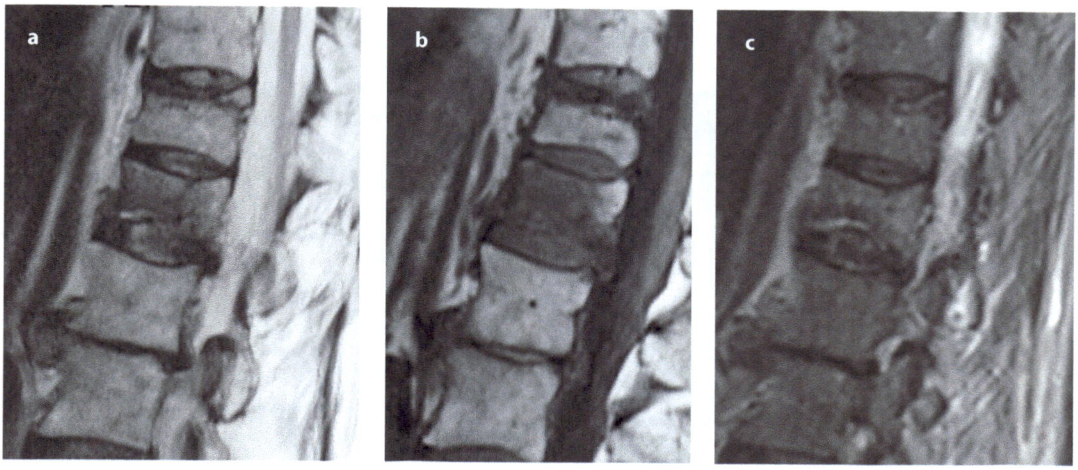

Fig. 2.8 Osteoporotic (benign) vertebral body compression fractures in a 73-year-old female patient with known osteoporosis. **a** On sagittal T2WI low-signal intensity and irregularity of vertebral endplates is noted in T12 vertebral body. Band-like hyperintensity ("fluid sign") is shown in the lower part, indicating recent collapse. Height decrease is also seen in T11 vertebral body with depression of the cover plate and band-like changes (old compression fracture). **b** On sagittal T1WI the affected vertebral body shows low-signal and blurred endplates. **c** Slightly higher signal in T12 is seen on sagittal STIR. Low signal is observed in T11 vertebra

osteoporosis [38]. Almost 50% of Caucasian females will develop osteoporotic fractures during their lifetimes [39]. If not treated aggressively, the mortality and morbidity are high.

The differentiation between osteoporotic and malignant fractures based on clinical and imaging findings in the acute setting is particularly challenging. Morphological signs (e.g., complete replacement of vertebral marrow; involvement of the posterior elements; epidural or paraspinal masses) can be used to improve the diagnostic accuracy for predicting metastatic disease but may be equivocal [40–42]. Up to one-third of fractures in patients with a known primary malignancy are benign, and approximately one-quarter of fractures in apparently osteopenic patients are due to metastases.

Results from recent studies have raised hopes that diffusion-weighted MRI (DWI) could be used to differentiate benign from malignant acute vertebral fractures. It has been hypothesized that proton diffusivity is increased in osteoporotic fractures because of bone-marrow edema. Conversely, metastatic lesions might change diffusivity only moderately (or even decrease) it. It has been postulated that the high cellularity of metastatic lesions (especially of actively growing tumors) reduces proton diffusivity. The first report of the clinical application of DWI of the spinal bone marrow focused on differentiation of benign osteoporotic and malignant vertebral compression fractures: it was published in 1997 by Baur et al. [7]. Benign osteoporotic fractures were hypointense or isointense on steady state free precession (SSFP)-based DWI, whereas malignant fractures exhibited hyperintensity (Figs 2.8 and 2.9). Most of the studies that followed confirmed these results [8, 9, 43, 44, 45]. Exceptions are sclerotic metastases and treated metastases that appear hypointense and give false-negative results [46, 47]. Low signals on DWI in treated metastases are due to tissue necrosis and increased diffusion of water protons. Subsequently, quantitative DWI has clearly shown the difference between normal and pathological vertebral bone marrow [48–52]. The apparent diffusion coefficient (ADC) of pathological bone is $0.7–1.0\times10^{-3}$ mm^2/s in metastatic and malignant fractures, and is $1.0–2.0\times10^{-3}$ mm^2/s in osteoporotic or traumatic fractures [53]. The diagnostic utility of DWI to differentiate benign from malignant acute compression fractures is controversial, primarily due to the considerable overlap in ADC values. Two or more images with different diffu-

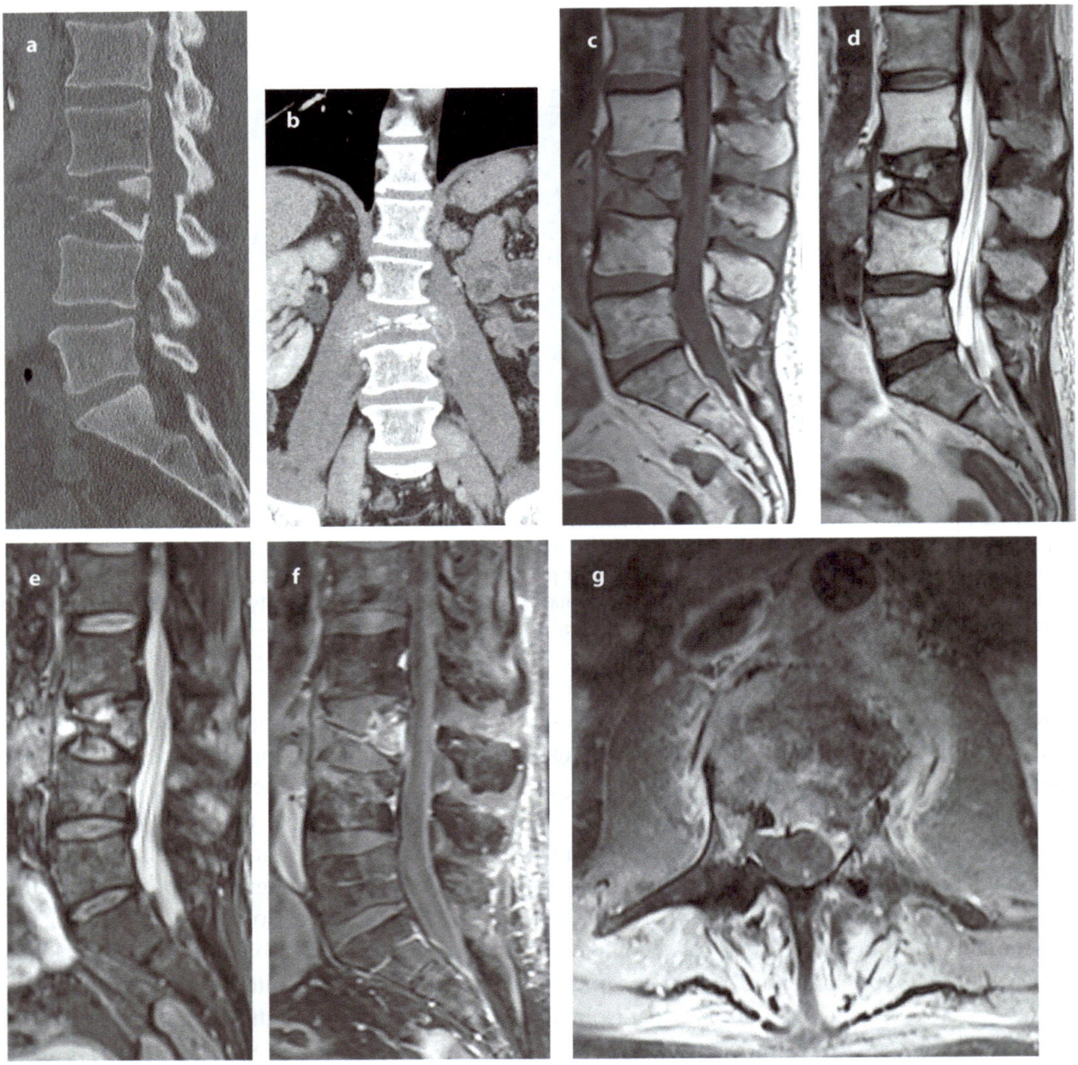

Fig. 2.9 Malignant vertebral body fracture in a 64-year-old male patient with known renal cancer. **a** CT scan (bone window setting) shows a compression fracture of the L3 vertebral body with height decrease and bone destruction. **b** Lytic bone lesion and paravertebral soft tissue masses are recognized on coronal CT scan. **c** On sagittal T1WI image of the lumbar spine low signal intensity is noted in affected vertebral body. **d,e** Mixed signal is observed on sagittal T2WI (**d**) and STIR (**e**). **f,g** On post-contrast T1WI in sagittal (**f**) and axial (**g**) planes intense enhancement of the collapsed vertebral body and paraspinal tumor masses

sion weightings are necessary to evaluate quantitatively the ADC. Typical values of the ADC in normal bone marrow are 0.2–0.5×10^{-3} mm^2/s.

The use of fat saturation is another important issue when obtaining ADC measurements in VBs. The calculated ADCs of normal bone marrow are systematically decreased if fat saturation is not applied. Typical values of the ADC determined without fat saturation [48, 49, 53–56] are 0.2–0.3×10^{-3} mm^2/s in contrast to 0.3–0.5×10^{-3} mm^2/s with fat saturation [51, 52, 57].

Hatipoglu et al. found positive correlation between the decrease of bone mineral density (BMD) and the ADC. This decrease was explained by accumulation of fatty bone marrow [39]. In their study, 51 patients underwent dual-energy X-ray absorptiometry (DEXA) and conventional MRI with diffusion and ADC measurements. In addition, ADC values were compared with BMD. In contrast, Griffith et al. found no correlation between BMD and ADCs [58]. All studies applied a fat-saturated sequence so there is no clear explanation of the contradictory results.

MR perfusion curves have received attention recently. Bone-marrow perfusion shows variations dependent on several factors. The appearance of the bone marrow on MRI is strongly dependent on the distribution of yellow marrow and red marrow. Yellow bone marrow has a sparse network of capillaries, venules, and thin-walled veins, whereas red bone marrow contains a rich vascular network [10]. Studies have shown that bone-marrow perfusion decreases with age and with increasing fat content [7, 58–60]. Chen et al. demonstrated that characterization of the lesions according to their time–intensity curve (TIC) patterns might be valuable [61]. Tokuda et al. found significant differences between perfusion parameters such as slope and maximum enhancement of benign and malignant fractures but not between TIC patterns [62].

A combined quantitative DWI and high-temporal-resolution dynamic contrast-enhanced MRI (DCEMRI) study in the vertebral bone marrow of patients with osteoporosis and acute vertebral compression was carried out recently [63]. Mean perfusion parameters and ADCs were significantly ($p<0.001$) different in the fractures compared to adjacent normal appearing vertebrae [63]. In-phase and out-of-phase gradient echo imaging is a promising new method suggested for distinguishing metastatic spread from acute osteoporotic fractures. The use of in-phase and out-of-phase imaging to differentiate benign from malignant lesions is based on the assumption that malignant lesions completely replace VB fat whereas VB fat is still present in benign lesions. Recently, Erly et al. showed that a signal intensity ratio for in- and out-of-phase images of >0.8 could be used to predict metastatic disease, whereas a ratio of <0.8 could predict benign compression fractures [64].

A recent study using vertebral T1 and T2 relaxation times of fat and water components as well as ADCs in patients presenting with vertebral lesions demonstrated significant differences between normal-appearing vertebral bone marrow and lesions [65]. Interestingly, only the ADCs determined with a diffusion-weighted-single shot turbo spin echo (DW-SS-TSE) method showed significant differences between osteoporotic fractures and malignant lesions.

2.6 Hemangioma

Vertebral body hemangiomas are benign lesions of the spinal column and represent 4% of all spinal tumors. The prevalence based on autopsy and imaging studies is 10–12% [66, 67] with a slightly increased prevalence with age and a slight female predominance. VB hemangiomas predominantly affect thoracic and upper lumbar VBs, although they may involve the pedicles (and rarely the spinous processes) or extend into soft tissue [68]; they are often discovered incidentally. The lesions vary in size and may be multiple in ≤30% of cases. Most VB hemangiomas are asymptomatic and do not cause pain or neurological sequelae. Symptomatic hemangiomas represent <1% of all hemangiomas. Typical symptoms are pain, myelopathy, and radiculopathy due to bone expansion compressing the thecal sac or nerve roots [69, 70]. Thoracic vertebral hemangiomas have been reported to produce neurological symptoms more often than lumbar vertebral hemangiomas. This is thought to be due to the smaller ratio of the spinal cord to the spinal canal in the thoracic segment, and the presence of normal thoracic kyphosis, both of which may facilitate early compression [71]. The management and treatment of symptomatic hemangiomas vary, and includes kyphoplasty, embolization or surgical stabilization.

Occasionally, hemangiomas may cause a pathological fracture, especially if they are: aggressive in nature; large; located posteriorly in the VB; extend into the pedicles.

Histologically, hemangiomas are hamartomatous proliferations of vascular tissue of endothelial origin, and appear as multiple small vessels and components of fatty tissue interspersed among bone trabeculae [72]. Two main types of hemangiomas most commonly present in osseous

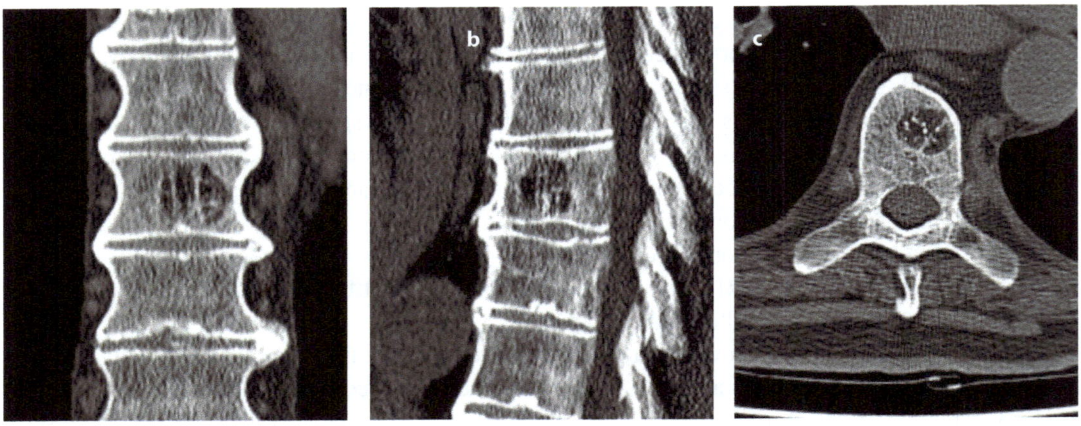

Fig. 2.10 Coronal (**a**), sagittal (**b**) and axial (**c**) CT with bone algorithms of a single vertebral body hemangioma in the thoracic spine. Multiple dots ("polka dots") representing a cross-section of reinforced trabeculae in the center of the vertebral body are seen

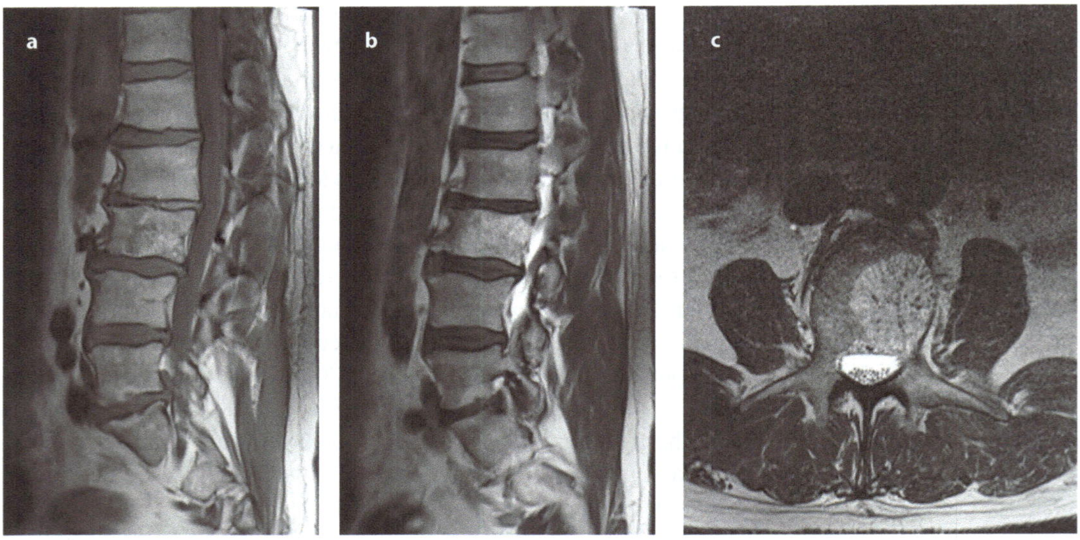

Fig. 2.11 Sagittal T1-weighted (**a**) and T2-weighted (**b**) as well as axial T2-weighted (**c**) MRI demonstrating a large hemangioma in the L3 vertebral body extending into the left pedicle. It presented as punctate areas of low or isointense signals compared with bone on T1-weighted MRI and high signal intensity on T2-weighted MRI

tissue, and are categorized as "capillary" or "cavernous" on the basis of the associated vessels.

Vertebral hemangiomas have typical imaging features. The radiographic appearance of hemangiomas is characteristic, with vertical trabeculae and soft-tissue stromas ("honeycomb" pattern), and the VB looks molted with a lower bone density [68, 73]. On CT, they have a multiple-dot pattern ("polka dots") representing a cross-section of reinforced trabeculae, and may demonstrate contrast enhancement (Fig. 2.10) [74]. On MRI, which is the gold-standard imaging, the imaging features of active hemangiomas are punctate areas of low or isointense signals compared with bone on T1-weighted images and high signal intensity on T2-weighted MRI. If the hemangiomas are inactive, they present with high signals on T1- and T2-weighted images (Fig. 2.11). They commonly demonstrate homogenous enhancement after contrast administration. Conventional digital angiography demonstrates the vascular nature of these lesions.

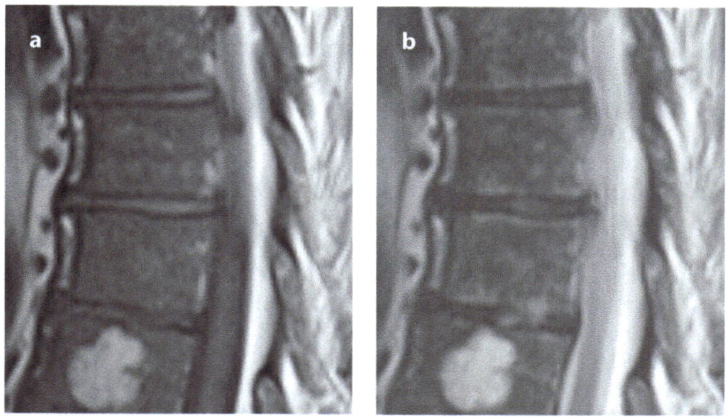

Fig. 2.12 Sagittal T1-weighted (**a**) and T2-weighted (**b**) MRI of an inactive hemangioma in the lower thoracic spine showing high signals

2.7 Summary

Imaging has an important role before and after spinal intervention. CT and MRI are the most used imaging modalities for the detection and differentiation of spinal lesions. CT and fluoroscopic imaging are used during interventional procedures.

Acknowledgements We would like to express our gratitude to Associate Professor Kasim Abul-Kasim (Senior Consultant in Neuroradiology, Skåne University Hospital, Malmoe, Sweden) for his help in processing the illustrations.

References

1. Tins B (2010) Technical aspects of CT imaging of the spine. Insights Imaging 1:349–359
2. Di Chiro G, Schellinger D (1976) Computed tomography of spinal cord after lumbar intrathecal introduction of metrizamide (computer assisted myelography). Radiology 120:101–104
3. Bartynski WS, Lin L (2003) Lumbar root compression in the lateral recess: MR imaging, conventional myelography, and CT myelography comparison with surgical confirmation. Am J Neuroradiol 24:348–360
4. Morita M, Miyauchi A, Okuda S et al (2011) Comparison between MRI and myelography in lumbar spinal canal stenosis for the decision of levels of decompression surgery. J Spinal Dis Tech 24:31–36
5. Grams AE, Gempt J, Förschler A (2010) Comparison of spinal anatomy between 3-Tesla MRI and CT-myelography under healthy and pathological conditions. Surg Radiol Anat 32:581–585
6. Naganawa T, Miyamoto K, Ogura H et al (2011) Comparison of magnetic resonance imaging and computed tomogram-myelography for evaluation of cross sections of cervical spinal morphology. Spine 36:50–56
7. Baur A, Stäbler A, Bartl R et al (1997) MRI gadolinium enhancement of bone marrow: age-related changes in normals and in diffuse neoplastic infiltration. Skeletal Radiol 26:414–418
8. Baur A, Huber A, Dürr HK et al (2002). Differentiation of benign osteoporotic and neoplastic vertebral compression fractures with a diffusion-weighted, steady-state free precession sequence. RöFo 174:70–75
9. Castillo M, Arbelaez A, Smith JK et al (2000) Diffusion-weighted MR imaging offers no advantage over routine noncontrast MR imaging in the detection of vertebral metastases. Am J Neuroradiol 21:948–95310. Biffar A, Sourbron S, Schmidt GP et al (2010) Measurement of perfusion and permeability from dynamic-contrast-enhanced MR imaging in normal and pathological vertebral bone marrow. Magn Reson Med 64:115–12411. Backes WH, Nijenhuis RJ (2008) Advances in spinal cord MR angiography. Am J Neuroradiol 29:619–631
12. Carrino JA, Lurie JD, Tosteson AN et al (2009) Lumbar spine reliability of MR imaging findings Radiology 250:161–170
13. Lurie JD, Tosteson AN, Tosteson TD et al (2008) Reliability of readings of magnetic resonance imaging features of lumbar spinal stenosis. Spine 33:1605–1610
14. Lurie JD, Tosteson AN, Tosteson TD et al (2008) Reliability of magnetic resonance imaging readings for lumbar disc herniation in the Spine Patient Outcomes Research Trial (SPORT). Spine (Phila Pa 1976) 33:991–998
15. Tyrrell PN, Cassar-Pullicino VN , McCall IW (1998) Gadolinium-DTPA enhancement of symptomatic nerve roots in MRI of the lumbar spine. Eur Radiol 8:116–122
16. Hoppe S, Quirbach S, Mamisch TC et al (2012) Axial T2* mapping in intervertebral discs: a new technique for assessment of intervertebral disc degeneration Eur Radiol 22: 2013–201917. Kettler A, Wilke H-J (2006)

Review of existing grading systems for cervical or lumbar disc and facet joint degeneration Eur Spine J 15:705–718
18. Pfirrmann CW, Metzdorf A, Zanetti M, Hodler J, Boos N (2001) Magnetic resonance classification of lumbar intervertebral disc degeneration. Spine 26:1873–1878
19. Bangert BA, Modic MT, Ross JS et al (1995) Hyperintense disks on T1-weighted MR images: correlation with calcification. Radiology 195:437–443
20. de Roos A, Kressel H, Spritzer et al (1987) MR imaging of marrow changes adjacent to end plates in degenerative lumbar disk disease. Am J Roentgenol 149:531–534
21. Modic MT, Steinberg PM, Ross JS et al (1988) Degenerative disk disease: assessment of changes in vertebral body marrow with MR imaging. Radiology166:193–199
22. Eguchi Y, Seiji Ohtori S Yamashita M (2011) Diffusion magnetic resonance imaging to differentiate degenerative from infectious endplate abnormalities in the lumbar spine. Spine 36:198–202
23. Emch TE, Modic MT (2011) Imaging of lumbar degenerative disk disease: history and current state. Skeletal Radiol 40:1175–1189
24. Jarvik JG, Deyo RA (2002) Diagnostic evaluation of low back pain with emphasis on imaging. Ann Intern Med 137:586–597
25. Lee IS, Kim HJ, Lee JS, et al (2009) Extraforaminal with or without foraminal disk herniation: reliable MRI findings. Am J Roentgenol 192:1392–1396
26. Heo DH, Lee MS, Sheen SH et al (2009) Simple oblique lumbar magnetic resonance Imaging technique and its diagnostic value for extraforaminal disc herniation. Spine 34:2419–2423
27. Zhang Z, Song L, Meng Q et al (2009) Morphological analysis in patients with sciatica: a magnetic resonance imaging study using three dimensional high-resolution diffusion-weighted magnetic resonance neurography techniques. Spine 34:245–250
28. Byun WM , Jang HW, Kim SW (2012) Three-dimensional magnetic resonance rendering imaging of lumbosacral radiculography in the diagnosis of symptomatic extraforaminal disc herniation with or without foraminal extension. Spine 37:840–844
29. Schellinger D, Wener L, Ragsdale BD et al (1987) Facet joint disorders and their role in the production of back pain and sciatica. Radiographics 7:923–944
30. Butler D, Trafimow JH, Andersson GBJ et al (1990) Discs degenerate before facets. Spine 15:111–113
31. Vernon-Roberts B, Pirie CJ (1977) Degenerative changes in the intervertebral discs of the lumbar spine and their sequelae. Rheumatol Rehabil 16:13–21
32. Varlotta GP, Lefkowitz TR, Schweitzer M et al (2011) The lumbar facet joint: a review of current knowledge: part 1: anatomy, biomechanics, and grading. Skeletal Radiol 40:13–23
33. Fujiwara A, Tamai K, Yamato M et al (1999) The relationship between facet joint osteoarthritis and disc degeneration of the lumbar spine: an MRI study. Eur Spine J 8:396–401
34. Epstein NE (2004) Lumbar synovial cysts: a review of diagnosis, surgical management, and outcome assessment. J Spinal Disord Tech 17:321–325
35. Schmid G, Willburger R, Jergas M et al (2002) Lumbar intraspinal juxtafacet cysts: MR imaging and CT-arthrography. RöFo 174:1247–1252
36. Wilmink JT (2011) The normal aging spine and degenerative spinal disease. Neuroradiology 53 (Suppl. 1):181–183
37. Fardon DF, Milette PC (2001) Nomenclature and classification of lumbar disc pathology. Recommendations of the combined task forces of the North American Spine Society, American Society of Spine Radiology, and American Society of Neuroradiology. Spine 26:93–113
38. National Osteoporosis Foundation (2002) America's bone health: the state of osteoporosis and low bone mass in our nation. National Osteoporosis Foundation, Washington DC39. Hatipoglu HG, Selvi A, Ciliz D et al (2007) Quantitative and diffusion MR Imaging as a new method to assess osteoporosis. Am J Neuroradiol 28:1934–1937
40. An HS, Andreshak TG, Nguyen C et al (1995) Can we distinguish between benign vs malignant compression fractures of the spine by magnetic resonance imaging? Spine 20:1776–178241. Rupp RE, Ebraheim NA, Coombs RJ (1995) Magnetic resonance imaging differentiation of compression spine fractures or vertebral lesions caused by osteoporosis or tumour. Spine 23:2499–2503 (discussion, 2504)
42. Yuh WT, Zachar CK, Barloon TJ et al (1989) Vertebral compression fractures: distinction between benign and malignant causes with MR imaging. Radiology 172:215–218
43. Spuentrup E, Bruecker A, Adam G et al (2001) Diffusion-weighted MR imaging for differentiation of benign fracture edema and tumor infiltration of the vertebral body. Am J Roentgenol 176:351–358
44. Abanoz R, Hakyemez B, Parlak M (2003) Diffusion-weighted imaging of acute vertebral compression: differential diagnosis of benign versus malignant pathologic fractures. Tani Girisim Radyol 9:176–183
45. Hackländer T, Scharwächter C, Golz R et al (2006) Value of diffusion-weighted imaging for diagnosing vertebral metastases due to prostate cancer in comparison to other primary tumors. RöFo 178:416–424
46. Byun WM, Shin SO, Chang Y et al (2002) Diffusion-weighted MR imaging of metastatic disease of the spine: assessment of response to therapy. Am J Neuroradiol 23:906–912
47. Otzekin O, Ozan E, Adibelli HZ et al (2009) SSH-EPI diffusion-weighted MR imaging of the spine with low b values: is it useful in differentiating malignant metastatic tumor infiltration from benign fracture edema? Skeletal Radiol 38:651–658
48. Zhou XJ, Leeds NE, McKinnon GC et al (2002) Characterization of benign and metastatic vertebral compression fractures with quantitative diffusion MR imaging. Am J Neuroradiol 23:165–170
49. Oner AY, Tali T, Celikyay F et al (2007) Diffusion-

weighted imaging of the spine with a non-carr-purcell-meiboom-gill single-shot fast spin-echo sequence: initial experience. Am J Neuroradiol 28:575–580
50. Herneth AM, Natude J, Philipp M et al (2000). The value of diffusion-weighted MRT in assessing the bone marrow changes in vertebral metastases. Radiologe 40:731–736
51. Chan JH, Peh WC, Tsui EY et al (2002). Acute vertebral body compression fractures: discrimination between benign and malignant causes using apparent diffusion coefficients. Br J Radiol 75:207–214
52. Herneth AM, Philipp MO, Naude J et al (2002) Vertebral metastases: assessment with apparent diffusion coefficient. Radiology 225:889–894
53. Dietrich O, Biffar A, Reiser MF et al (2009) Diffusion-weighted imaging of bone marrow. Semin Musculoskelet Radiol 13:134–144
54. Byun WM, Jang HHW, Kim SW et al (2007) Diffusion-weighted magnetic resonance imaging of sacral insufficiency fractures: comparison with metastases of the sacrum. Spine 32:820–824
55. Bammer R, Herneth AM, Maier SE et al (2003) Line scan diffusion imaging of the spine. Am J Neuroradiol 24:5–12
56. Raya J, Dietrich O, Birkenmaier C et al (2007) Feasibility of a RARE-based sequence for quantitative diffusion-weighted MRI of the spine. Eur Radiol 17:2872–2879
57. Piu MH, Mith A, Rae WI, et al (2005) Diffusion-weighted magnetic resonance imaging of spinal infection and malignancy. J Neuroimaging 15:164–170
58. Griffith JF, Yeung DK, Antonio GE et al (2005) Vertebral bone mineral density, marrow perfusion, and fat content in healthy men and men with osteoporosis: dynamic contrast-enhanced MR imaging and MR spectroscopy. Radiology 236:945–951
59. Chen WT, Shih TT, Chen RC et al (2001) Vertebral bone marrow perfusion evaluated with dynamic contrast-enhanced MR imaging: significance of aging and sex. Radiology 220:213–218
60. Montazel JL, Divine M, Lepage E et al (2003) Normal spinal bone marrow in adults: dynamic gadolinium-enhanced MR imaging. Radiology 229:703–709
61. Chen WT, Shih TT, Chen RC et al (2002) Blood perfusion of vertebral lesions evaluated with gadolinium-enhanced dynamic MRI: in comparison with compression fracture and metastasis. J Magn Reson Imaging 15:308–314
62. Tokuda O, Hayashi N, Taguchi K et al (2005) Dynamic contrast-enhanced perfusion MR imaging of diseased vertebrae: analysis of three parameters and the distribution of the time-intensity curve patterns. Skeletal Radiol 34:632–638
63. Biffar A, Dietrich O, Sourbron S et al (2010) Diffusion and perfusion imaging of bone marrow. Eur J Radiol 76:323–328
64. Erly WK, Oh ES, Outwater EK (2006) The utility of in-phase/opposed-phase imaging in differentiating malignancy from acute benign compression fractures of the spine. Am J Neuroradiol 27:1183–1188
65. Biffar A, Baur-Melnyk A, Schmidt GP et al (2010) Multiparameter MRI assessment of normal-appearing and diseased vertebral bone marrow. Eur Radiol 20:2679–268966. Barzin M, Maleki I (2009). Incidence of vertebral hemangioma on spinal magnetic resonance imaging in Northern Iran. Pak J Biol Sci 12:542–544
67. Fox MW, Onofrio BM (1993) The natural history and management of symptomatic and asymptomatic vertebral hemangiomas. J Neurosurg 78:36–45
68. Greenspan A (2004) Orthopedic imaging: a practical approach. 4th ed. Lippincott Williams & Wilkins, Philadelphia 69. Acosta FL Jr, Sanai N, Chi JH et al (2008). Comprehensive management of symptomatic and aggressive vertebral hemangiomas. Neurosurg Clin N Am 19:17–29
70. Templin CR, Stambough JB, Stambough JL (2004) Acute spinal cord compression caused by vertebral hemangioma. Spine J 4:595–600
71. Vinay S, Khan SK, Braybrooke JR (2011) Lumbar vertebral haemangioma causing pathological fracture, epidural haemorrhage, and cord compression: a case report and review of the literature. J Spinal Cord Med 34:335–339
72. Fletcher CDM (1995) Diagnostic histopathology of tumors. Churchill Livingstone, Edinburgh73. Ross JS, Masaryk TJ, Modic MT et al (1987) Vertebral hemangiomas: MR imaging. Radiology 165:165–169
74. Rodallec MH, Feydy A, Larousserie F et al (2008) Diagnostic imaging of solitary tumors of the spine: what to do and say. Radiographics 28:1019–1041

Radiological Anatomy and Approaches to the Spine

3

Alvaro Antonio Diano, Gianluigi Guarnieri
and Mario Muto

3.1 Introduction

The fundamental concept of normal anatomy of the spine is crucial for a correct approach to minimally invasive spinal treatments. In this chapter, the spinal anatomy and paravertebral soft tissue will be discussed because they represent the "roadmap" during the percutaneous procedures carried out under fluoroscopic or computed tomography (CT) guidance.

The goal of a minimally invasive interventional procedure in the spine (irrespective of which one is employed) is to reach a particular "target" located in the vertebral body (VB) or the posterior arch by the least traumatic and safest way possible. However, the approach must permit valid diagnostic or therapeutic results.

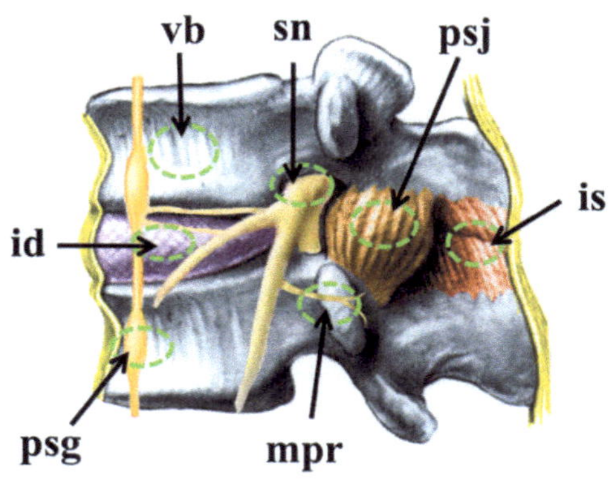

Fig. 3.1 Main targets of percutaneous interventional procedures in the spine. Vertebral body (*vb*); intervertebral disks (*id*); ganglion and spinal nerve (*sn*); paraspinal sympathetic ganglion (*psg*); posterior spinal facet joint (*psj*); interspinous space (*is*); medial branch posterior ramus (*mpr*)

3.2 General Points to Consider

The *rationale* of percutaneous treatment is to reach a specific target under radiographic guidance in the safest possible way. It is possible to design precisely the route to reach the anatomical location desired, as well as constant monitoring during execution of the procedure and the immediate verification of the results obtained.

In the specific case of the spine, the target is anatomical landmarks such as facet joints, intervertebral disks, posterior arch, lamina, and paraspinal nerve structures (Fig. 3.1). These regions are readily identified by fluoroscopy or CT. Fluoroscopy is characterized by a wide field of view and sufficient spatial resolution only on skeletal parts. CT also provides detailed information on soft paravertebral tissue (especially on muscle or fatty tissue and often about vascular and nerve structures). To carry out minimally invasive percutaneous procedures, summarizing

M. Muto (✉)
Neuroradiology Department, A. Cardarelli Hospital,
Naples, Italy
e-mail: mutomar2@gmail.com

M. Muto (ed.), *Interventional Neuroradiology of the Spine*,
DOI 10.1007/978-88-470-2790-9_3, © Springer-Verlag Italia 2013

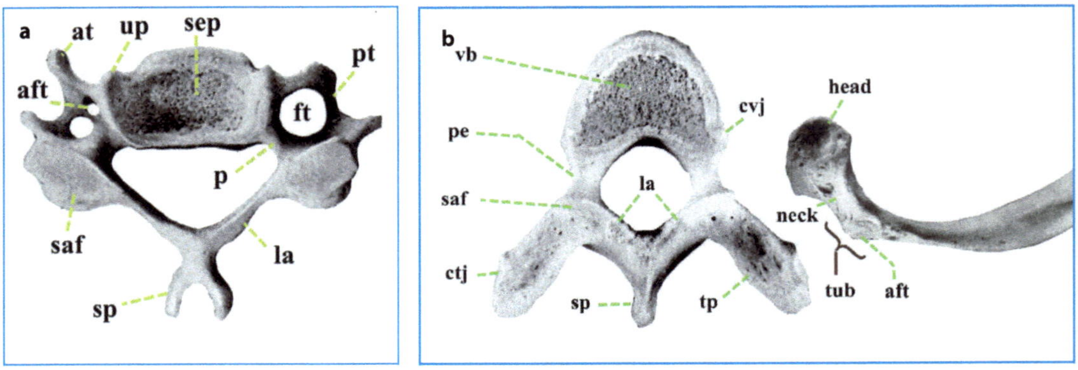

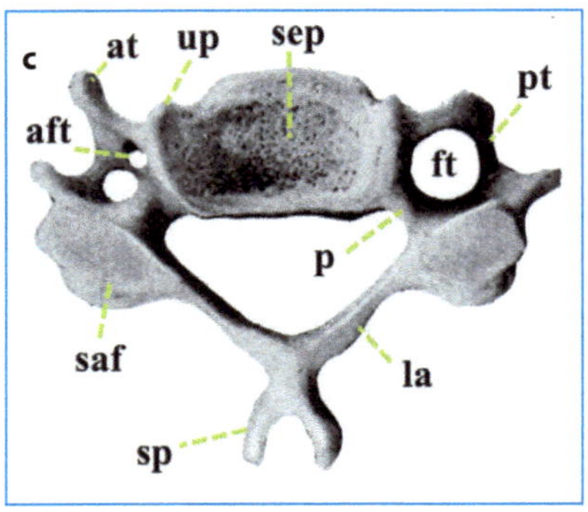

Fig. 3.2 Axial view of anatomical preparations of cervical vertebrae (**a**), corresponding to the dorsal portions (**b**) and cervical portions (**c**). Superior vertebral endplate (*sep*); hooked process (*up*); anterior tubercle of transverse process (*at*); posterior tubercle of the transverse process (*tp*); posterior superior articular facet joint (*saf*); spinous process (bifid at the cervical level) (*sp*); lamina (*la*); accessory foramen transversarium (*aft*); pedicle (*p*); foramen transversarium (*ft*); vertebral body (*vb*); costotransverse joint (*ctj*); costovertebral joint (*cvj*); tubercle (*tub*); articular facet for transverse process (*aft*); mammillary process (*mp*); central spinal canal (*sc*)

the normal spinal anatomy and radiographic elements of the spine is important.

3.3 Normal Anatomy of the Spine

The spinal column is divided in five segments: cervical, thoracic, lumbar, sacral and coccyx. The spinal column comprises thirty-three individual segments: the vertebrae. They consist of an anterior bony block, the body and a posterior element, as well as the neural arch (which contains the articular, transverse and spinous processes). The VB is a cylindrical formation of cancellous bone enclosed in a thin shell of compact bone, which is in correspondence with the upper and lower surface.

The basic architecture is similar in the different regions of the spinal column. However, the mass and size of the vertebrae increases gradually proceeding from the first cervical vertebra up to the last lumbar vertebra as a natural adaptation in response increases in mechanical loading. Other major differences are the presence of the foramina for both vertebral arteries in the transverse processes at the cervical level, the facet joints in the ribs at the thoracic vertebrae, and the mammary processes at the lumbar level (Fig. 3.2).

The first two cervical vertebrae are considerably different from the others. The atlas (C1) does not have an anterior body. It corresponds to the odontoid process of the second cervical vertebra and is formed by an anterior arch that is joined to the posterior arch by two lateral masses (the articular processes) to which there are the transverse processes. The surface of the upper articular processes has an ellipsoid, irregular and concave shape (Fig. 3.3) with an axis directed forward and laterally (the inclination is about 40° from the median sagittal plane), also known as the “glenoid cavity”, that receives the occipital condyles.

The posterior arch corresponds to the lamina of the remaining vertebrae where, on its upper surface, is located the sulcus for the vertebral artery. The posterior tubercle is the vestigial remnant of the spinous processes. The second cervical vertebra is characterized by the odontoid process or dens, which is derived from the central nucleus of ossification of the atlas (C1). The dens

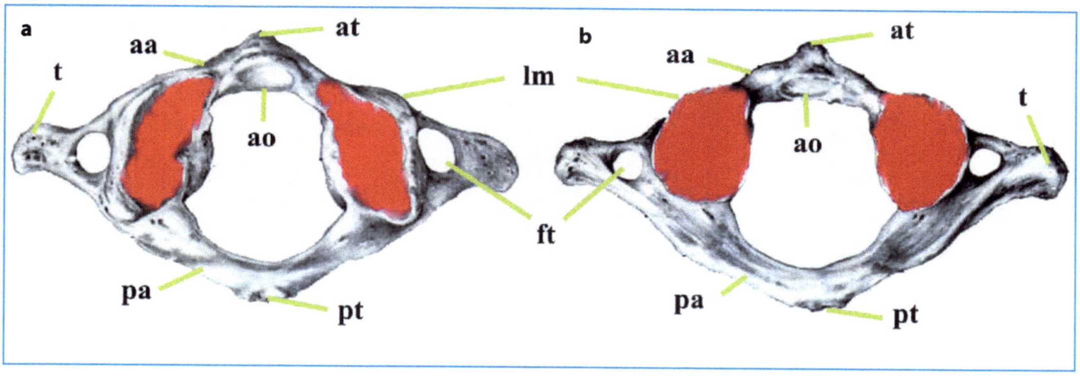

Fig. 3.3 The atlas. Upper (**a**) and lower view anatomical detail (**b**). Articular surface for odontoid process of C2 (*o*); anterior arch (*aa*); posterior neural arch (lamina) (*pa*); lateral mass (*lm*) for vertebral artery foramen transversarium/veins (*ft*); posterior tubercle (*pt*); anterior tubercle (*Pt*); transverse process (*t*)

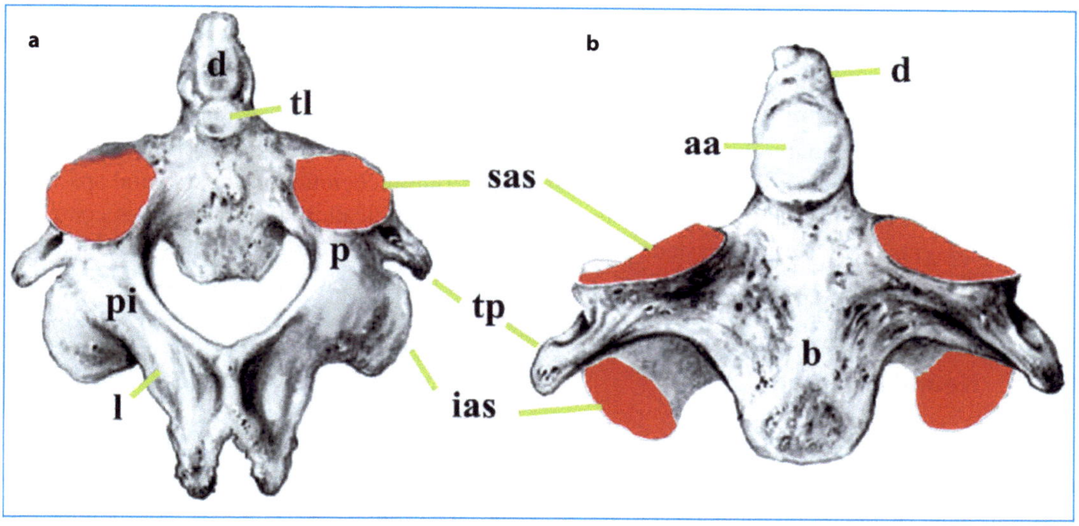

Fig. 3.4 Axis. Anatomical detail of C2: three quarters posterior superior view (**a**) and frontal view (**b**). Dens (*d*); point of insertion of transverse axial ligament (posterior articular facet) (*tl*); anterior articular facet for median atlanto-axial joint (*aa*); superior articular facet (*sas*); inferior articular facet (*ias*); pars interarticularis (*pi*); pedicle (*p*); lamina (*L*); transverse process (*tp*); body of C2 (*b*)

is a bony, conical-shaped process that extends up almost to the inferior end plate of the clivus and is provided with two articular facets: a ventral one in contact with the anterior arch of the atlas and a dorsal one that comes into contact with the transverse ligament (Fig. 3.4). By each side of the dens are two articular apophyses which support the weight of the head.

The upper facet joints overflow outside, below and behind with respect to the body of C2, standing midway between the two structures on which the load is shared: the diskal and articular processes. Their surface is flat in the transverse direction but can be also slightly convex, and they have a thin edge of compact bone along which a ring on left lateral (LL) radiographic projection can be defined. The peduncles are particularly large, more vertical and less oriented with respect to other cervical vertebrae, and delimit the vertebral artery canal. The posterior arch appears to be disproportionate with respect to the body because it must distribute the forces of the muscle inserted on the spinous C2 apophysis. The transverse processes are short, the laminae have a

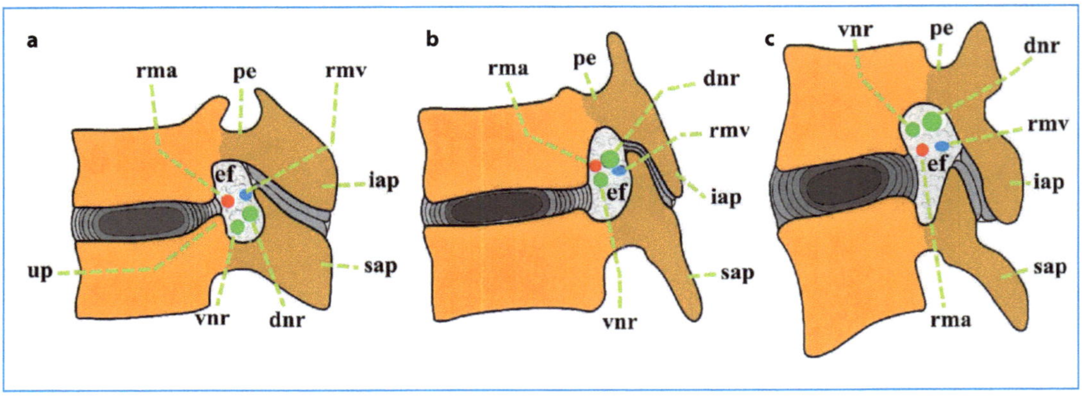

Fig. 3.5 Schematic view in the sagittal section of the foramen and nerve vascular structures at cervical (**a**), thoracic (**b**) and lumbar (**c**) levels. Ventral nerve root (*vnr*); dorsal nerve root (*dnr*); epidural fat (*f*); hooked process (*up*); radiculomedullary artery (*rma*); radiculomedullary vein (*rmv*); superior articular process (*sap*); inferior articular process (*iap*), pedicle (*pe*)

rectangular shape, and the spinous processes are often long and stout [1–7]

To carry out minimally invasive interventional procedures, knowing four key spinal elements is important: neural foramen, posterior facet joints, sympathetic nervous system, and the spinal nerve.

3.3.1 Neural Foramen

The neural foramen is also called the "intervertebral foramen". It contains primarily the nerves (with an anterior motor root and posterior sensitive root plus its ganglion), the vascular structures, and some fatty cells primarily distributed in its upper portion. The neural foramen is delimited: by the articular process posteriorly; by the VB with the disk anteriorly; on the upper side by the inferior margin of the pedicle of the cranial vertebra; and inferiorly by the upper margin of the pedicle of the vertebra below. At the cervical level, the anterior nerve root is related to the unciform processes and the vertebral artery. At the cervical level, the nerve root occupies the lower part of the foramen, whereas in the upper portion are placed the vessels and fat (Fig. 3.5a). At the thoracic level, the nerves and vessels are in the middle portion of the foramen (Fig. 3.5b). At the lumbar level they are in the upper portion of the foramen (Fig. 3.5c).

These neural elements (particularly those at the cervical level) are surrounded by numerous veins that, on CT after injection of contrast media, permit recognition of the epidural space, allowing identification of the structures contained therein. The cervical nerve roots are numbered from C1. The first nerve root leaves the spinal canal at the space between the occipital bone and C1, up to the C8 nerve root that emerges from the neural foramen of C7–D1. Consequently, the numbering of the nerve roots in the remaining thoracic and lumbar segments is staggered by one level down compared with the corresponding VB (the twelfth thoracic nerve engages the intervertebral foramen D12–L1, whereas the fifth lumbar nerve engages the foramen L5–S1). The extent of inclination of the foramina changes in the various segments of the spine compared with the sagittal plane. The channel is directed obliquely in the anterolateral side in the cervical and laterally in the thoracolumbar level [8–9] (Fig. 3.6).

3.3.2 Posterior Facet Joints

At the cervical level, the articular apophyses have a cylindrical shape with an angle of 45° with respect to the horizontal plane. On their surface are the facet joints, which are inclined downwards by about 45°. Because of their spatial orientation they seem to have a "parallelogram" appearance

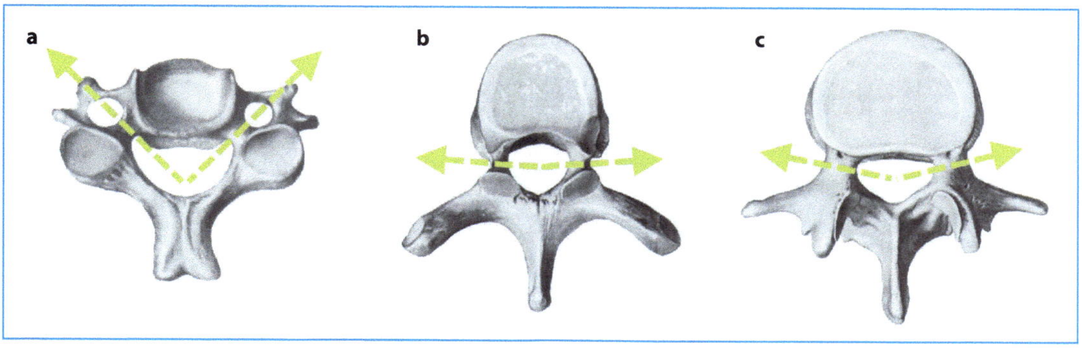

Fig. 3.6 Orientation in the axial plane of the channel of conjugation in the cervical (**a**), thoracic (**b**) and lumbar (**c**) levels

Fig. 3.7 Lateral view of cervical and thoracic spinal segments and oblique view of lumbar segments with demonstration of the facet joints

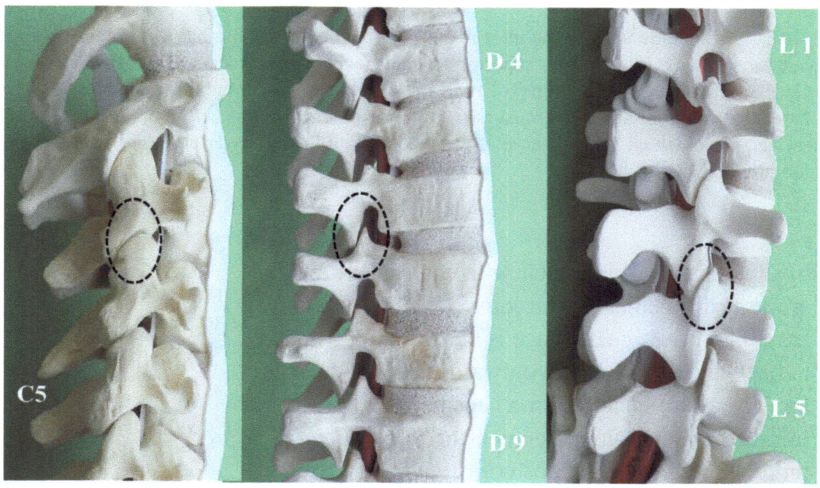

with a cone shape on the LL view on radiographs, whereas on all other radiographic projections they assume an oval appearance with margins that are more or less rounded. At the thoracic level, the facet joints have a flat surface and are directed back and forth over the lower ones. At the lumbar level, the articular processes appear as flattened bone formations located at the junction between the lamina and pedicles and posteriorly with respect to the transverse processes. The superior articular apophyses have an internal joint surface in the form of a vertical shower, covered with cartilage. Their outer surface shows a small bone on the back edge called the mammillary tubercle. The inferior articular apophyses are implanted on the lower edge of the lamina, and are directed obliquely downwards and backwards.

The convex articular surface of the inferior articular apophyses is in contact with the upper articular apophysis of the vertebra below. At the sagittal plane they form an angle that increases progressively from L1 to L5, being nearly a sagittal line from L1 to L4 and almost a frontal line at L4–L5 and L5–S1. However, the orientation changes from one subject to another or in the same subject, and often there is an asymmetry between the two sides. At the L4–L5 and L5–S1 joint space, the right side is more sagittal than the left in 70% of cases [10–13]. In the sagittal plane, the orientation of the joint is almost vertical (Fig. 3.7). To understand the important role of this articulation during interventional procedures, its anatomy must be specified. The interapophyseal articulation is a synovial joint that is often associated (as with all other joints) with inflammatory–degenerative processes. The folds of the synovial membrane may extend between the articular surfaces and cause pain if they are inflamed. The articular surfaces are covered with

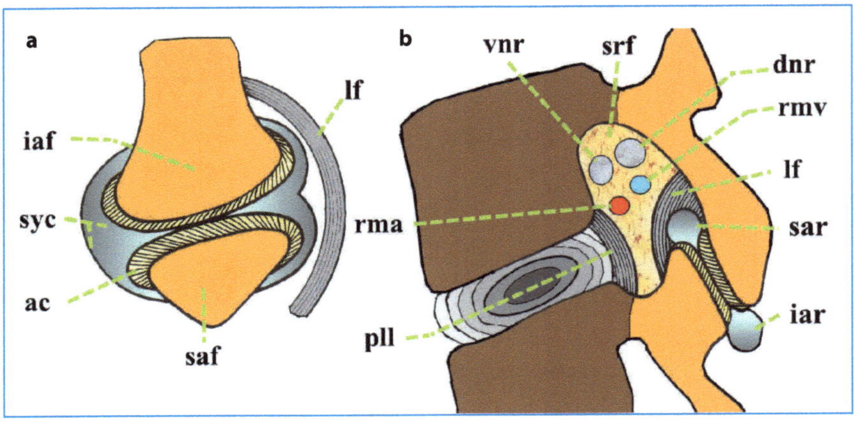

Fig. 3.8 Schematic view of the inter-apophysis junction at the lumbar level in axial (**a**) and sagittal (**b**) sections. Ligamentum flavum (*lf*); posterior superior articular facet joint surface (*saf*); posterior inferior articular facet joint surface (*iaf*); articular cartilage (hyaline) of facet joint (*ac*); synovial membrane and capsular ligament of posterior spinal joint face (*syc*); superior articular recess (*sar*); inferior articular recess (*iar*); superior recess of the neural foramen (*srf*); dorsal nerve root (*dnr*); ventral nerve root (*vnr*); radiculomedullary artery (*rma*); radiculomedullary vein (*rmv*); posterior longitudinal ligament (*pll*)

hyaline cartilage, interlock with each other, and are joined together by the joint capsule. In general, the interarticular space is curved from front to back and forwards and outwards. The articular apophyses are enclosed in a capsule, and are reinforced by the lateral segment of the ligamentum flavum and by the posterior ligament. There are two joint recesses: the higher one is located anteriorly and is in proximity to the spinal canal and neural elements, and can be up to the neural foramen (Fig. 3.8).

Two other small recesses can be found. They are inconstant and extend the full height of the joint: the anterior-medial recess and posterolateral recess [14]. The size of the inferior recess varies based on the static lumbar spine. An increase in lumbar lordosis tends to widen the upper recess, whereas an increase in kyphosis determines a wider inferior recess. Hence, it is desirable to place a pillow under the abdomen of the patient to reduce the lordosis and facilitate puncture of the inferior recess.

The innervation of the posterior vertebral joints is rich and complex (Fig. 3.9). On each side there is a sensory nerve from the ipsilateral posterior branch of the same level of the spinal nerve, and sensory branches of the spinal nerve arise from those above.

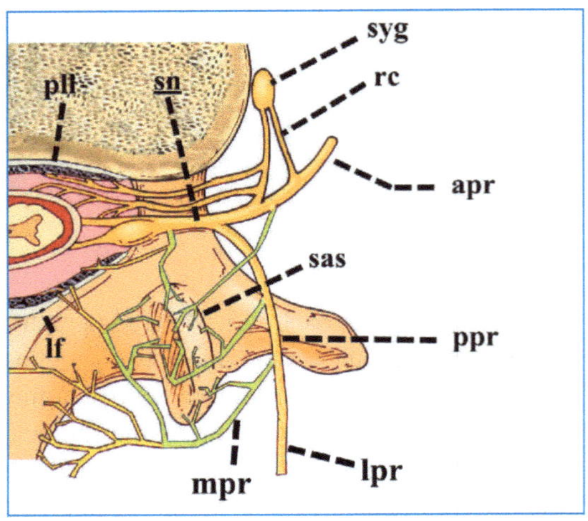

Fig. 3.9 Innervation of the facet joints and spinal nerve. The nerve branches directed to the articular apophyses are highlighted. Sympathetic ganglion (*syg*); branches comunicantes (*rc*); anterior primary ramus (*apr*); posterior primary ramus (*ppr*); medial branch posterior ramus (*mpr*); ramus posterior lateral branch (*lpr*); posterior longitudinal ligament (*pll*); ligamentum flavum (*lf*); superior articular facet (*sas*); spinal nerve (*sn*)

3.3.3 Sympathetic Nervous System in the Spine

Pre-ganglion cells of the anterior horn of the nerve fibers of the spinal cord originate in the passing ventral root of the spinal nerve and are

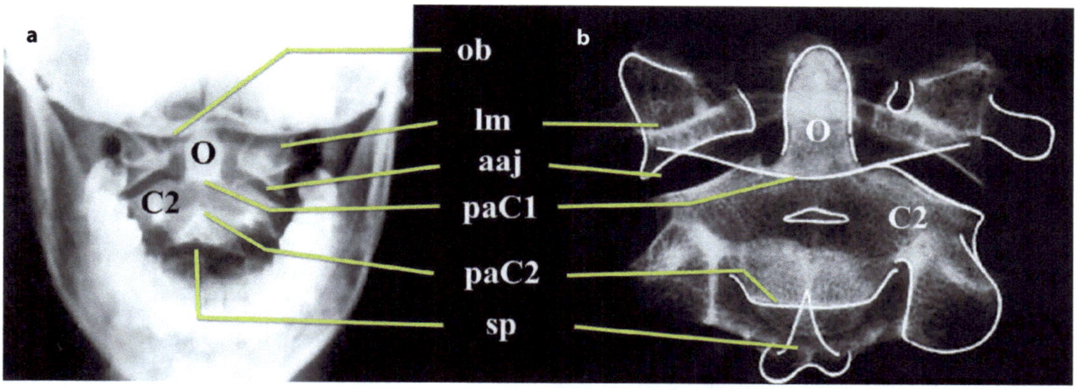

Fig. 3.10 Plain radiograph (anteroposterior projection) of the occipito-vertebral hinge (**a**) and anatomical preparation of dry bone (**b**). Odontoid process (dens) (*O*); body of C2 (*C2*); occipital bubble (*b*); lateral mass of C1 (*lm*); atlanto-axial joint (*aaj*); posterior arch of C1 (*inferior edge*); posterior arch of C2 (*superior edge*); spinous process of C2 (*sp*)

conveyed through gray communicating branches to form a sympathetic chain. Their nerve impulses produce contraction of smooth muscle cells (e.g., the muscular coats of the intestine, bronchi, vessels), and determine the secretory effects (glands) or trophic effects on the connective tissue of the organs. The two chains of sympathetic ganglia or trunks located in the paravertebral space extend from the base of the skull to the coccyx and divide into complexes. A detailed description of the sympathetic chain and spinal nerve is beyond the scope of this chapter.

3.4 Radiographic Anatomy of the Spine

3.4.1 Cervical Spine

The radiographic study is undertaken with a transoral projection for the first two cervical vertebrae and with the anteroposterior (AP), LL and oblique projections for the lower cervical segments.

In the transoral projection it is possible to reduce the overlap of most of the skeletal structures of the face. The central X-ray beam affects the center of the mouth and flows out to the height of the inion (or just below). The degree of forward head tilt should be well balanced because it can cause a pronounced overlap of the upper alveolar processes of the teeth, and a slight extension can cause a similar overlap due to the occipital bone. Anatomical radiographic findings start from the midline and proceed outwards: the odontoid process, the lateral masses of the atlas, and the transverse processes of the atlas. The inferior articular facets of C1 are increasingly evident with a well-defined lower edge and acute infero-external angle. The anterior lamina of C1 is projected on the lateral mass as an opaque ring. On the inner face of the lateral masses, tubercles that give attachments to the transverse ligament are clearly visible. The C2 pedicles are projected onto the VB with an external concavity. The posterior arch of C2 is evident through the body as well as the spinous process. The superior articular facets of C1 and the occipital condyles are more or less evident in relation to the maxilla and occipital bone (Fig. 3.10).

The cervical spine from C3 to C7 can be examined with three projections: AP; LL; and right and left 45° oblique.

AP projection: The cervical spine from C3 to T1 is represented, and shows the VBs, interbody space, unciform apophyses and uncovertebral joints (Fig. 3.11). Because of their orientation, the peduncles are not clearly shown in AP projection. They are reduced to two small opacities situated at the sides of the body which can be appreciated only in the upper and lower outlines. In general, it is not possible to distinguish the upper and lower edges of the posterior arch, of which only the spinous process is evident. Due to their orienta-

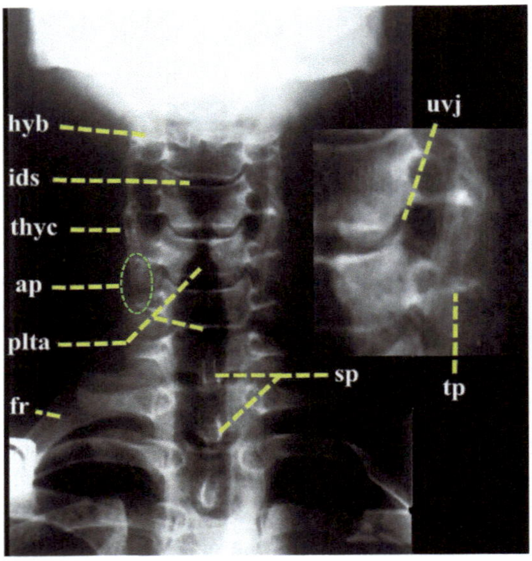

Fig. 3.11 Conventional radiographic anatomy of the cervical spine in the anteroposterior projection. Hyoid bone (*hyb*); uncovertebral joint (*uvj*); intervertebral disk space (*ids*); thyroid cartilage (*thyc*); laryngo–pharyngo–tracheal airway (*plta*); tansverse process (*tp*); articular process (*ap*); spinous process (*sp*); first rib (*fr*)

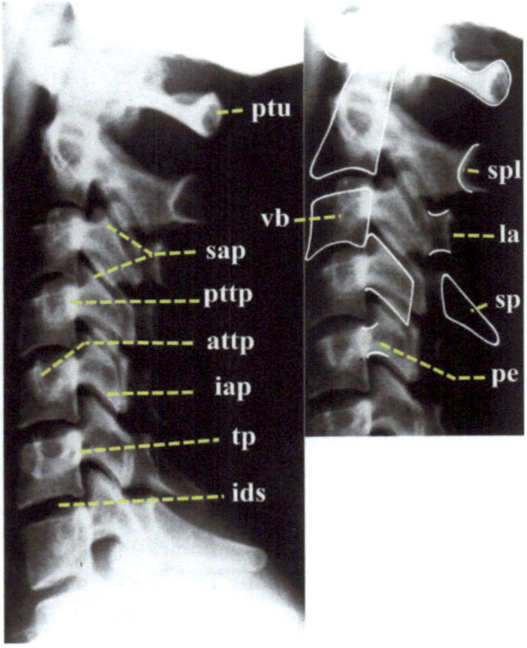

Fig. 3.12 Plain radiograph (left lateral projection) of the cervical spine. Posterior tubercle of the posterior arch of C1 (*ptu*); posterior tubercle of the transverse process (*pttp*); anterior tubercle of the transverse process (*attp*); superior articular process of the posterior spinal facet joint (zygapophyseal) (*sap*); inferior articular process of the posterior spinal facet joint (zygapophyseal) (*iap*); lamina (*la*); pedicle (*pe*); spinolaminar line (*spl*); transverse process (*tp*); intervertebral disk space (*ids*); spinous process (*sp*); vertebral body (*vb*) (C3)

tion and subtlety, the articular apophyses are not clearly visible and appear as an "elephant's ear". Only the VBs are clearly visible along with the uncus and uncovertebral joints. The articular processes are overlapped as a double opacity with a vertical course, almost constant, at the sides of the soma. The first ribs and first dorsal vertebrae can be seen clearly. False images at the C4 and C5 levels can be created due to: the transparency of the tracheo–pharyngeal–laryngeal axis; the epiglottis; the opacity of the larynx cartilage; the hyoid bone; overlapping of the spine.

LL projection: VBs and the interbody space can be assessed on the LL projection. With regard to the atlas, the profile of the anterior arch (like a signet ring) and the posterior arch (in which the cortex is very clear) can be evaluated clearly.

The space between the odontoid and anterior arch of the atlas is usually ≤2.5 mm in adults. The lateral masses of the atlas are projected on the odontoid and, in general, are poorly analyzed. The posterior margin of the soma of C2 is in continuity with that of the dens, but sometimes it can form an angle as an anatomical variant. In the section below the atlo-occipital joint, the VBs have a rectangular appearance with an antero-inferior "beak" with overlapping of the transverse process. Posterior to the body are the articular processes with a parallelogram shape. Posterior to the articular processes are projected the laminae, which form the "spinolaminar space" (used to evaluate stenosis of the spinal canal). Behind the laminae are the spinous processes, non-existent only for C1, whereas they are more developed from C6 to C7 (Fig. 3.12).

The 45° oblique projection is used to evaluate the conjugation foramen, so the orientation of the X-ray beam must be the same as that of the conjugation foramen: 40° in relation to the frontal plane and 15–20° in relation to the horizontal

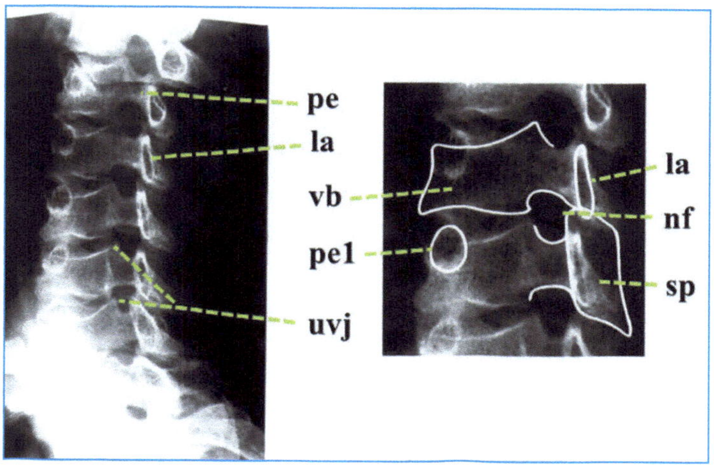

Fig. 3.13 Plain radiograph (oblique projection) of the cervical spine. Pedicle (*pe*); lamina (*la*); vertebral body (*vb*); neural foramen (*nf*); spinous process (*sp*); pedicle side in the examination (*pe1*); uncovertebral joint (*uvj*)

plane. In this projection, the foramina have an oval shape that is delimited anteriorly by the posterolateral angle of the VBs, disk and uncus, and posteriorly by and the articular apophysis. The peduncles can be seen clearly; those which are ipsilateral are seen according to their major axis. The contralateral laminae are projected in the foramen whereas the ipsilateral laminae appear as vertical opacities. The facet joints are not seen clearly: they appear as partially overlapping oval formations. More posteriorly, spinous processes can be observed [2] (Fig. 3.13).

3.4.2 Thoracic Spine

The radiographic views used to study the thoracic spine, unlike the other segments of the spine, are the AP and LL projections. In some cases, these projections are supplemented by detailed projections studying the VBs and interbody space.

AP projection (Fig. 3.14a): VBs are rectangular and their volume increases progressively if proceeding in a caudal direction. The endplates are regular but the lateral edges are slightly concave. The peduncles are of very variable form, often rounded, and projected in the top half of the vertebral VB near the lateral angle. They are quite small at the level of the first thoracic vertebrae and reach maximum size at the T11–T12 level. The inter-pedicular distance remains almost constant throughout the thoracic spine. The spinous processes are projected onto the VB below. The intervertebral space has a nearly constant height throughout the thoracic segment. The anatomical structures that are most difficult by radiography are the: upper edges of the laminae (on AP projection they overlap with the superior endplate of the vertebra below because they are concave); upper and lower facet joints; transverse processes (which are masked by overlapping of the head of the ribs).

LL projection (Fig. 3.14b): VBs are rectangular and the endplates slightly concave. The front edge of the soma is vertical or slightly concave, the back wall is straight and less defined. The peduncles are implanted on the upper half of the VB and have an upper edge that is almost in continuity with the upper somatic plate; the lower edge is concave. The shape of the neural foramina is oval. The articular apophysis is just behind the foramina as an isosceles triangle. The interbody spaces for each level are the same height from back to front and increase up to the lumbar level. The spinous processes as well as the transverse and inferior articular processes are more difficult to analyze because of the overlap of the ribs and lungs [10].

3.4.3 Lumbar Spine

AP projection: VBs have a rectangular shape with straight endplates and lateral margins that

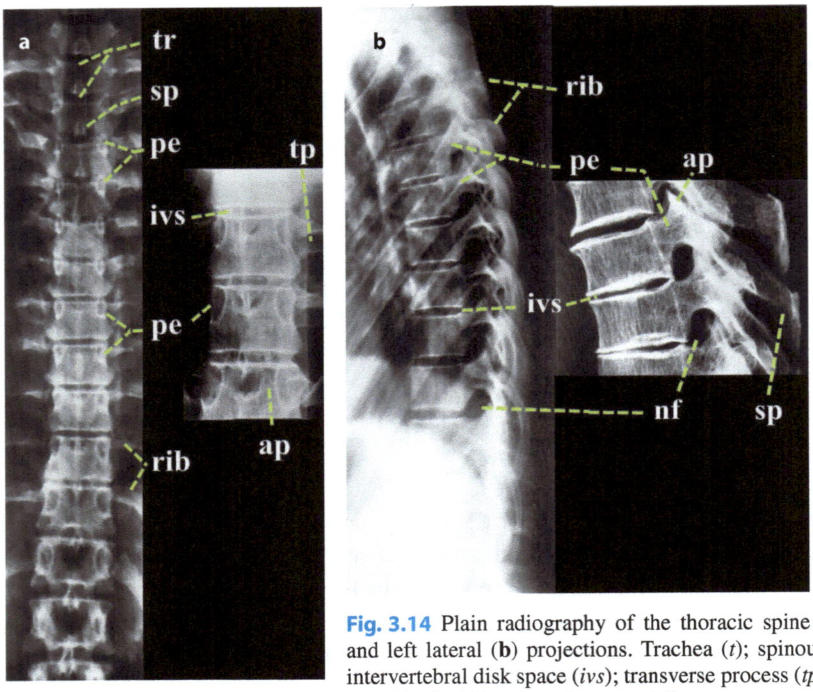

Fig. 3.14 Plain radiography of the thoracic spine showing anteroposterior (**a**) and left lateral (**b**) projections. Trachea (*t*); spinous process (*sp*); pedicle (*pe*); intervertebral disk space (*ivs*); transverse process (*tp*); articular process (*ap*); vertebral body (*vb*); neural foramen (*nf*)

are often concave. The image of the VB can be deformed depending on the angle of incidence of the radiation beam. The peduncles are projected on the supero-external angles of the soma and aligned symmetrically in the AP direction, thereby defining the outer boundaries of the spinal canal. The inter-pedicular distance increases gradually from L1 to L5.

Recognizing the inter-apofiso–laminar space (a diamond shape flanked by two adjacent vertebrae) is important. Its boundaries are arranged from the bottom edge of the laminae and the spinous process of the vertebra above, laterally from the inner surface of the articular apophyses, and downwards from the upper edge of the laminae of the underlying vertebra. This airspace increases progressively in amplitude caudally and is important for evaluation of stenosis of the spinal canal (Fig. 3.15a). The interbody space is occupied by the intervertebral disk and looks like a transparent band when assessing the height. Sometimes, this transparency is reduced by disk calcification or increased in the presence of vacuolar degeneration by accumulation of gas in the disk.

LL projection (Fig. 3.15b): VBs have a quadrangular shape with a central portion of cancellous bone bounded by cortical bone. The front profile of the VB is, in general, straight or slightly concave forward; the posterior profile is concave (sometimes quite pronounced). The soma of L5 shows slight deformation of the posterior wedge. The pedicles overlap perfectly with the upper and lower edge, and are slightly concave. The posterior articular apophyses overlap with each other to form a column of relative opacity in which the superior and inferior processes can be recognized. The foramina are bordered on the posterior margin of the intervertebral disk and corresponding vertebral soma, posteriorly by the surface of the articular processes, up from the bottom edge of the vertebra above and below the upper edge of the one below.

LL projection: The neural foramina between L1 and L4 are displayed without deformation as a large oval shape that decrease progressively in size proceeding downwards and which have a small indentation caused by the posterior superior articular process of the underlying vertebra.

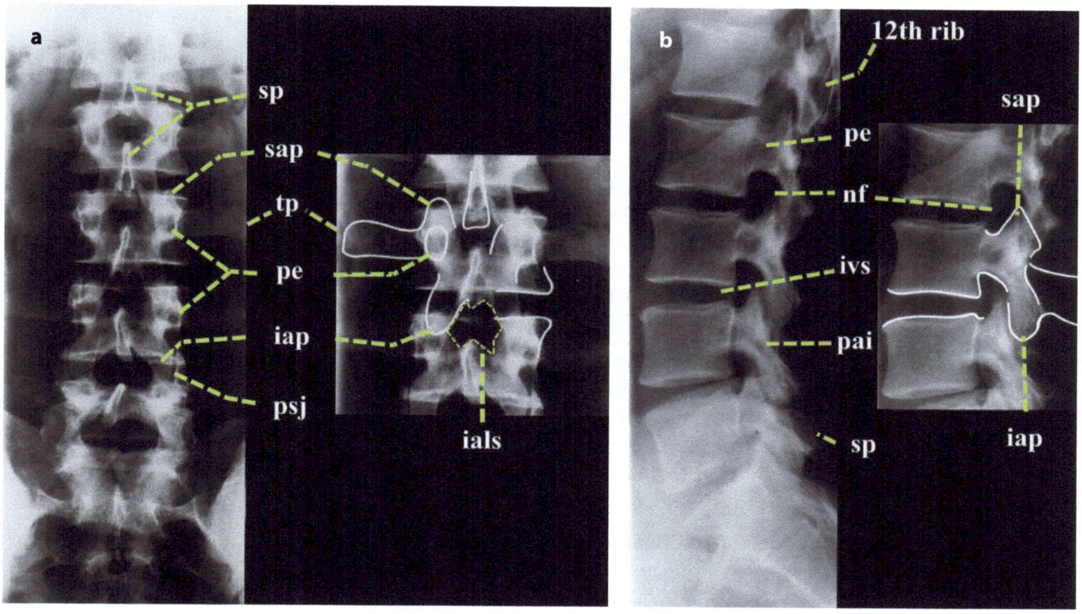

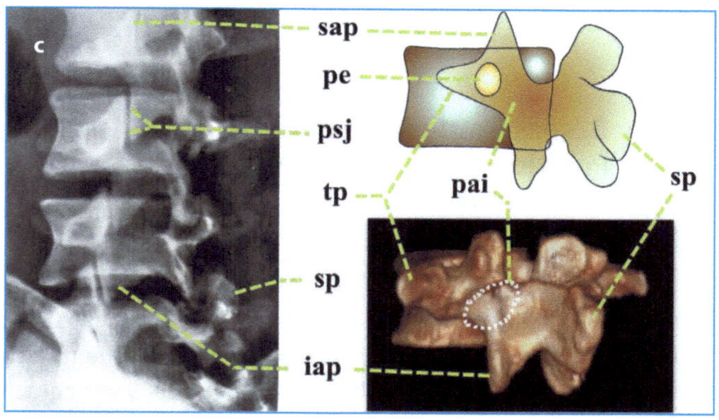

Fig. 3.15 Plain radiography of lumbosacral segments in anteroposterior (**a**), left lateral (**b**) and oblique projections with three-dimensional volume-rendered multidetector row CT reconstruction of the lumbar vertebra (**c**). Inter-apophyseal laminar space (*ials*); transverse process (*tp*); twelfth rib (12th rib); pedicle (*pe*); intervertebral disk space (*ivs*); spinous process (*sp*); inferior articular process (*iap*); superior articular process (*sap*); pars interarticularis (*pai*); vertebral body (*vb*); neural foramen (*nf*); posterior spinal facet joint (zygapophyseal) (*psj*)

At L5–S1 the foramen appears to be smaller and flattened because it has a different orientation than those situated above. Narrowing in the AP position of the foramina can result from congenital shortness of the pedicles, hypertrophy of the posterior facet joint, arthrosis, or degenerative spondylolisthesis. A reduction in height can be an indicator of disk degeneration (which undergoes thinning) or by an increase of the thickness of the pedicle.

The oblique view (Fig. 3.15c) is still used frequently in the lumbar spine for exploration of the posterior arch. It has the classic appearance of the "Scottie dog" in which the: face corresponds to the transverse apophysis; ear to the superior articular apophysis; eye to the pedicle; neck to the inter-joint isthmus; front leg to the inferior articular apophysis; body to the lamina. The main interest of this projection lies in the study of the isthmus inter-articular and posterior joints because the spacing and articular surface can be seen.

3.4.3.1 Anatomical Variations in the Lumbar Spine

During percutaneous treatment, to avoid complications or mistakes, knowing the anatomical variations in the lumbar spine is extremely important [12]. These variations are detailed in Table 3.1.

Table 3.1 Anatomical variations in the lumbar spine

• Costiform process at L1. The transverse apophysis of L1 can assume a morphology similar to that of a rib and be unilateral or bilateral.
• Persistence of accessory ossification nucleus. This is sometimes present in correspondence with the transverse processes or joints, which are situated distally.
• Persistence of the epiphyseal center of ossification. This is most often observed on the anterior superior margin of L1 or, more rarely, L2 and L3. It should not be confused with marginal bone trauma.
• Persistence of a "vascular window" of the vertebral body that is manifested as an area of segmental radio-transparency (front or back).
• Net linear opacities and somatic courses parallel to the plates with the same meaning as metaphyses of long bones, and which correspond to growth striae;
• Lumbar styloid apophysis. Corresponds to hypertrophy of the tubercle accessory located below the mammillary tubercle and behind the superior articular apophysis. On AP projection it appears as a bone of varying length originating (apparently) from the superior articular apophysis heading down and out (where it crosses the transverse process).
• Constitutional hypertrophy of the pedicles or vertebral joints that can cause narrowing of the conjugation foramen.
• Presence of "eyes" in the classic image of a Scottie dog caused by hypertrophy of the mammillary process.
• Partial or complete sacralization of L5. This is very common and characterized by a transverse mega-apophysis (unilateral or bilateral L5) associated with neo-articulation with the sacral bone. The distinction between a sacralization of L5 or S1 lumbarization is not straightforward and may require an exact definition for the full count of the individual vertebrae of the entire vertebral spine.

3.5 Access Routes and Patient Positioning for Percutaneous Treatments

The percutaneous route is chosen based on the location and depth of the target so as to reach it with a route as short as possible while respecting sensitive anatomical structures. Recognition of the main landmarks in the skin (normally used for the execution of conventional radiography) which correspond in depth to a given vertebral spine are useful for the choice of the decubitus position (Fig. 3.16). The prone position is the most commonly used and allows access to almost any target in the dorsal and lumbosacral segments. Placement of a pillow under the abdomen reduces lumbar lordosis, and facilitates access to the most caudal intervertebral disks and the lower termination of the vertebral posterior articular synovium. The entry point of the skin for the decubitus position is, in general, posterolateral and at a variable distance from the interspinous line (or may coincide with this line in specific cases) (Fig. 3.17a). The lateral decubitus position is sometimes employed, especially in the lumbosacral segments, to reach the intervertebral disk [13–15]. Also, in this case, placement of a pillow under the side support can align the vertebrae in the median plane (Fig. 3.17b). For percutaneous treatment at the cervical spine, a supine decubitus position with slight hyperextension of the head is the most commonly used. The salience of the muscle bundle of the sternomastoid is the reference for access to lower-middle cervical vertebrae (Fig. 3.18).

The mouth as the "gateway" to the second cervical vertebra was employed by surgeons of various disciplines for many years [16–19]. More recently it has been used to undertake percutaneous vertebroplasty due to vertebral collapse caused by osteoporosis or cancer. Vertebroplasty of C2 can be achieved with an equal probability of success under radiographic or CT guidance [20–24].

Accesses route for percutaneous procedures that can create particular difficulties are the high thoracic region and cervical–thoracic transition. This is due to the overlap of the scapulohumeral crack and small size of the pedicles of the upper thoracic vertebrae. Good visualization of the vertebrae and the paraspinal soft tissue is of fundamental importance because of the close relationship with the spinal canal, pleural cavity

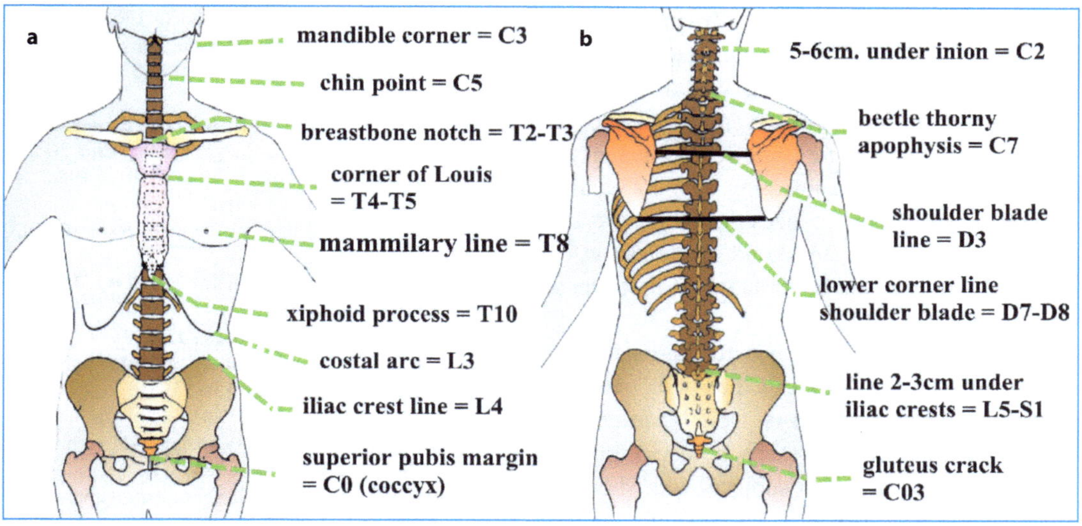

Fig. 3.16 Points of reference to locate the vertebral level in skin according to anterior (**a**) and posterior (**b**) projections

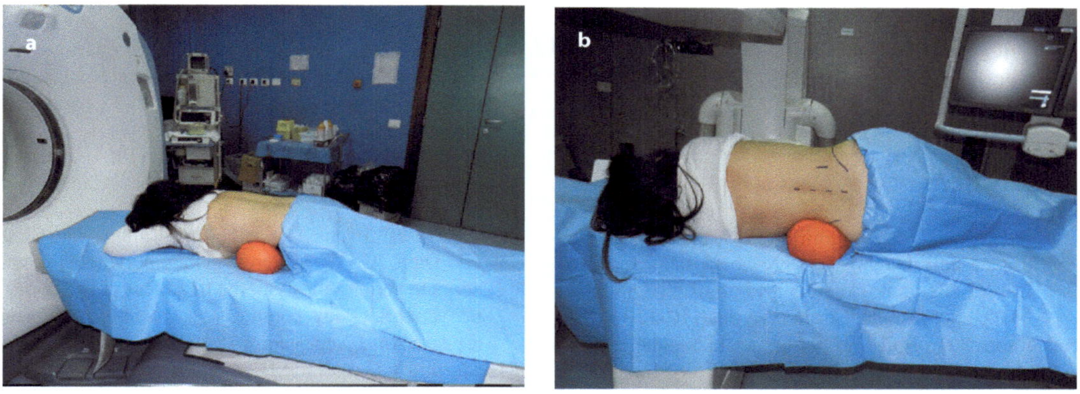

Fig. 3.17 Patient positioning for access to the thoracic–lumbar–sacral region. Supine (**a**) and lateral decubitus (**b**) positions are shown

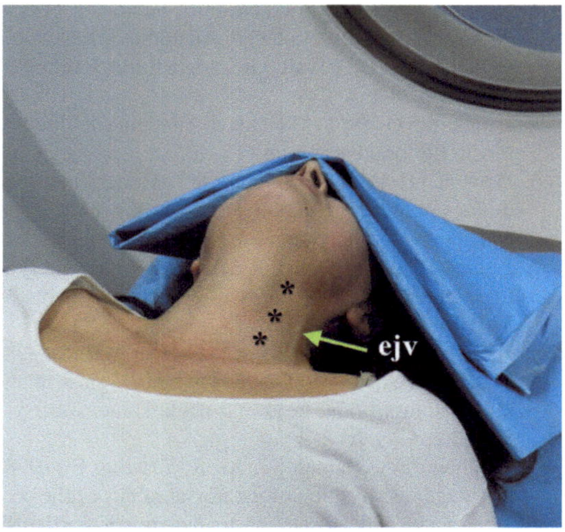

Fig. 3.18 Patient positioning for percutaneous access to the cervical spine (C3–C7). External jugular vein (*ejv*)

and major vascular structures. To improve the accuracy of radiological visualization, various measures should be adopted, including ensuring that the arms are abducted and elbows flexed forward if the procedure is carried out under sedation. This results in lowering of the shoulder blades, which greatly reduces the image overlay in the LL projection and good visualization of T2, resulting in easier undertaking of percutaneous treatments [25].

When using CT guidance for percutaneous treatments, the "swimmer's position" can be adopted to reduce artifacts from "hardening" of the radiation beam present at cervicothoracic junction (especially in subjects with short or thick necks). The patient is placed supine on the CT table and one of his/her arms placed behind the head. This position has been shown to elicit a net reduction of artifacts with clearer evidence of pathological processes at the base of the neck and cervicothoracic junction [26–27].

References

1. Rabischong R, Salvolini U (1987) La "logica" anatomica dell'imaging vertebro-nevrassiale. In: Pistolesi GF, Bergamo Andreis IA (eds) L'imaging diagnostico del rachide. Cortina, Verona 110–120
2. Rabischong P (1989) Anatomie functionnelle du rachis et de la moelle. In: Manelfe C (ed) Imagerie du rachis et de la moelle. Vigot, Paris, 109–134
3. Koritke JG, Sick H (1983) Atlas of sectional human anatomy. Urban & Schwarzenberger, Baltimore-Munich, pp 65–95
4. Zaccaria F, Marinozzi G, Nesci E, Santoro A (1973) Atlante fotografico a colori di Anatomia macroscopica dell'uomo. Dr. F. Vallardi Società Editrice Libraria, Roma, pp 75–90
5. Lambertini G (1968) Manuale di Anatomia dell'uomo. Piccin Editore, Padova pp 115–135
6. Newton TH, Potts DG (eds) (1983) Modern neuroradiology volume 1: computed tomography of the spine and spinal cord. Clavadel Press, San Anselmo
7. Jinkins JR (2000) Atlas of neuroradiologic embryologic anatomy and variants. Lippincott Williams & Wilkins, Edinburgh, pp 15–25
8. Harnsberger HR, Salzman KL, Osborn AG, Ross JS, Macdonald AJ (2006) Diagnostic and surgical imaging anatomy: brain, head and neck, spine. Amirsys, Salt Lake City, pp 2–4
9. Ebraheim NA, Haman ST, Xu R, Yeasting R (1998) The anatomic location of the dorsal ramus of the cervical nerve and its relation to the superior articular process of the lateral mass. Spine 23:1968–1971
10. Runge M (1988) Rachis dorsal. Encycl Med Chir (Paris, France), Radiodiagnostic 1, 30650 B10.12-1988
11. Runge M (1988) Rachis lombar. Examen radiographique standard. Encycl Med Chir (Paris, France), Radiodiagnostic 1, 30600 A10.12-1988
12. Runge M (1988) Rachis lombar. Données anatomique. Encycl Med Chir (Paris, France), Radiodiagnostic 1, 30650 A10.12-1988
13. Fabris G, Lavaroni A, Leonardi M (1991) Discography. Del Centauro, Udine
14. Benoist M, Deburge A, Busson J. (1984) La chimonucleolyse dans le traitment des sciatique par hernie discale. La Press Medicale 13:733–736
15. Boneville J-F, Clarisse J (1984) Radiologie interventionelle. In: Manelfe C (ed) Imagerie du rachis et de la moelle. Vigot, Paris, 761–784
16. Bonney G, Williams JP (1985) Trans-oral approach to the upper cervical spine. A report of 16 cases. J Bone Joint Surg Br 67:691–698
17. Merwin GE, Post JC, Sypert GW (1991) Transoral approach to the upper cervical spine. Laryngoscope 101:780–784
18. Menezes AH, VanGilder JC (1988) Transoral–transpharyngeal approach to the anterior craniocervical junction: ten-year experience with 72 patients. J Neurosurg 69:895–903
19. Fang HS, Ong GB, Hodgson AR (1964) Anterior spinal fusion: the operative approaches. Clin Orthop 35:16–33
20. Jensen ME, Evans AJ, Mathis JM, Kallmes DF, Cloft HJ, Dion JE (1997) Percutaneous polymethylmethacrylate vertebroplasty in the treatment of osteoporotic vertebral body compression fractures: technical aspects. Am J Neuroradiol 18:1897–1904
21. Martin JB, Gailloud P, Dietrich PY et al (2002) Direct transoral approach to C2 for percutaneous vertebroplasty. Cardiovasc Intervent Radiol 25:517–519
22. Gailloud P, Martin JB, Olivi A, Gailloud P, Martin JB (2002) Transoral vertebroplasty for a fractured C2 aneurysmal bone cyst. J Vasc Interv Radiol 13:340–341
23. Tong FC, Cloft HJ, Joseph GJ Rodts GR, Dion JE (2000) Transoral approach to cervical vertebroplasty for multiple myeloma. Am J Roentgenol 175:1322–1324
24. Arra S. Reddy, Mary Hochman, Shaun Loh et al (2005) CT guided direct transoral approach to C2 for percutaneous vertebroplasty. Pain Physician 8:235–238
25. Bayley E, Clamp J, Bronek MB (2009) Percutaneous approach to the upper thoracic spine: optimal patient positioning. Eur Spine J 18:1986–1988
26. Kane AG, Reilly KC, Murphy TF (2004) Swimmer's CT: improved imaging of the lower neck and thoracic inlet. Am J Neuroradiol 25:859–862
27. Bartynski WS Whitt DS, Sheetz MA, Jennings RB, Rothfus WE (2007) Lower cervical nerve root block using CT fluoroscopy in patients with large body habitus: another benefit of the swimmer's position. Am J Neuroradiol 28:706–708

Clinical Evaluation of Spinal Disease 4

Luigi Genovese and Pasqualino De Marinis

4.1 Introduction

Neurodiagnostic evaluation of spinal diseases is based upon accurate clinical assessment. Perfect accordance between clinical and neuroradiological assessment guarantees a correct diagnosis and, finally, optimal management of the disease.

4.2 Clinical Examination

Clinical evaluation offers the opportunity to address neuroradiological and neurophysiological examinations and to define the diagnosis. Clinical evaluation comprises accurate documentation of the medical history and neurological examination.

4.2.1 Medical History

Taking an accurate medical history is extremely important and should include ascertaining:

- history of cancer;
- duration of symptoms;
- history of trauma;
- history of infection;
- psychological and social aspects.

4.2.2 Neurological Examination

Spinal disease can involve the spinal cord and/or the nerve roots. Spasticity with hyperreflexia, hypertonicity and weakness distal to the lesion are signs of upper motor neuron involvement. Hypotonia, hyporeflexia and weakness with radicular distribution are typical signs of a lower motor neuron lesion. The most common symptom is pain: its characteristics and distribution help in delineation of the type and level of lesion. According to Byrne et al. (see Recommended Reading), pain can be of five types:

- *local pain* is deep and exacerbated by movements; it occurs in the case of spondylosis and metastatic lesions;
- *referred pain* is coupled with local pain. This diffuse, troublesome pain affects the shoulder and chest in the case of chronic spondylosis;
- *radicular pain* is acute, lancinating and often associated with paresthesia. It is caused by compression/irritation of dorsal nerve roots and has a radicular distribution. The cause can be a herniated disk, metastatic tumor, or schwannoma;
- *cruralgia with testicular referred pain*, in general, diffuses to the trunk and extremities. It is due to involvement of the sensitive

L. Genovese (✉)
Neurosurgery Unit, A. Cardarelli Hospital,
Naples, Italy
email: luigi_genovese@hotmail.com

M. Muto (ed.), *Interventional Neuroradiology of the Spine*,
DOI 10.1007/978-88-470-2790-9_4, © Springer-Verlag Italia 2013

intramedullary pathways. An example is the "electric shock" (Lhermitte's sign) felt due to neck flexion. It is observed in syringomyelia, intramedullary tumors and myelitis;
- *muscular spasm* is the most frequent cause of neck pain. Limitation of neck movements and positive Valleix points are commonly present.

Dysfunctions of sensitivity (paresthesia, dysesthesia, numbness) and hyposthenia can be associated with different levels of severity.

4.3 Cervical Spine

4.3.1 Upper Segment (C0–C4)

Symptomatology is dependent upon involvement of anatomical structures (medulla oblongata, upper cervical cord, lower cranial nerves, cervical nerve roots, vessels). There are various symptoms and signs that can be insidious and lead to mis-identifying the localization:
- Neck pain and limitation of neck motion
- Vertigo
- Basilar migraine
- Nystagmus
- Dysphagia
- Tinnitus
- Hearing loss
- Quadriparesis/paraparesis/monoparesis
- Sensory abnormalities.

4.3.2 Middle and Lower Segments (C5–T1)

Cervical pain and muscular spasms are localized in the posterior region of the neck.

Lesional signs are dependent upon the involved level. Disease at the C5–C6 level causes pain in the shoulder; external surface of the arm, forearm, thumb and index finger; paresis and hypotrophy of the deltoid, brachial, biceps, and supinator longus muscles; and reduction of bicipital and styloradial reflexes. Lesions at the C7 level result in pain and hypoaesthesia of the posterior surface of the arm and forearm as well as the second, third and fourth finger; paresis and hypotrophy of the triceps, extensor muscles of the fingers and thenar eminence; and reduction of the tricipital reflex. The clinical aspects of disorders at the C8–T1 level are pain and hypoaesthesia of the internal surface of the arm and forearm up to fourth and fifth finger; paresis and hypotrophy of the flexor muscles of the fingers and hypothenar eminence; and reduction of the cubitopronator reflex (Table 4.1).

Sublesional signs are characterized by spastic paralysis of the lower and upper extremities whose centers are below the compression; hypoaesthesia; and dysfunction of the bladder and bowel.

4.4 Thoracic Spine

Diseases of the dorsal column can affect the osseous and the spinal compartment. Diseases of the osseous compartment include: deformities, arthrosis, herniated disks, traumatic fractures, vertebral tumors, and infections. Diseases of the spinal cord include: tumors (extradural, intradural extramedullary, intramedullary), atrioventricular malformations and syringomyelia. Signs and symptoms include pain, numbness as well as motor and sensory disturbances.

Lesional syndrome is constituted by girdle pain, atrophic paresis of the intercostal muscles and

Table 4.1 Characteristics of lumbar disk syndrome

	Pain Location	Weakness	Reflex	Sensory Loss
L3–L4	Anterior thigh	Posterior lower	Patellar	Medial malleolus
L4–L5	Posterior lower extremity	Extensor hallicus longus, anterior tibialis		Dorsum of foot
L5–S1	Index finger, middle finger	Gastrocnemius	Achilles	Lateral foot

suppression of abdominal reflexes that allows identification of the lesion level. The T4 level refers to a sensory deficit of the mammary region; the T6 of the xiphoid region; the T9–T10 of the omphalic region; and the T12 of the inguinal region. Suppression of the superior abdominal reflex is referred to the T7–T8 level; of the middle abdominal reflex to the T9–T10 level; and of the inferior abdominal reflex to the T11–T12 level.

Sublesional signs suggest spastic paraparesis, hypoaesthesia as well as dysfunction of the bladder and bowel.

4.5 Lumbar Spine

The lumbosacral segment can be affected by degenerative, traumatic, tumor-based, infectious or psychiatric disorders. Clinical evaluation of this tract is difficult because the vertebral levels do not correspond to the metameric levels and the relevant dermatomes: the spinal cord ends at the L1–L2 level and consequently the nerve roots run caudally, following a vertical direction down to the neural foramina. For this reason topographic localization of the spino-radicular impairment is more complex. Pain remains the most relevant symptom, followed by sensory and motor disturbances. In accordance with the non-correspondence between the vertebral and metameric levels, clinical signs can be schematized as shown below.

Lesion of the T11 vertebra: The L1 and L2 metameres as well as the nerve roots T11, T12, L1 and L2 are involved. The lesional syndrome is characterized by pain and dysesthesia of the inguinal region as well as the antero-external thigh; reduction of the cremasteric reflex; and hypotony and hypotrophy of the psoas and quadriceps muscles. Sublesional signs are spastic paraparesis and sphincter dysfunction.

Lesion of the T12 vertebra: The L3, L4 and L5 metameres and lumbar roots are involved. The lesional signs are pain and hypoaesthesia of the anterior thigh and leg; hypotony and hypotrophy of the quadriceps and adductor muscles; and reduction of the patellar reflex. The sublesional syndrome is characterized by Achilles hyperreflexia, Babinski sign, as well as early and severe sphincter dysfunction.

Lesion of the L1 vertebra: The S1, S2 and S3 metameres as well as lumbosacral roots are impaired. Clinical signs are: crural and perianal pain; sciatica; perianal and genital dysesthesia; motor and trophic disturbances of the crural and sciatic area; reduction of patellar and Achilles reflexes; sphincter incontinence; and impotence.

Lesion of the medullary sacral metameres: This causes the conus medullaris syndrome with sphincter incontinence as well as perianal, genital and gluteal anesthesia without motor disturbances.

Lesion below the L1 vertebra: The lumbosacral nerve roots are involved. Radiculopathies are frequently observed syndromes related to osteodiscoarthrosic degenerative processes and, in particular, herniated disks and spinal stenosis. The most widespread radiculopathies in increasing order with corresponding symptoms are detailed below (also see Table 4.2).

- *L4 radiculopathy*: pain and numbness of the anterior thigh and medial malleolus, with weakness of the quadriceps and resulting difficulty in knee extension. The patellar reflex is reduced;

Table 4.2 Characteristics of cervical disk syndrome

	Pain Location	Weakness	Reflex	Sensory Loss
C4–C5	Shoulder	Deltoid		Shoulder
C5–C6	Upper arm, radial forearm	Biceps	Biceps	Upper arm, thumb, radial forearm
C6–C7	Index finger, middle finger	Triceps	Triceps	Index finger, middle finger

- *S1 radiculopathy*: pain and numbness of the posterior lower extremity, weakness of the gastrocnemius muscle with deficit of the plantar flexion of the foot, sensory loss of the lateral foot, and reduction of the Achilles reflex;
- *L5 radiculopathy*: pain of the postero-external lower extremity, weakness of the tibialis and the extensor hallicus longus muscles with deficit of the dorsiflexion of the foot, sensory loss of the dorsum of the foot, with no change in reflexes;
- *cauda equina syndrome* is due to pluriradicular involvement and is characterized by flaccid paraparesis, bilateral absence of patellar and Achilles reflexes, hypoaesthesia of posterior-superior thighs and perineum ("saddle anesthesia"), sphincter incontinence and impotence.

4.6 Summary

Clinical evaluation is extremely important for the correct management of spinal disease. Accurate documentation of medical history provides information about potential etiology. Neurological examination (sensory and motor examination, reflexes) can provide information about the level and type of lesion. Accordance between clinical aspects and neuroradiological/neurophysiological data will result in the correct diagnosis and aid management planning.

Suggested Reading

Bassewitz HL, Fischgrund JS (2003) Thoracic degenerative disc disease. In: Vaccaro AR, Betz RR, Zeidman SM (eds) Principles and practice of spine surgery. Mosby, Philadelphia, p 333–345

Byrne T, Benzel E, Waxman S (2000) Clinical pathophysiology of spinal signs and symptoms. In: Byrne T, Benzel E, Waxman S (eds) Diseases of the spine and spinal sord. Oxford University Press, Oxford, p 40–90

Hanson MR, Galvez N (2005) Neurological evaluation of the cervical spine. In: Clark CR (ed) The cervical spine, 4th edn. Lippincott Williams & Wilkins, Philadelphia, p 166–174

Lemma MA, Herzka AS, Tortolani PJ, Carbone JJ (2003) Cauda equina syndrome secondary to lumbar disc prolapse. In: Vaccaro AR, Betz RR, Zeidman SM (eds) Principles and practice of spine surgery. Mosby, Philadelphia, p 347–353

Menezes AH (2006) Abnormalities of the craniocervical junction. In: Fessler RG, Sekhar L (eds) Atlas of neurosurgical techniques. Spine and peripheral nerves. Thieme, New York, p 3–11

Patten J (1977) Neurological differential diagnosis. Springer-Verlag, New York

Perez-Cruet MJ, Samartzis D (2006) Lumbar degenerative disk disease. In: Fessler RG, Sekhar L (eds) Atlas of neurosurgical techniques. Spine and peripheral nerves. Thieme, New York, p 555–566

Post N, Frempong-Boadu AK (2006) Disk disease of the thoracic and thoracolumbar spine. In: Fessler RG, Sekhar L (eds) Atlas of neurosurgical techniques. Spine and peripheral nerves. Thieme, New York, p 378–381

How and When to Carry Out Spinal Biopsy

5

Giannantonio Pellicanò, Arturo Consoli, Massimo Falchini and Ernesto Mazza

5.1 Introduction

Spinal biopsies are carried out to obtain specimens of vertebral bodies or vertebral lesions. This provides biological samples for cytological and histopathological analyses. Primary and secondary tumors and infectious diseases are the most common causes for which vertebral biopses are required.

In the last decade, percutaneous biopsy of the spine has replaced open biopsy. This has been possible mainly because of: (i) a growing need for minimally invasive procedures and (ii) the development of diagnostic imaging methods used to carry out percutaneous biopsies. These include MRI, CT, fluoroscopy and ultrasonography. Several materials have been proposed for the sampling of vertebral lesions and for the therapeutic procedures (drainages) that may be undertaken.

G. Pellicanò (✉)
Radiodiagnostic 2-3, Azienda Ospedaliero-Universitaria Careggi, Florence, Italy
e-mail: gianni.pellicano@unifi.it

5.2 Indications for Spinal Biopsy

As stated above, the most common situations that necessiate a vertebral biopsy are vascular or infectious diseases and spinal or paraspinal tumors. Metabolic diseases also represent an indication to carry out a biopsy, paricularly if a differential diagnosis is necessary. These procedures are done to: discriminate the nature of spinal or paraspinal lesions; evaluate atypical or incidental findings; study lytic isolated vertebral lesions without specific radiological features in the absence of a known primary disease. In some rare cases, a percutanous biopsy of the spine may be essential to provide a differential diagnosis of vascular lesions that may mimic other diseases, thereby influencing the treatment strategy and prognosis [1]. Conversely, a spinal biopsy is frequently required in cases of osteomyelitis, spondylitis, spondylodiscitis and other infectious diseases. In these cases, a percutaneous approach may be considered to be the "diagnostic gold standard" and a therapeutic approach. The specimens obtained are the object of cytological and histological analyses and are useful to determine the pathological agent of the infection, and prebioptic antibiotic exposure does not seem to influence outcome [2]. A standardized algorithm for the optimal management of pyogenic and non-tuberculous diskitis has not been accepted, but the value of percutaneous disk biopsy has been established [3–7]. It has been described as a safe,

M. Muto (ed.), *Interventional Neuroradiology of the Spine*,
DOI 10.1007/978-88-470-2790-9_5, © Springer-Verlag Italia 2013

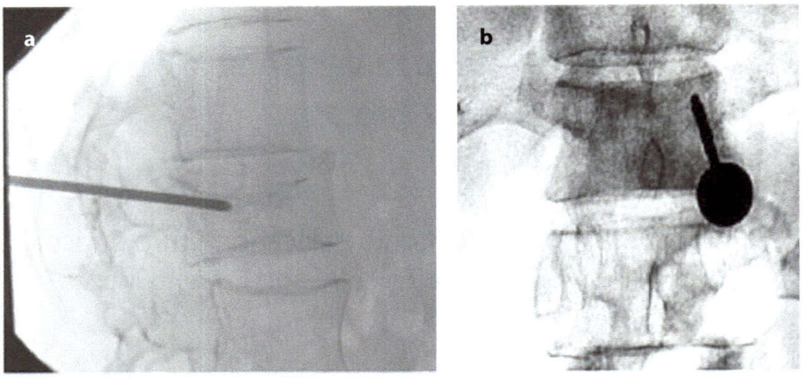

Fig. 5.1 A transpedicular approach under fluoroscopic guidance: lateral (**a**) and anteroposterior (**b**) view

recommended, minimally invasive and accurate procedure, with the advantage of avoidance of diagnostic delays in these cases [8–10]. The accuracy of percutaneous biopsy of the spine in the diagnosis of tumoral lesions has been evaluated in several series, and ranges between 72% and 95%, with higher values observed in more recent studies (particularly with respect to malignant tumors) [11–14]. In cases in which a vertebral metastasis is present, percutaneous biopsy of the vertebral spine has been shown to be a useful tool, particularly for the evaluation of unknown primary tumors [15]. The indication to perform a percutaneous vertebral biopsy before treatment in case of metabolic disease, such as osteoporosis, in very controversial. Vertebral demineralization may be identified with conventional radiology, CT and MRI. Therefore, a percutaneous biopsy is indicated only in those patients with other suspected diseases, such as osteolytic tumors or metastases [16]. Percutaneous biopsies of the spine at thoracic and lumbar levels are thought to have a significant role, but the advantages in the sacro-coccygeal region have not been presented thoroughly [17,18].

5.3 Imaging Methods and Devices

Diagnostic imaging (fluoroscopy, CT, MRI, ultrasonography) is essential for guiding spinal biopsies. MRI provides fast real-time monitoring (in MRI-guided biopsies). Useful information such as multiplanar analyses with respect to a percutaneous approach (even if open magnets and dedicated equipment are necessary) can be obtained. Ultrasonography also allows real-time monitoring and multiplanar analyses, but artifacts due to bone and air limit the acoustic window. Fluoroscopy is particularly useful for transpedicular approaches and is a safe approach, especially with respect to access to the thoracic spine [19, 20] (Fig. 5.1). However, the first-choice technique remains CT. CT allows guidance of the percutaneous approach in axial planes with high spatial resolution to control progression of the needle in critical regions and reduces the risk of complications.

CT-guided vertebral biopsies are carried out in the prone position (less frequently in the oblique or lateral position, (Fig. 5.2). This is after having achieved preliminary "scout scans" of 2.5-mm thickness with a relatively small field of view to achieve optimal visualization of the spine and to control the needle direction (Fig. 5.3). A 0° gantry slope is recommended, and access should be perpendicular to the bed to achieve latero-vertebral access by directing the needle in a latero-medial direction (Fig. 5.4). In transpedicular approaches, perpendicular access is preferred. If the biopsy is carried out in the cervical region, use of a contrast agent for greater accuracy of vascular structures is recommended.

A critical issue is the correct choice of needle and devices that should be made in relation to the type of bony lesion (osteolytitc/osteo-thickened) to the level (cervical, dorsal, lumbar, sacral) to the type of analysis (18-G needle for histological biopsy; 20–22-G needle for cytological with-

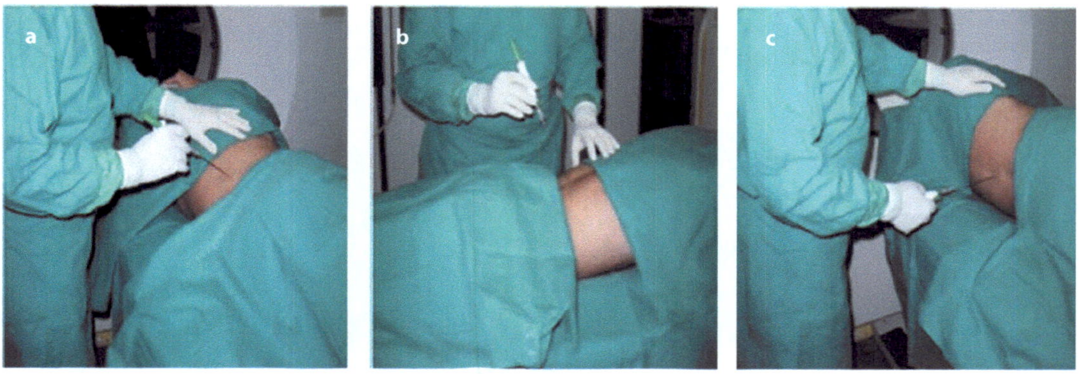

Fig. 5.2 Different approaches under CT guidance: oblique (**a**), anteroposterior (**b**) and lateral (**c**)

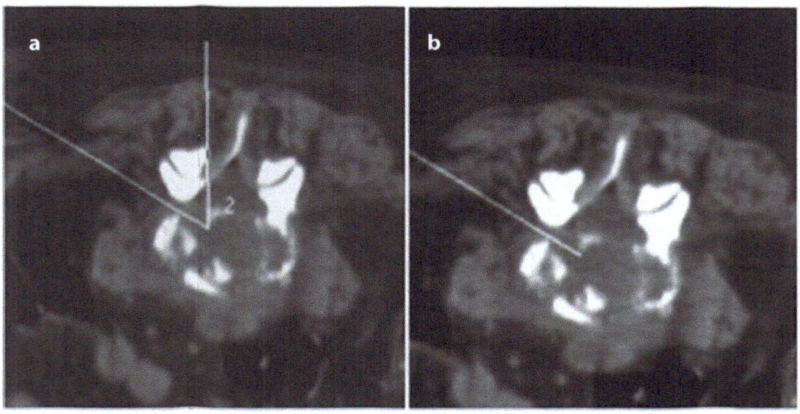

Fig. 5.3 **a** CT scan, scout image: measurement of distance from skin surface to the vertebral body and to the pedicle; **b** CT scan, scout image: needle correctly directed

drawal). Trocar-like devices of different gauges (4 mm for lumbar biopsies; 2–3 mm for cervical and dorsal regions) should be cosidered in thickened lesions, whereas Tru-Cut® devices or fine 14–20-G needles with manual or automatic devices are often used.

A small cutaneous incision is made. A needle with a guidewire is inserted and successive sleeves containing "toothed" cannules are employed. Clockwise and counterclockwise rotations provide satisafctory and repeatable positioning of the needle. Vertebral biopsies usually represent the first phase of therapeutic neuroradiological CT-guided treatments (Figs. 5.5–5.9) such as radiofrequency vertebroplasty (Fig. 5.10). Some complications may occur. These could be pneumo-hemothorax in dorsal approaches, paraspinal hematomas, sepsis, and radiculopathies with transitory anesthesia in cases of trauma to nerve roots. Severe coagulopathy, drugs that interfere with platelet function, epidural/intradural extension with signs of spinal compression, severe kyphosis and vertebral instability are considered to be extraordinary contraindications and may require further investigation. However, CT-guided biopsy is considered to be safe, accurate and inexpensive procedure with good diagnostic accuracy (Figs. 5.11–5.12). Patients undergoing a vertebral biopsy should be admitted for close observation after the procedure.

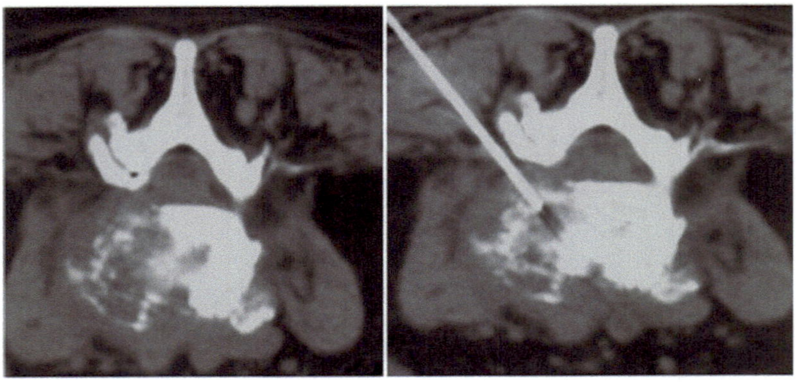

Fig. 5.4 CT scan: percutaneous spinal biopsy of a secondary vertebral tumor

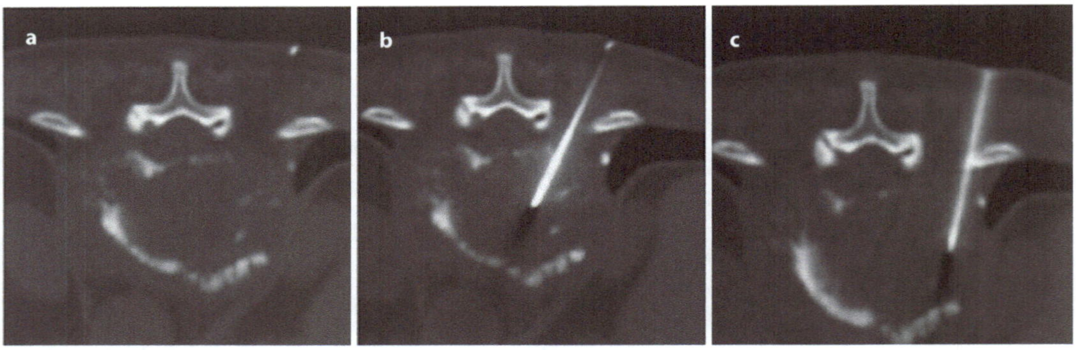

Fig. 5.5 CT-guided multiple sampling of a secondary tumor in the vertebral body. Different positions of the needle: on the skin surface (**a**), in the medial part of the vertebral body (**b**) and in left lateral position within the vertebral body (**c**)

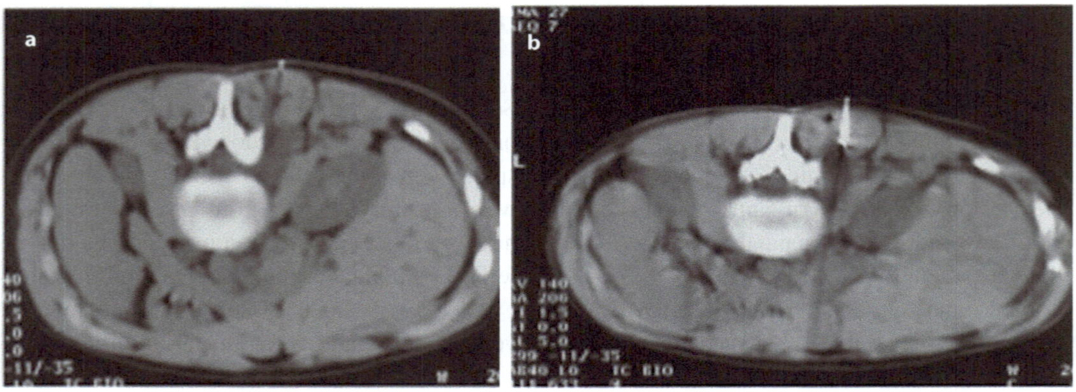

Fig. 5.6 CT-guided approach to identify a flogistic collection in a case of spondylodiscitis. Different position of the needle: on skin surface (**a**) and within the collection (**b**)

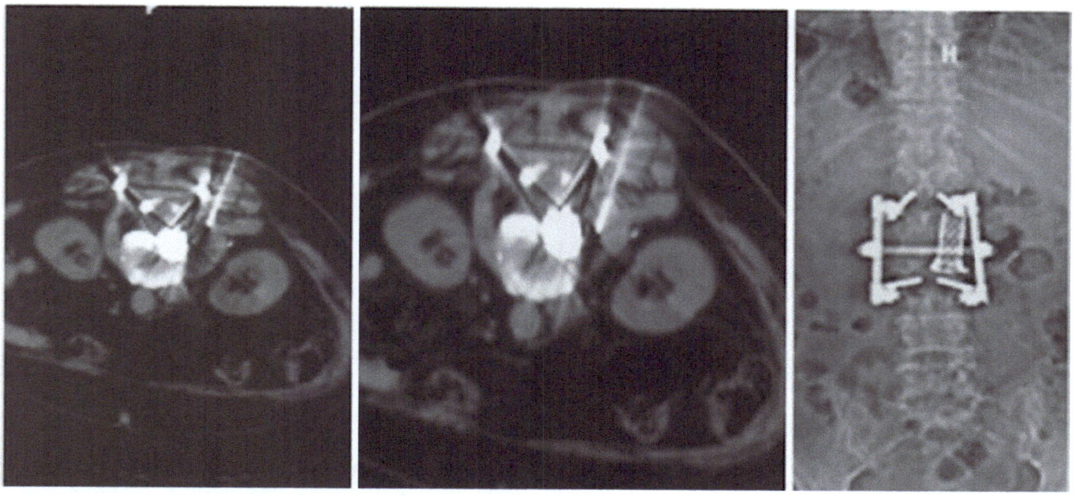

Fig. 5.7 CT image showing correct positioning of the needle. Drainage of paravertebral liquid is feasible even in the presence of orthopedic devices

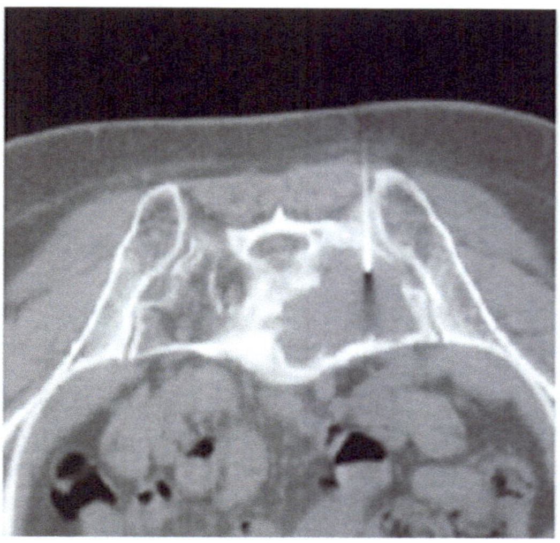

Fig. 5.8 CT image showing the needle position in a tumor in the sacral spine

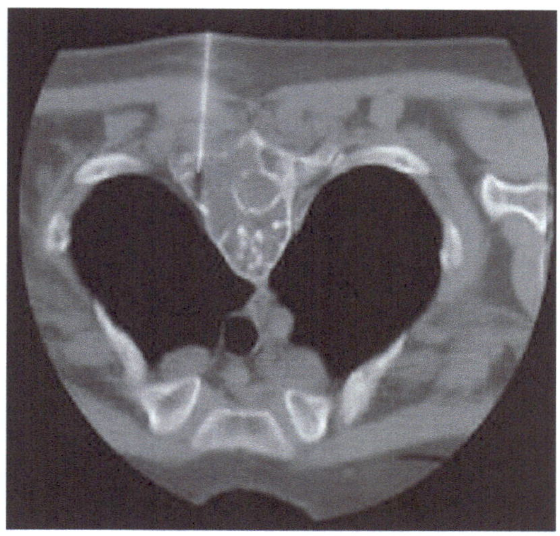

Fig. 5.9 CT-guided needle position in dorsal vertebral tumors. CT guidance allows precise and safe sampling even in the proximity of the pleura and lung

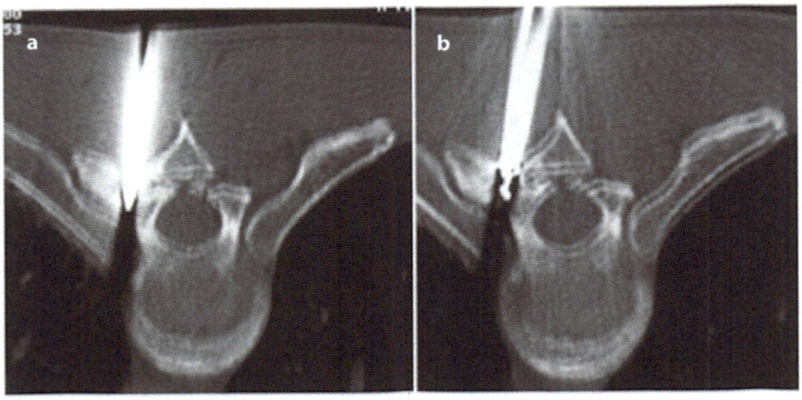

Fig. 5.10 Bone sampling during percutaneous radiofrequency ablation for an osteoid osteoma. CT-guided positioning of the needle (**a**) and its final position (**b**)

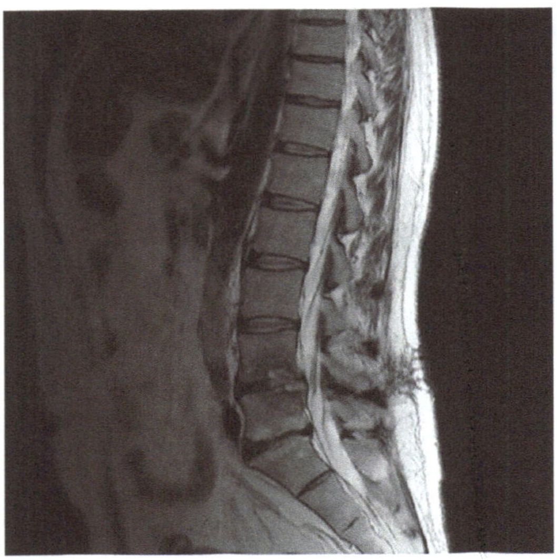

Fig. 5.11 MRI after surgical discectomy. A hyperintense area on T2-weighted images inside the disk and along the surgical approach

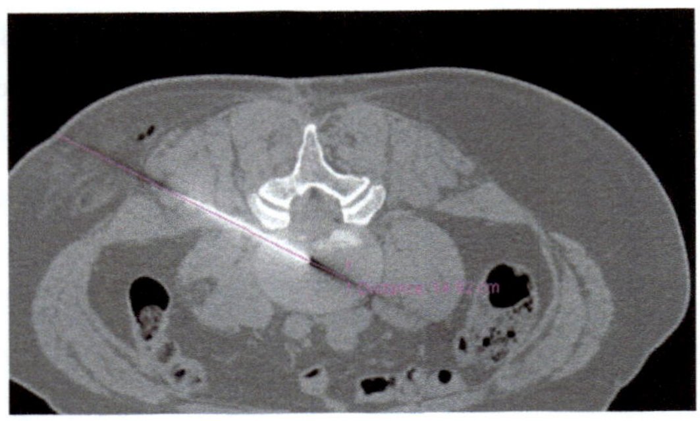

Fig. 5.12 Disk biopsy in two points of the disc with distance calculation

References

1. Kulcsár Z, Veres R, Hanzély Z, Berentei Z, Marosfoi M, Nyáry I, Szikora I (2012) Rare angioproliferative tumors mimicking aggressive spinal hemangioma with epidural expansion. Ideggyogy Sz 65:42–47
2. Marschall J, Bhavan KP,Olsen MA, Fraser VJ, Wright NM, Warren DK (2011) The impact of prebiopsy antibiotics on pathogen recovery in hematogenous vertebral osteomyelitis. Clin Infect Dis 52:867–872
3. Chew FS, Kline MJ (2001) Diagnostic yield of CT-guided percutaneous aspiration procedures in suspected spontaneous infectious diskitis. Radiology 218:211–214
4. Hadjipavlou AG, Kontakis GM, Gaitanis JN et al (2003) Effectiveness and pitfalls of percutaneous transpedicle biopsy of the spine. Clin Orthop Relat Res 411:54–60
5. Rankine JJ, Barron DA, Robinson P et al (2004) Therapeutic impact of percutaneous spinal biopsy in spinal infection. Postgrad Med J 80:607–609
6. Enoch DA, Cargill JS, Laing R et al (2008) Value of CT-guided biopsy in the diagnosis of septic discitis. J Clin Pathol 61:750–753
7. Kornblum MB, Wesolowski DP, Fischgrund JS et al (1998) Computed tomography-guided biopsy of the spine. A review of 103 patients. Spine (Phila Pa 1976) 23:81–85
8. Cottle L, Riordan T (2008) Infectious spondylodiscitis. J Infect 56:401–412
9. Cebrián Parra JL, Saez-Arenillas Martín A, Urda Martínez-Aedo AL, SolerIvañez I, Agreda E, Lopez-Duran Stern L (2012) Management of infectious dis-

citis. Outcome in one hundred and eight patients in a university hospital. Int Orthop 36:239–244
10. Legrand E, Flipo RM, Guggenbuhl P, Masson C, Maillefert JF, Soubrier M, Noël E, Saraux A, Di Fazano CS, Sibilia J, Goupille P, Chevalie X, Cantagrel A, Conrozier T, Ravaud P, Lioté F; Rheumatology Network Organization (2001) Management of nontuberculous infectious discitis. treatments used in 110 patients admitted to 12 teaching hospitals in France. Joint Bone Spine 68:504–509
11. Brugieres P, Gaston A, Heran F et al (1990) Percutaneous biopsies of the thoracic spine under CT guidance: transcostovertebral approach. J Comput Assist Tomogr 14:446–448
12. Saad RS, Clary KM, Liu Y et al (2004) Fine needle aspiration biopsy of vertebral lesions. Acta Cytol 48:39–46
13. Akhtar I,Flowers R,Siddiqi A et al (2006) Fine needle aspiration biopsy of vertebral and paravertebral lesions: Retrospective study of 124 cases. Acta Cyto 150:364–371
14. Phadke DM,Lucas DR,Madan S (2001) Fine-needle aspiration biopsy of vertebral and intervertebral disc lesions: specimen adequacy, diagnostic utility, and pitfalls. Arch Pathol Lab Med 125:1463–1468
15. Buyukbebeci O, Karakurum G, Tutar E, Gulec A, Arpacioglu O (2010) Biopsy of vertebral tumour metastasis for diagnosing unknown primaries. J Orthop Surg (Hong Kong) 18:361–363
16. Pneumaticos SG, Chatziioannou SN, Savvidou C, Pilichou A, Rontogianni D, Korres DS (2010) Routine needle biopsy during vertebral augmentation procedures. Is it necessary? Eur Spine J 19:1894–1898
17. Syed R, Bishop JA, Ali SZ (2012) Sacral and presacral lesions: cytopathologic analysis and clinical correlates. Diagn Cytopathol 40:7–13
18. Ozerdemoglu RA, Thompson RC, Jr, Transfeldt EE et al (2003) Diagnostic value of open and needle biopsies in tumors of the sacrum. Spine 28: 909–915
19. Dave BR, Nanda A, Anandjiwala JV (2009) Transpedicular percutaneous biopsy of vertebral body lesions: a series of 71 cases. Spinal Cord 47:384–389
20. Clamp JA, Bayley EJ, Ebrahimi FV, Quraishi NA, Boszczyk BM (2012) Safety of fluoroscopy guided percutaneous access to the thoracic spine. Eur Spine J 21(Suppl 2): S207–211

Percutaneous Treatment of Cervical and Lumbar Disks

6

Gianluigi Guarnieri, Matteo Bonetti, Mario Muto, Cosma Andreula and Marco Leonardi

6.1 Introduction

Cervical pain and low back pain (LBP) with/without radiculopathies are the most common spinal disorders. They are the leading cause of absence from work in "developed" countries. Around 80% of adults suffer from LBP during their lifetime and 55% suffer from back pain associated with radicular syndrome [1]. The most common cause of LBP with classical irradiation along the nerve root course is disk herniation.

The natural history of herniated disks at cervical and lumbar levels has been described by several epidemiological studies, and with correlation with magnetic resonance imaging (MRI) findings [2–5]. It is characterized by the disappearance of clinical symptoms in ≤60% with conservative treatment through rest for about 6 weeks as well as shrinkage of disk herniation as revealed by computed tomography (CT) or MRI within 8–9 months after the onset of back pain [6–8]. It has also been demonstrated that the mean space-occupying ratio of herniation is significantly reduced during 2-year MRI follow-up, with progression of degeneration of the intervertebral disk and morphologic changes of lumbar disk herniation [9]. About 88% of patients with herniated disks have >50% reduction of the hernia 3–12 months after onset, with morphologic changes of the herniated mass that are well correlated with clinical outcome [10].

Surgery is the first-line treatment for extruded, migrated and free-fragment herniated disks associated with cauda-conus syndrome, progressive foot droop, and hyperalgic radiculopathy. The success rate in the short term for such treatment is around 85–90% [11]. This rate drops to around 80% in the long-term (>6 months) and is related to failed back surgery syndrome (FBSS). FBSS is characterized by relapse and/or hypertrophic scarring with severe symptoms in 20% of cases and with real FBSS in 15% of patients [12]. Currently, the prevelance of recurrence of herniated disks after surgery is approximately 2–6% [13].

The approach taken by neurosurgeons has become increasingly less aggressive. In the USA it is estimated that, among all patients suffering from back pain/sciatica, only 3–4% undergo surgery. Patients with small or contained herniated disks who do not derive benefit from simple medical treatment can be candidates for a minimally invasive percutaneous preocedures. The outcome of such procedures is dependent upon the characteristics of the hernia and on the selected procedure [14].

M. Muto (✉)
Neuroradiology Department, A. Cardarelli Hospital, Naples, Italy
e-mail: mutomar2@gmail.com

M. Muto (ed.), *Interventional Neuroradiology of the Spine*,
DOI 10.1007/978-88-470-2790-9_6, © Springer-Verlag Italia 2013

6.2 Pathogenesis of LBP

The pathogenesis of LBP is multifactorial. It is characterized by mechanical causes (nerve-root compression) and by the associated inflammatory factors [15]. The direct mechanical factors are:

- direct compression of herniated disks on spinal ganglia (intra- and extraforaminal herniation);
- mechanical deformation of the posterior longitudinal ligament and annulus with nociceptor stimulation of the recurrent laryngeal nerve.

There are four main indirect mechanical factors. The first factor is ischemia due to compression of afferent arterioles and the microcirculation of nerve bundles (with consequent anoxic demyelination of nerve fibers). The second is venous stasis. The third is neural and peri-neural inflammation. It plays an important part in the pathogenesis of pain of herniated disks from cell-mediated inflammatory reactions to disk protrusion. Also, herniated fragments may trigger inflammatory processes with autoimmune cell-mediated responses led by macrophages. The fourth factor is biohumoral immunological responses due to phospholipase A2, which produces prostaglandin (PG)E2 and leukotrienes from arachidonic acid. Also, matrix metalloproteinase (MMP)-1, MMP-2, MMP-3 and MMP-9 degrade disk tissue and increase the inflammatory reaction. In addition, interleukin (IL)-1, IL-6 and tumor necrosis factor (TNF)-alpha cause degradation of the cellular matrix.

In this context, the *rationale* for use of these minimally invasive methods is to act upon compressive mechanical factors and the inflammatory responses to herniated disks.

6.3 Methods

Long-term follow-up studies suggest that conservative treatments can offer better results than surgery. It has been reported that only one-third of patients with lumbar pain treated conservatively need surgery. This finding has stimulated research into minimally invasive techniques to improve outcome [16]. Multiple methods are available:

- automated percutaneous lumbar diskectomy (APLD);
- percutaneous laser disk decompression (PLDD);
- intradiskal electrothermal therapy (IDET);
- percutaneous coblation nucleoplasty (PCN);
- decompressor percutaneous diskectomy (DPD);
- chemodiskolysis with a mixture of oxygen (O_2) and ozone (O_3) with periradicular and periganglionic infiltration;
- radiopaque gelified ethanol (Discogel®).

The basics of percutaneous diskal treatment are:

- correct and complete clinical evaluation to distinguish radicular pain from articular facet syndrome or piriformis syndrome, and to discern a diskal origin from a vertebral source of pain;
- evaluation with high-quality imaging (radiographs, CT, MRI) and electromyography (EMG);
- involvement of a multidisciplinary team (interventional and diagnostic neuroradiologist, neurosurgeon, pain therapist, physiotherapist, psychologist) working together to assess the best treatment.

In general, these treatments offer good results with good patient compliance and low costs. Patients will need a short period of hospitalization. Correct employment of these methods will reduce the risk of complications such as infections or hypertrophic scarring, which are often responsible for pain recurrence [12]. The aim of all percutaneous treatments is to reduce intradiskal pressure to create the space required for retropulsion or digestion of the disk.

6.3.1 APLD

Hijkata et al. were the first to describe percutaneous diskectomy with a fenestrated probe [11]. On the basis of this experience, in 1985 Onik et al. [17] introduced "automated percutaneous lumbar diskectomy" or "nucleo-diskal aspiration" using a "nucleotome". This instrument comprised a pneumatic pump working with an air compressor connected to an "aspirating-cutting" probe with an external diameter of 2 mm. The probe was

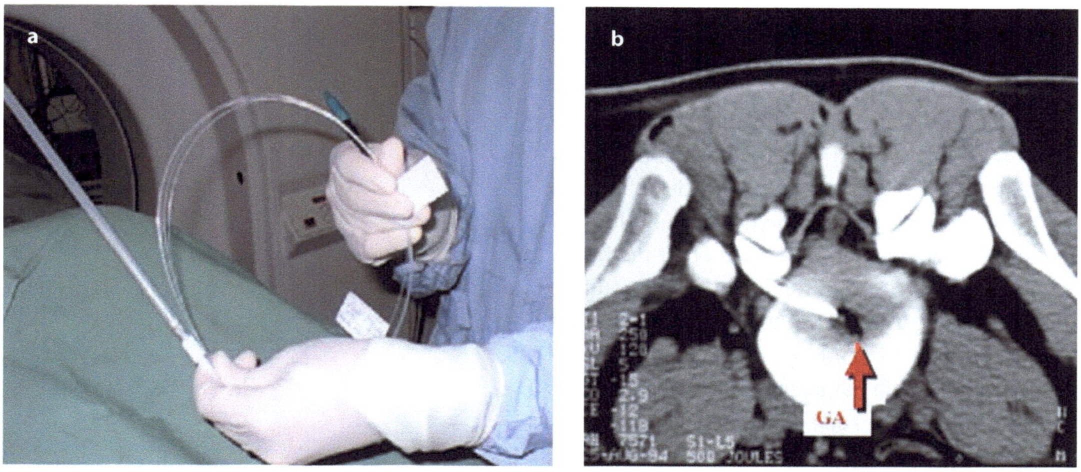

Fig 6.1 Patient with left posterolateral herniated disk at the L5–S1 level being treated by percutaneous laser disk decompression under CT guidance (**a**). Post-treatment axial CT in a patient in the prone position using a posterolateral approach (**b**)

introduced in the disk through a needle (diameter, 2.5 mm) under fluoroscopic guidance. The nucleus pulposus was aspirated through a lateral window of the probe while a blade moving in a coaxial direction in the probe destroyed it and allowed it to be drained externally.

The success rate is around 70–80% (17–20) but, if the exclusion criteria are not considered, this drops to 49.4% [18]. Supporters of this technique believe that it carries fewer risks than percutaneous laser diskectomy and IDET [20]. If the procedure is carried out incorrectly, nerve roots or dural tissue may be damaged. The most serious complication of this procedure is cauda equina syndrome, which is characterized by "saddle anesthesia" in the perianal region, retention of urine/feces, urine/fecal incontinence, and bilateral hyposthenia [21–22]

6.3.2 PLDD

Daniel Choy introduced percutaneous laser diskectomy in the 1980s. The procedure was carried out for the first time in Graz, Austria, in February 1986. The Food and Drug Administration (FDA) in the USA approved its use in clinical practice in 1991.

PLLD is carried out under local anesthesia. It involves introducing (under fluoroscopic guidance) a soft needle (caliber, 0.8 mm) inside the nucleus pulposus of the herniated disk. The operator uses a laser on the nucleus pulposus to vaporize the water of a small part of the nucleus pulposus to enable decompression of diskal pressure.

The action of PDLL is based on the idea that the vertebral disk is a "closed hydraulic system" comprising the nucleus pulposus (which is made of water) surrounded by a fibrous annulus. The increasing water content of the nucleus pulposus causes a disproportionate increase in the intradiskal pressure [23] (Fig. 6.1).

The power of the single laser pulse, the number of pulses, the intervals among each pulse and the total power allocated must be individualized for each patient [24].

PDLL has been quoted as being successful in 75–87% of cases [25–28].

However, the high temperature created by the laser can cause pain and spasms in patients after surgery, and is responsible for a high prevalence of complications (26). Septic and aseptic discitis is the most common complication, and causes recurrence in 0–1.2% of cases [26–29]. Aseptic diskitis is caused by the action of the laser on the disk and on the adjacent vertebral plate, but studies evaluating the efficacy and safety of one type of laser compared with another are lacking [31–33].

6.3.3 IDET

IDET is a minimally invasive method for the therapy of LBP of diskal origin invented by Saal et al. in 1997. It is indicated in percutaneous treatment of bulging or contained herniated disks. It acts on the posterior aspect of the fibrous annulus and not on the nucleus pulposus as in other methods.

IDET involves introducing a needle (under fluoroscopic guidance) into the intervertebral disk to be treated. Through the needle, an electrothermic flexible catheter is introduced around the periphery between the nucleus pulposus and annulus. The tip of the catheter has a resistance that, once placed near the posterior margin of the annulus, is warmed at 90° for 16–17 min and is then removed (Fig. 6.2). It is believed that warming of the fibrous annulus reduces the symptoms and stabilizes the diskal lesion through: reorganization of the collagen fibers; strengthening of the disk; the ablation of pain receptors [34].

The outcome of IDET is controversial [35]. Pauza at al. [36] evaluated the therapeutic effects of IDET on pain of diskal origin in a randomized trial, and showed improvement in pain symptoms in most of the treated patients. However, at 6-month follow-up, only 40% of patients had a reduction of symptoms of >50%. Saal et al. [37–39] detailed their experience with patients who underwent IDET with a follow-up at 6, 12 and 24 months: they reported pain resolution in 71% of cases.

In an analysis from 1998 to 2005, IDET was shown to cause a mean reduction of pain of about 2.9 points as measured using a visual analog scale (VAS). A mean improvement in physical activity of 21.1 points related to the Short Form (SF)-36, and a mean improvement in disability of 7.0 points related to the Oswestry Disability Index (ODS) was noted. The mean prevalence of complications was 0.8%, and the complication associated with the poorest prognosis and highest prevalence was osteonecrosis [40].

6.3.4 PCN

PCN is another minimally invasive method indicated for the treatment of symptomatic herniated (and not extruded) disks. PCN was approved for general use in 1999.

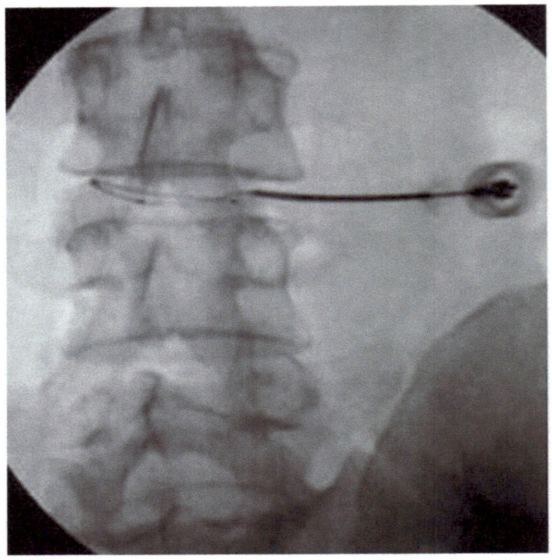

Fig. 6.2 Anteroposterior view under fluoroscopic control shows the IDET catheter at the L3–L4 level after a right posterolateral approach

PCN is carried out at low temperatures (50–70°C), different from conventional radiofrequency ablation (RFA), which uses higher temperatures (150–200°C) to obtain identical results in a shorter time (2–3 min *versus* 15–17 min, respectively). This feature leads to less invasiveness of tissue and lower risks for patients.

RFA is done by percutaneous introduction (under fluoroscopic guidance) of a thermal coagulator (Perc-D coblation Probe) into the nucleus pulposus. By application of a bipolar current on the extremity of an electrode it produces a radiofrequency field that breaks collagen bonds in the area it reaches. It creates "ionic plasma" inside the nucleus comprising simple molecules and ionized gases such as O_2, hydrogen (H) and nitric oxide (NO) that are removed through the needle used to introduce the electrode. The heat produced does not exceed 70°C and has a limited diffusion of 2 mm and creates a "canal" of "thermal lesions" in the nucleus pulposus. Rotating the probe 360° six times creates six channels of thermal lesions with rapid dehydration of the nucleus, resulting in reduction of disk volume of 10–20%. Subsequent contraction of the collagen fibers allows reduction of the protruded portion of the disk with decompression of the compressed root.

The complete integrity of the fibrous annulus must be guaranteed otherwise retraction will be unsuccessful. An intervertebral disk is like a closed hydraulic system in which removal of even a small amount of material causes a considerable decrease in internal hydraulic pressure. Results obtained from controlled trials have reported resolution of pain symptoms in 70% of cases with duration of pain relief of ≥6 months.

The risk of complications is very low. Complications such as diskitis and perforation of the anterior disk caused by the probe, as well as cauda equina syndrome have been reported [41–44].

PCN has been extended to the treatment of cervical disk protrusion. Bonaldi et al. studied outcome in 55 patients affected by herniated disks. They reported good or excellent outcome with regard to the symptoms of nerve-root compression and myelopathy in 80% of cases at 2–6 months, with an incidence of diskitis of 1 in 55 [45].

6.3.5 DPD

An improvement in diskectomy has been obtained with the introduction of decompressor probes (diameter, 1.5 mm) that allow removal of the nucleus pulposus of intervertebral disks through tiny canals. DPD can be carried out with CT or fluoroscopic guidance under local anesthesia. The decompressor probe is introduced through the coaxial trocar that, with continuing movement like a "screw", is inserted in the nucleus pulposus. After switching on the rotating engine, the radiologist moves the probe back and forth. The tissue removed from the herniated nucleus pulposus goes up through the probe and it is expelled externally (Fig. 6.3). DPD is complete if there is no more material to be extracted or if the radiologist feels satisfactory decompression has obtained.

DPD was introduced by Kennet Robert and offers several advantages:

- the caliber of the probe is only 16 G with a diameter of 1.5 mm. This reduces the risk of damaging the longitudinal posterior ligament and the annulus;
- the probe and the trocar can be curved manually in a difficult approach is envisioned;
- the rotation system of the probe allows aspiration of the nucleus not only in cases of central or paramedian herniation but also in cases of foraminal and extraforaminal herniated disks. Decompressing the intraforaminal hernia with no risk of root damage is therefore achievable.

Removal of a small amount of disk material results in a significant decrease in pressure on the peripheral portion of the disk. A reduction in pain symptoms of >70% among 70–72% of patients treated with DPD has been reported [46–47]. The location of the hernia is, however, the most important parameter for the efficacy of therapy. The reduction of symptoms is >70% in 79% of foraminal posterolateral or extraforaminal hernias. Similar results can be obtained in only 50% of patients with middle-posterior hernias [48]. Complications such as broken probes have been reported [49] (the probe can break in proximal and caudal directions).

6.3.6 Chemodiskolysis

Chemodiskolysis using a mixture of O_2 and O_3 as well as periradicular and perigangliar infiltrations is a recently introduced percutaneous method for treating herniated disks that is widespread in Europe (especially Italy, Germany, Spain).

O_3 is an unstable, colorless, irritating gas with a thorny smell as well as antiseptic, disinfectant and anti-viral properties. It is prepared and used in real time, transforming a small percentage of O_2 to O_2–O_3 by the use of special generators. The O_2–O_3 mixture is injected into the intradiskal space (3–4 mL) and the foramen (10 mL). The administrated dose for treating the disk is 30–40 µL; this is the best concentration to dehydrate the nucleus as well as to reduce inflammation and the risk of complications according to experimental studies [50]. The *rationale* for this treatment is that the pain is due to mechanical compression on the nerve root with associated inflammatory

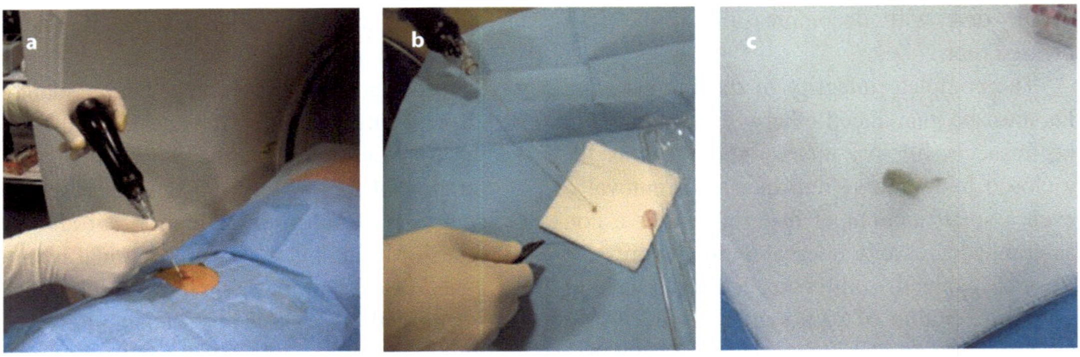

Fig. 6.3 The decompressor percutaneous diskectomy system under CT guidance (**a**) Removal of tissue from the herniated nucleus pulposus through the Dekompressor probe (**b** and **c**)

changes in peri-gangliar and peri-radicular spaces [51–52].

Chemodiskolysis can be carried out under fluoroscopic or CT guidance. Under the latter, better evaluation of gas distribution is possible, with intradiskal and perigangliar diffusion; intra- and extraforaminal injection is suggested for a mildly compressed, highly inflamed root.

After CT shows the disk level, a needle (18–20 G) is inserted into the nucleus pulposus using an oblique paravertebral approach by targeting the specific disk space (Fig. 6.4). Sometimes, for anatomical reasons, the "classic" oblique approach can be difficult (especially at the L5–S1 level). Hence, further inclination of the needle of 30° in a cranio-caudal direction is needed to reach the specific disk space. If this approach remains difficult, a translaminar medial approach should be used without fear of crossing the dural sac to reach the vertebral disk (Fig. 6.5).

Once the needle has been positioned in the center of the disk, the gas mixture is injected slowly into the nucleus pulposus, then into the epidural and intraforaminal spaces using a local anti-inflammatory effect.

Different from other percutaneous methods, infiltration of a mixture of O_2–O_3 can be undertaken safely at the cervical level with some differences compared with that at the lumbar level. The indications are very restricted and selective. Only a soft herniated disk without calcified elements, a central spinal stenosis or lateral foraminal stenosis can be treated. Symptomatic herniated disks with important motor deficits in the upper limb are contraindicated, and surgery is indicated. Pretreatment imaging (CT, MRI, EMG) is recommended. Then, for treatment at the cervical level, there are technical differences:

- the needle used for treatment at the cervical level is thinner and smaller than the one used at the lumbar level;
- chemodiskolysis is done with the patient in the supine position and can be carried out under CT or fluoroscopic guidance;
- chemodiskolysis is undertaken with a right anterolateral approach with manual alteration of the carotid axis (Fig. 6.6);
- the amount of the O_2–O_3 mixture used at the cervical level is less than that used at the lumbar level: only 1–2 cm^3 is injected into cervical disks;
- chemodiskolysis is not associated with injection of anesthetic drugs (so as to avoid breathing disturbances);
- as for the lumbar level, a periforaminal injection of corticosteroid may be associated.

The mechanisms of action of the O_2–O_3 mixture are being investigated and include [53]:

- anti-inflammatory effects due to oxidative actions on the chemical mediators of pain;
- improvement in capillary blood perfusion, resolution of venous stasis with better tissue oxygenation in the site of compression, as well as reduction of ischemic pain and root edema;
- direct actions through oxygenation.

If O_2–O_3 moves into cerebrospinal fluid (CSF) or the subarachnoid space, it does not damage

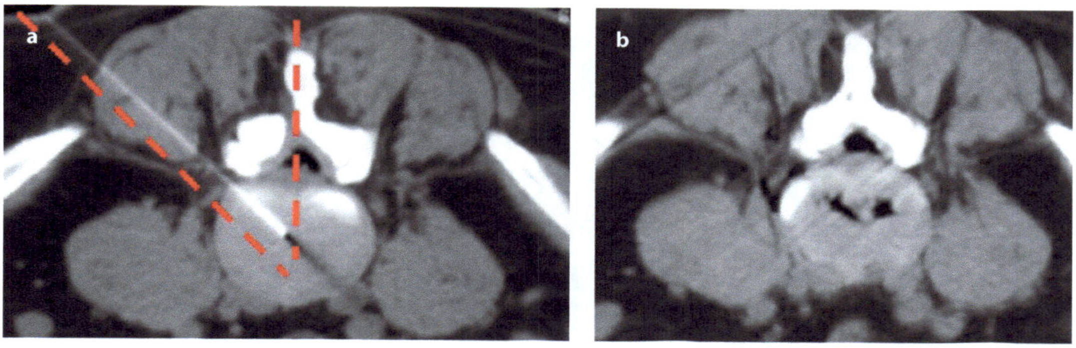

Fig. 6.4 Axial CT during intradiskal infiltration of an O_2–O_3 mixture at the L4–L5 level using a left posterolateral approach in a patient in the prone position shows good positioning of the needle in the center of the disk (**a**). Final axial CT shows gas distribution in the center of the disk and periganglial space (**b**)

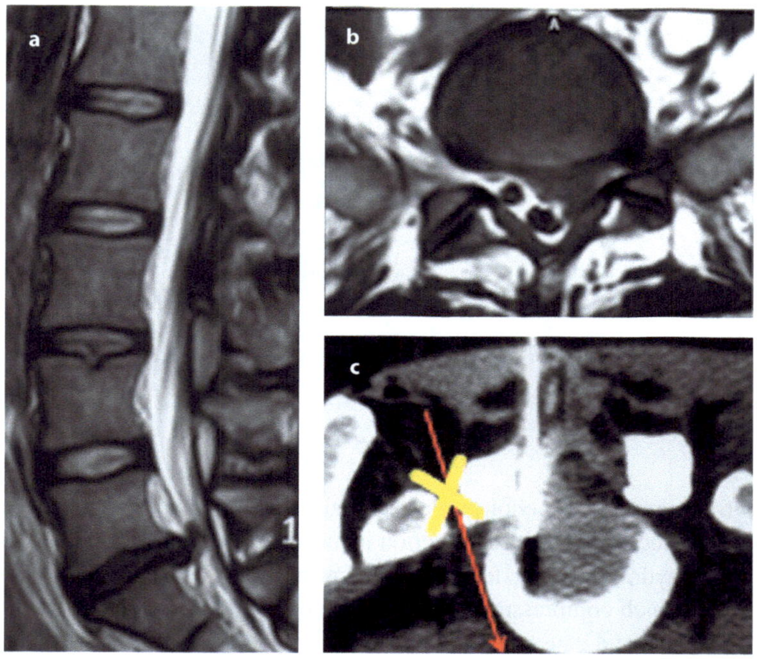

Fig. 6.5 Sagittal and axial T2-weighted MRI show left posterolateral herniated disks at the L5–S1 level (**a** and **b**). Axial CT during intradiskal infiltration of an O_2–O_3 mixture using a left translaminar approach in a patient in the prone position shows the needle position in the disk (**c**)

structures, as reported by Tian et al. in an experimental study on pigs using high doses of O_3 [54]. Experimental studies have demonstrated an O_2–O_3 mixture at a concentration used for intradiskal injection produces the same results upon the production of steroids and cytokines, and so reduces pain [55]. The therapeutic efficacy of an O_2–O_3 mixture in the treatment of root–disk conflict from herniated disks is largely known. Reports of a success rate of 70–80% without complications in randomized studies evaluating conservative treatment *versus* treatment with a O_2–O_3 mixture have been documented. Early or late neurological or infectious complications have not been reported after injection with an O_2–O_3 mixture [55–65].

6.3.7 Discogel

Discogel is a sterile viscous solution containing ethyl alcohol and cellulose derivative products added to a radiopaque element (tungsten). It is injected into the vertebral disk and relieves LBP as well as radicular and lumbar–radicular pain. The

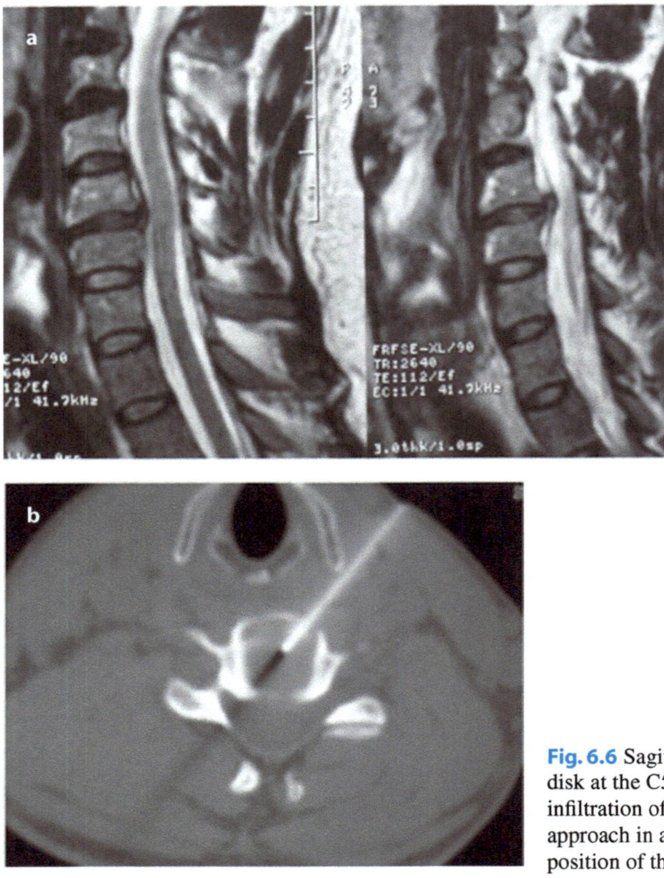

Fig. 6.6 Sagittal T2-weighted MRI shows a herniated disk at the C5–C6 level (**a**). Axial CT during intradiskal infiltration of an O_2–O_3 mixture using a right anterolateral approach in a patient in the supine position shows the position of the needle in the disk (**b**)

96%-pure ethyl alcohol produces local necrosis of the nucleus pulposus. Its action is mechanical *via* dehydration of the turgescent and protruding disk (which compresses the peripheral nerves of the rachis and causes extreme pain). Discogel is injected into the nucleus pulposus under imaging (CT or fluoroscopy) with a postlateral approach for thoracic or lumbar levels and an anterolateral approach for the cervical level.

In general, a small (18 G) needle is used for thoracic and lumbar levels, whereas a 20-G needle is employed for the cervical level. The quantity of Discogel injected varies according to the dimension of the disk and extent of the hernia. In general: 0.2 mL is injected for cervical disks; 0.3–0.5 mL for thoracic disks; and 0.6–0.8 mL for lumbar disks.

At the beginning of the injection, the patient may experience a transitional "scalding" sensation at the injection site which disappears during the course of the injection. To minimize this risk, Discogel must be injected very slowly. Once it has been injected, the needle is left for 2 min before being withdrawn.

The viscosity of Discogel is dependent upon the temperature. Avoidance of administration of Discogel that is warmer than room temperature is important because the gel becomes more liquid and is below its optimum viscosity. To increase its viscosity, Discogel can be refrigerated immediately before injection (Fig. 6.7).

Discogel is not indicated in pregnancy, for patients known to be allergic to any one of the components, or for patients in severe depression (or any other condition making the interpretation of pain difficult).

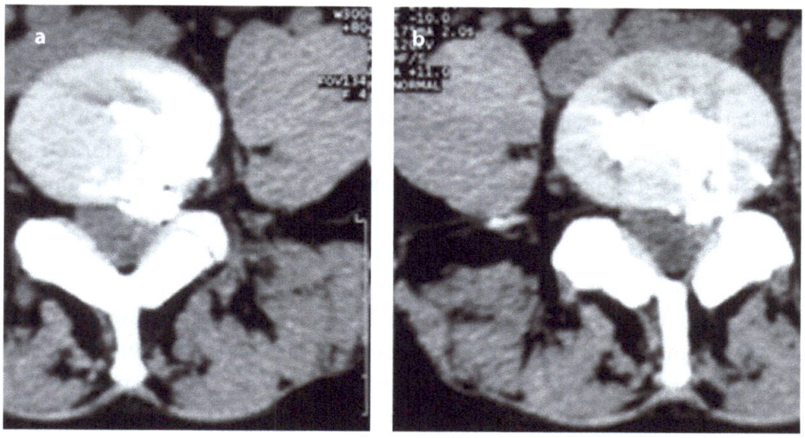

Fig. 6.7 Axial CT after infiltration of Discogel® at the L3–L4 level shows the distribution of radiopaque gelified ethanol in the center of the disk (**a**) and a herniated canal in the disk (**b**)

Experimental studies using Discogel on pigs demonstrated that it does not produce morphological/structural changes when in contact with nerves or muscles. No tissue alteration was found. However, some inflammatory cells (lymphocytes, monocytes) and venous stasis with some granular material colored black by hematoxylin & eosin staining (tungsten) in paravertebral, muscular and connective tissue were observed. The nucleus pulposus, disk, chondromixoid fibromas and root ganglia were normal, without morphological/structural changes in nuclear tissue and the annulus in contact with Discogel [66]. Successful outcome in 89–91% of cases without minor or major complications has been reported [67–69].

6.3.8 Patient Selection: Indications and Contraindications

The selection of patients undergoing minimally invasive treatments is the most important factor for the success of the methods described above. This is primarily because they are alternative treatments to classical surgery, which has already been standardized by guidelines validated by international surgical associations. In general, the exclusion criteria are:

- extruded herniated disks;
- free herniated fragments;
- recent infection of disks or vertebral bodies;
- progressive motor deficits in the arms and feet;
- conus-cauda syndrome;
- hyperalgic sciatica.

The last three conditions are absolute indications for surgery. Failure in IDET treatment may be due to obesity, wide herniated disks, significant reduction of intradiskal space and a complex syndrome dependent upon three or more diskal spaces. Chemodiskolysis using a mixture of O_2 and O_3 has the advantage of having no absolute contraindications

The best results are reported for small and medium-sized herniations with a normal spinal canal without calcifications. Prognostic factors for an unsuccessful outcome are: a calcified herniated disk; a high grade of spinal stenosis; a small descending herniated disk in the lateral spinal recess; FBSS; and recurring herniation.

The clinical criteria are LBP and sciatica resistant to conservative medical therapy, physical therapy and others manipulations (e.g., needle puncture for ≥2–3 months). For IDET, the indication is for patients with LBP without root-compression symptoms and resistance to pharmacological therapy and physiotherapy for >6 months.

With respect to neurological criteria, paresthesia or hypoesthesia over the dermatome involved, as well as weakness and signs of root-ganglion irritation, must be considered. Another important criterion is psychological. It is important to understand if the pain is real or is an expression of psychological disturbances. Also, one must ascertain if the patient wishes to cooperate and undergo subsequent physiotherapy with postural and motor rehabilitation.

With regard to neuroradiological criteria, one must consider (using CT and MRI):

- evidence of small and medium-sized herniated disks correlating with symptoms with or without degenerative disk/vertebral disease complicated by changes in intervertebral disks (protrusion, herniation);
- pain evoked by low-pressure injection of contrast in the compromised disk during IDET, nucleoplasty and APLD;
- residual surgical (micro)diskectomy with herniation recurrence and/or hypertrophic fibrous scarring.

DPD is indicated for central and posterolateral herniated disks as well as for cases of foraminal and extraforaminal herniation. Chemodiskolysis using a mixture of O_2 and O_3 seems to more useful, easier to undertake, and less traumatic than the other methods. It is also useful in patients with: FBSS (because O_3 is effective against chronic inflammation and venous stasis); large or free fragments without significant symptoms.

6.3.9 Choice of Imaging Guidance: CT or Fluoroscopy?

All the methods described in this chapter require imaging support, whether it be CT or fluoroscopy. The choice is dependent upon the operator and equipment availability.

IDET, nucleoplasty and APLD are undertaken using fluoroscopy, whereas therapy using O_2–O_3 mixtures is under CT. This choice allows the radiologist to evaluate the presence of a bowel segment behind the muscle psoas; an absolute contraindication for treatment and intradiskal gas distribution. If the hernia is contained, PLDD under fluoroscopic guidance is possible by releasing laser energy at the center and posterior portion of the vertebral disk. If the hernia is not contained but is connected to the intervertebral disk, it is better to carry out PLDD under CT guidance to better assess the connection between the disk and hernia. In this way, the laser energy can be released along multiple sites of the herniated disk, resulting in better vaporization and greater retraction of the hernia with root decompression and symptom resolution. PLDD can be done under CT or fluoroscopic guidance without limitations to the procedure. APLD and IDET require previous diskography to obtain better evaluation of the: contained hernia; disk compression; disk pressure. For therapy using O_2–O_3 mixtures, diskography is not required because it does not provide diagnostic information. CT guidance allows the operator to avoid intradiskal administration of contrast that even at low doses reduces O_3 absorption and causes obstruction to intraforaminal injection of the O_2–O_3 mixture.

6.4 Conclusions

Percutaneous methods can be good alternatives to surgery for herniated disks for patients affected by LBP and sciatica. Each method has a low prevalence of complications and is relatively easy to undertake. The duration of hospitalization is quite short and surgery is possible if the percutaneous procedure is unsuccessful.

Of all the percutaneous methods described here, chemodiskolysis with O_2–O_3 mixtures and periradicular and periganglionic infiltration elicits the best therapeutic results, has the lowest prevalence of complications, and is the least expensive. Surgery is indicated in emergency cases of conus-cauda syndrome, progressive neurologic deficits, hyperalgic sciatica, and upper-arm radiculopathy.

References

1. Long MD (2001) Decision making in lumbar disc disease. Clin Neurosurg 39:36–51
2. Bozzao A, Gallucci M, Masciocchi C, Aprile I, Barile A, Passariello R. (1992) Lumbar disk herniation: MR imaging assessment of natural history in patients treated without surgery. Radiology 185:135–141
3. Splendiani A, Puglielli E, De Amicis R, Barile A, Masciocchi C, Gallucci M. (2004) Spontaneous reso-

lution of lumbar disk herniation: predictive signs for prognostic evaluation. Neuroradiology 46:916–922
4. Casey E (2011) Natural history of radiculopathy. Phys Med Rehabil Clin N Am 22:1–5
5. Awad JN, Moskovich R.(2006) Lumbar disc herniations: surgical versus nonsurgical treatment. Clin Orthop Relat Res. 443:183–197
6. Muto M, De Maria G, Izzo R, Fucci G (1997) Nondiscal lumbar radiculopathy: combined approach by CT and MR. Riv Neuroradiol 10:165–173
7. Bush K, Cowan N, Katz DE, Gishen P. (1992) The natural history of sciatica associated with disc pathology. A prospective study with clinical and independent radiologic follow-up. Spine 17:1205–1212
8. van de Velden J, de Bakker DH (1990) Basis rapport: morbiditeit in de huisartsenpraktijk. Nivel, Utrecht
9. Masui T, Yukawa Y, Nakamura S et al (2005) Natural history of patients with lumbar disc herniation observed by magnetic resonance imaging for minimum 7 years. J Spinal Disord Tech 18:121–126
10. Takada E, Takahashi M, Shimada K (2001) Natural history of lumbar disc hernia with radicular leg pain: spontaneous MRI changes of the herniated mass and correlation with clinical outcome. J Orthop Surg 9:1–7
11. Singh V Piryani C Liao K (2002) Percutaneous disc decompression using coblation in the treatment of chronic discogenic pain Pain Physician 5: 250–259
12. Gangi A, Dietemann JL, Mortazavi R et al. (1998) CT-guided interventional procedures for pain management in the lumbosacral spine. Radiographics 18:621–633
13. Gallucci M, Splendiani A, Masciocchi C (1997) Spine and spinal cord: neuroradiological funcional anatomy. Riv Neuroradiol 11:293–304
14. von Tulder MW, Koes BW, Bouter LM (1997) Conservative treatment of acute and chronic non-specific low back pain. Spine 22:2128–2156
15. Saal J (1995) The role of inflammation in lumbar spine Spine 20:1821–1827
16. Wilco CP, van Houwelingen H, van der Hout WB et al for the Leiden–The Hague Spine Intervention Prognostic Study Group (2007) Surgery versus prolonged conservative treatment for sciatica. New Engl J Med 356:2245–2256
17. Onik G, Helms CA, Ginsberg L et al. (1985) Percutaneous lumbar discectomy using a new aspiration probe Am J Neuroradiol 6:290–296
18. Kaps H, Cotta H (1989) Early results of automated percutaneous lumbar discectomy. In: Mayer HM and Brock M (eds) Percutaneous lumbar discectomy. Springer-Verlag, Berlin, p 153–156
19. Hammon W (1989) Percutaneous lumbar nucleotomy. Western Neurological Society 635
20. Onik G, Mooney V, Maroon JC, Wiltse L et al (1990) Automated percutaneous discectomy: a prospective multi-institutional study. Neurosurgery 26:228–232 (discussion 232–233)
21. Mathews RS (2000) Automated percutaneous lumbar discectomy. In: Savitz MH, Chiu JC, Rauschning W et al (eds) The practice of minimally invasive spinal techniques. Wyndham Hall, Ohio p 97–100
22. Onik G, Maroon J, Jackson R (1992) Cauda equina syndrome secondary to an improperly placed nucleotome probe. Neurosurgery 30:412–414
23. Choy DSJ, Michelsen J, Getrajdman D et al (1992) Percutaneus laser disc decompression: an update: spring 1992. J Clin Laser Med Surg 10:177–184
24. Schenk B, Brouwer PA, Peul WC, van Buchem MA (2006) Percutaneous laser disk decompression: a review of the literature. Am J Neuroradiol 27:232–235
25. Choy DSJ, Case RB, Fielding W et al (1992) Percutaneous laser disc decompression, a new therapeutic modality. Spine 17:949–956
26. Choy DS (1998) Percutaneous laser disc decompression (PLDD): twelve years experience with 752 procedures in 518 patients. J Clin Laser Med Surg 16:325–331
27. Gupta AK, Bodhey NK, Jayasree RS et al (2006) Percutaneous laser disc decompression: clinical experience at SCTIMST and long term follow up. Neurol India 54:164–167
28. Nerubay J, Caspi I, Levinkopf M (1997) Percutaneous carbon dioxide laser nucleolysis with 2- to 5-year follow-up. Clin Orthop 337:45–48
29. Agarwal S, Bhagwat AS (2003) Ho:YAG laser-assisted lumbar disc decompression: a minimally invasive procedure under local anesthesia. Neurol India 51:35–38
30. Ohnmeiss DD, Guyer RD, Hochschuler SH (1994) Laser disc decompression: the importance of proper patient selection. Spine 19:2054–2058
31. Turgut M (2007) Extensive damage to the end-plates as a complication of laser discectomy: an experimental study using an animal model. Acta Neurochir Wien 139:404–410
32. Takeno K, Kobayashi S, Yonezawa T et al (2006) Salvage operation for persistent low back pain and sciatica induced by percutaneous laser disc decompression performed at outside institution: correlation of magnetic resonance imaging and intraoperative and pathological findings. Photomed Laser Surg 24:414–423
33. Gibson JNA, Grant IC, Waddell G (2003) Surgery for lumbar disc prolapse (Cochrane Review). In: The Cochrane Library. Oxford: Update Software, Issue 2
34. Eckel TS (2002) Intradiscal electrothermal therapy. In: Williams AL, Murtagh FR (eds) Handbook of diagnostic and therapeutic spine procedures. Mosby, St. Louis, 229 –244
35. Boswell MV, Shah RV, Everett CR, Sehgal N et al. (2005) Interventional techniques in the management of chronic spinal pain: evidence-based practice guidelines. Pain Physician 8:1–47
36. Pauza KJ, Howell S, Dreyfuss P. (2004) A randomized, placebo-controlled trial of intradiscal electrothermal therapy for the treatment of discogenic low back pain. Spine J 4:27–35
37. Saal JA, Saal JS. (2000) Intradiscal electrothermal treatment for chronic discogenic low back pain: a pro-

spective outcome study with minimum 1-year follow-up. Spine 25:2622–2627
38. Saal JA, Saal JS (2002) Intradiscal electrothermal treatment for chronic discogenic low back pain: Prospective outcome study with a minimum 2-year follow-up. Spine 27:966–974
39. Saal JA, Saal JS (2002) Intradiscal electrothermal treatment for chronic discogenic low back pain. Clin Sports Med 21:167–187
40. Appleby D, Andersson G, Totta M (2006) Meta-analysis of the efficacy and safety of intradiscal electrothermal therapy (IDET). Pain Med 7:308–316
41. Singh V Piryani C, Liao K, et al (2002) Percutaneous disc decompression using coblation (Nucleoplasty) in the treatment of chronic discogenic pain. Pain Physician 5:250–259
42. Sharps LS, Isacc Z (2002) Percutaneous disc decompression using nucleoplasty. Pain Physician 5:121–126
43. Hellinger J (1999) Technical aspects of the percutaneous cervical and lumbar laser-disc decompression and nucleotomy. Neurol Res 21:99–102
44. Kelekis AD, Somon T, Yilmaz H et al (2005) Interventional spine procedures. Eur J Radiol 55:362–383
45. Bonaldi G, Baruzzi F, Facchinetti A, Facchinetti P, Lunghi S (2006) Plasma radio-frequency–based diskectomy for treatment of cervical herniated nucleus pulposus: feasibility, safety, and preliminary clinical results. Am J Neuroradiol 27:2104–2111
46. Aco KM, Wrigiat RE, Brandt SA (2004) Percutaneous lumbar discectomy: clinical response in an initial cohort of fifty consecutive patients with chronic radicular pain. Pain Pract 4:19–29
47. Amoretti N, Huchot F, Flory P et al (2005) Percutaneous nucleotomy: preliminary communication on a decompression probe (Dekompressor) in percutaneous discectomy. Ten case reports. Clin Imaging 29:98–101
48. Amoretti N, Davida P, Grimaud A et al (2006) Clinical follow-up of 50 patients treated by percutaneous lumbar discectomy. Clin Imaging 30:242–244
49. Domsky R, Goldberg ME, Hirsh RA et al (2006) Critical failure of a percutaneous discectomy probe requiring surgical removal during disc decompression. Regional Anesthesia Pain Med 31:177–179
50. Muto M (2004) Alterazioni indotte da infiltrazioni intradiscali e intramuscolari di ossigeno-ozono: studio anatomo-patologico. Risultati preliminari. Riv. Italiana di Ossigeno-Ozonoterapia 3:7–13
51. Andreula C, Muto M, Leonardi M (2004) Interventional spinal procedures Eur J Radiol 50:112–119
52. Muto M, Andreula C, Leonardi M (2004) Treatment of herniated lumbar disc by intradiscal and intraforaminal oxygen-ozone injection. J Neuroradiol 31:183–189
53. Andreula CF, Simonetti L, Leonardi M (2003) Minimally invasive oxygen-ozone therapy for lumbar disk herniation. Am J Neuroradiol 24:996–1000
54. Tian JL Zhang JS, Xiao YY et al (2007) Changes of CSF and spinal path-morphology after height concentration ozone injection into the subarachnoid space: an experimental study in pigs. Am J Neuroradiol 28:1051–1054
55. Muto M, Avella F (1998) Percutaneous treatment of herniated lumbar disc by intradiscal oxygen-ozone injection. Interv Neuroradiol 20:279–286
56. Iliakis E (1995) Ozone treatment in low back pain. Orthopaedics 1:29–33
57. Fabris G, Tommasini G, et al (1999) Oxygen-ozone therapy in percutaneous treatment of lumbar HNP. Riv Neuroradiol 12:23
58. D' Erme M, Scarchilli A, Lasagni M, et al (1999) Ozone therapy in lumbar sciatic pain. Radiol Med 95:21–24
59. Muto M, Guarnieri G, Rotondo A et al (2008) Low back pain and sciatica: treatment with intradiscal-intraforaminal O_2-O_3 injection. Our experience. Radiol Med_113:695–706
60. Bonetti M, Cotticelli B et al (2000) Oxygen-ozone therapy versus epidural steroid injection. Riv Neuroradiol 13:203–206
61. Leonardi M, Barbara C et al. (2001) Percutaneous treatment of lumbar herniated disk with intradiscal injection of ozone mixture. Riv Neuroradiol 14:51–53
62. Andreula C (2002) Lumbar herniated disk and degenerative changes. Interventional spinal treatment with chemiodiscolysis with nucleoptesis with O_2-O_3 and perigangliar infiltration in 150 cases. Riv Neuroradiol 14:81–88
63. Andreula CF, Simonetti L, Leonardi M et al (2003) Minimally invasive oxygen-ozone therapy for lumbar disk herniation. Am J Neuroradiol 24:996–1000
64. Gallucci M, Limbucci N, Masciocchi C et al (2007) Sciatica: treatment with intradiscal and intraforaminal injections of steroid and oxygen-ozone versus steroid only. Radiology 242:907–917
65. Bonetti M, Fontana A, Leonardi M et al (2005) Intraforaminal O_2-O_3 versus periradicular steroidal infiltrations in lower back pain: randomized controlled trial. Am J Neuroradiol 26:996–1000
66. Guarnieri G, de Dominicis G, Muto M (2010) Intradiscal and intramuscular injection of discogel® - radiopaque gelified ethanol: pathological evaluation. Neuroradiol J 23:249–252
67. Theron J, Cuellar H, Sola T, Casasco A, Courtheoux P (2010) Percutaneous treatment of cervical disk hernias using gelified ethanol. Am J Neuroradiol 31:1454–1456
68. Theron J, Guimaraens L, Casasco A, Sola T, Cuellar H, Courtheoux P (2007) Percutaneous treatment of lumbar intervertebral disk hernias with radiopaque gelified ethanol: a preliminary study. J Spinal Disord Tech 20:526–532
69. Stagni S, Simonetti L, Stafa A et al (2012) A minimally invasive treatment for lumbar disc herniation: DiscoGel® chemonucleolysis in patients unresponsive to chemonucleolysis with oxygen-ozone. Interv Neuroradiol 18:97–104

7 Treatment of Facet Joints

Stefano Marcia, Salvatore Masala,
Mariangela Marras and Alberto Cauli

7.1 Introduction

Lumbar zygapophysial joints are also called "facet joints". They are often cause of chronic back pain because of rich innervation of the articular structures. In 1933, Ghormley named the spectrum of symptoms arising from its pathological involvement as "facet joint syndrome" (FCS). FCS represents ≤15% of chronic pain in the lower back. It is characterized by joint pain which is usually insidious in its onset and which may derive from almost any structure in the zygapophysial joints (fibrous capsule, synovial membrane, hyaline cartilage, tendons, bone) due to mechanical or inflammatory stimulation of nociceptors. Standard treatments for pain in lumbar facet joints are mainly intra-articular injections of corticosteroids and radiofrequency denervation (RFD) of the medial branches which innervate the zygapophysial joint. We review here the anatomy and physiology of the lumbar zygapophysial joints as well as diagnostic tools and treatments.

7.2 Anatomy

Lumbar zygapophysial joints connect posteriously the vertebral arch of adjacent vertebrae. They present hyaline cartilage surfaces, a synovial membrane and a fibrous capsule. Their main function is to support and protect intervertebral disks from loads and to limit vertebral movement. In the cervical spine, the articular rim is oriented to the coronal plane at 30°–45° with respect to the horizontal plane. In the dorsal tract the angle is 60°, whereas at the lumbar level the articular rims are sagittal and oblique. Constitutional asymmetry in the orientation of the articular surfaces may predispose to osteoarthritis. Each facet joint is innervated by two medial branches arising from the posterior primary rami of the same level and from one level above the zygapophysial joint [1,2]. According to this rule, the inferior articular surface of the L4–L5 facet joint is innervated by the L4 medial branch, and its superior articular surface is innervated by the L3 medial branch. The medial branches of L1–L4 dorsal rami run from their respective transverse processes to one level below through the inter-transverse ligament. Each nerve then runs downward, dividing into multiple branches as it crosses the vertebral lamina (Fig. 7.1) [3–5]. The L5 nerve differs because it is the dorsal ramus itself that runs along the sacral ala, whereas its medial branch arises opposite the infero-lateral corner of the lowest facet joint. This anatomical difference must be considered if treating disor-

S. Marcia (✉)
Radiology Department, SS. Trinità Hospital,
ASL Cagliari, Cagliari, Italy
e-mail: stemarcia@gmail.com

M. Muto (ed.), *Interventional Neuroradiology of the Spine*,
DOI 10.1007/978-88-470-2790-9_7, © Springer-Verlag Italia 2013

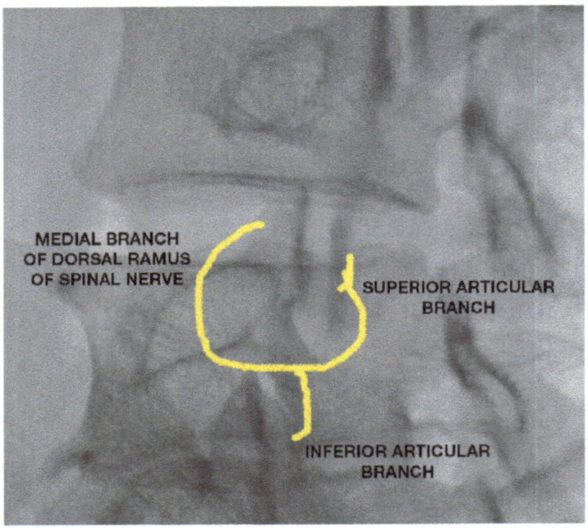

Fig. 7.1 The medial branch runs downward between transverse and articular processes. It then splits into two articular branches: the superior for the inferior articular process, and the inferior for the superior articular process of the same vertebra

ders at this level because the dorsal ramus itself rather than its medial branch has to be the target of the therapeutic intervention.

7.3 Patient Selection for Percutaneous Procedures

Lumbar FCS is a classical indication for interventional procedures on zygapophysial joints. The syndrome has a high incidence in the elderly because it is frequently caused by osteoarthritic degenerative lesions secondary to abnormal articular load or to repetitive stress injury. Less frequently, FCS is associated with synovitis and joint effusion (due to non-specific inflammation or after trauma); entrapment of meniscal structures; synovial impingement; articular subluxation; chondromalacia; mechanical trauma to joint capsules; or compression. Sometimes, lumbar pain resembling FCS may be associated with instability of the posterior arch.

This syndrome is not easy to diagnose because of its similarity to other painful spinal conditions and, above all, because lumbar pain is, in general, multifactorial in origin. The most common symptom is median lumbar pain, which may be irradiated to gluteal regions and posteriously in a tight, imprecise dermatomeric distribution. In general, it does not irradiate to the inferior limb below the knee. The pain is usually worst in the morning and after rest, worsening also after hyperextension and torsion movements to the involved side. Neurological examination and electromyography are usually normal. In some patients, para-articular synovial cysts are detected, and they can determine radicular compression. In these cases, aspiration under CT guidance is recommended. Patients with disease in cervical facet joints complain of paravertebral pain which worsens with twisting movements and which may radiate to the shoulder and cause headaches.

Classically, radiography reveals degenerative changes and limitations in the range of flexion/extension. CT and MRI can be used to detect spondylitis and asymmetry in orientation of the articular rim (if present). In subjects with pain exacerbation, MRI may show joint effusion (especially in patients with joint instability) and bone edema. Paramagnetic contrast enhancement may show uptake not only in the involved joints but also in the surrounding soft tissue. In patients with lumbar pain and joint instability, MRI undertaken with the patient in the standing position may reveal joint subluxation and/or join effusion (Fig. 7.2).

The clinical picture, together with imaging data, will lead to the correct diagnosis. In difficult cases, a diagnostic anesthetic nerve block may be needed. In most cases, anesthetic injections are given to alleviate pain (and may be repeated if the pain is persistent). Medial branch neurotomy is reserved for patients with chronic pain derived from facet joints to achieve long-lasting analgesia. This procedure follows a positive diagnostic block [5]. Contraindications are rare, but can include hypersensitivity to the medication, coagulation disorders or local infections. Relative contraindications include hypersensitivity to corticosteroids or iodine contrast (which can be avoided in most cases).

Injections are administered in Outpatient Clinics or in Day Surgery Centers under local anesthesia; specific preparations for patients are not needed. Neurolytic procedures may require sedation and therefore should be carried out in hospital.

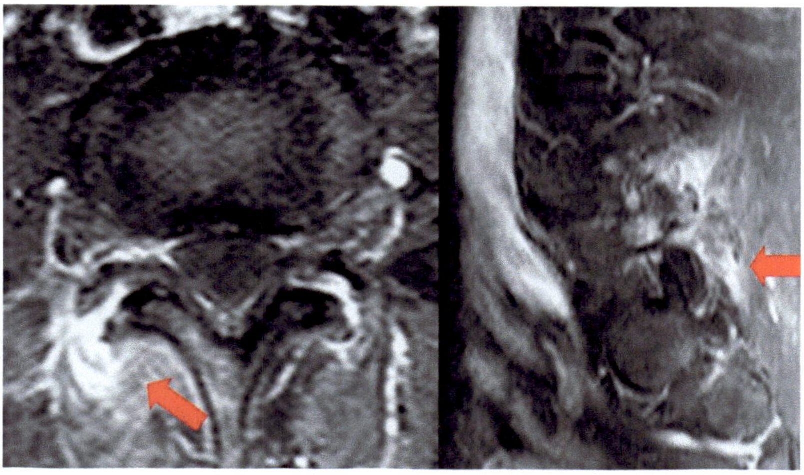

Fig. 7.2 MRI after administration of gadolinium contrast agent shows enhancement in the right facet joint and closer soft tissues (arrows)

7.4 Diagnostic Blocks

Nerve block tests can be done by injection of 1 mL of lidocaine in the tender joint. Pain relief in two repeated blocks (1 week apart) is considered to be a good prognostic factor for successful RFD. Numerous guidelines and reviews have asserted that diagnostic blocks are very important for the diagnosis of facet-related pain [6–8] even though false-positive [9, 10] and false-negative blocks have been described [10, 11].

7.5 Corticosteroid Injections

The use of intra-articular corticosteroid injections to treat facet-related pain is controversial. Injections into facet joints can be done under guidance by fluoroscopy or CT. The C-arm has to be positioned approximately 30–40° on the side of the target joint; this ensures that the X-ray beam is perpendicular to the zygapophysial joint. A 25-G needle is introduced to the lower part of the articular rim (where the synovial recess is wider). Injection of contrast agent (0.1–0.3 mL) into the joint is done to assess the position of the needle. Then 1–2 mL of a solution of corticosteroid and local anaesthetic can be injected. To avoid rupture of the joint capsule, ≤2 mL of this solution is injected. An para-articular injection can be carried out and, in such cases, a higher volume of solution can be injected. However, similar results between intra- and para-articular injections have been demonstrated in the literature. Under CT or fluoroscopic guidance, facet joints can be approached readily for corticosteroid injections.

7.6 RFD

RFD is carried out as day surgery under CT or fluoroscopic guidance. The patient lies in the prone position. The oblique view under fluoroscopic guidance allows good visualization of the target point for needle positioning: the groove between the transverse and articular process (Fig. 7.3).

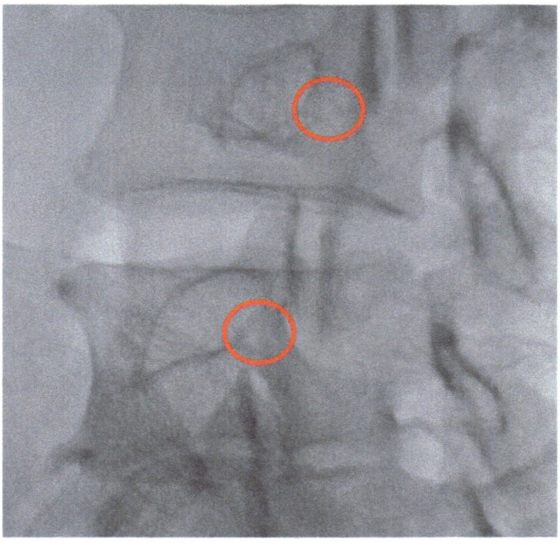

Fig. 7.3 Oblique view: red circles show the correct point to introduce the exposed tip of the needle: between the transverse and articular process

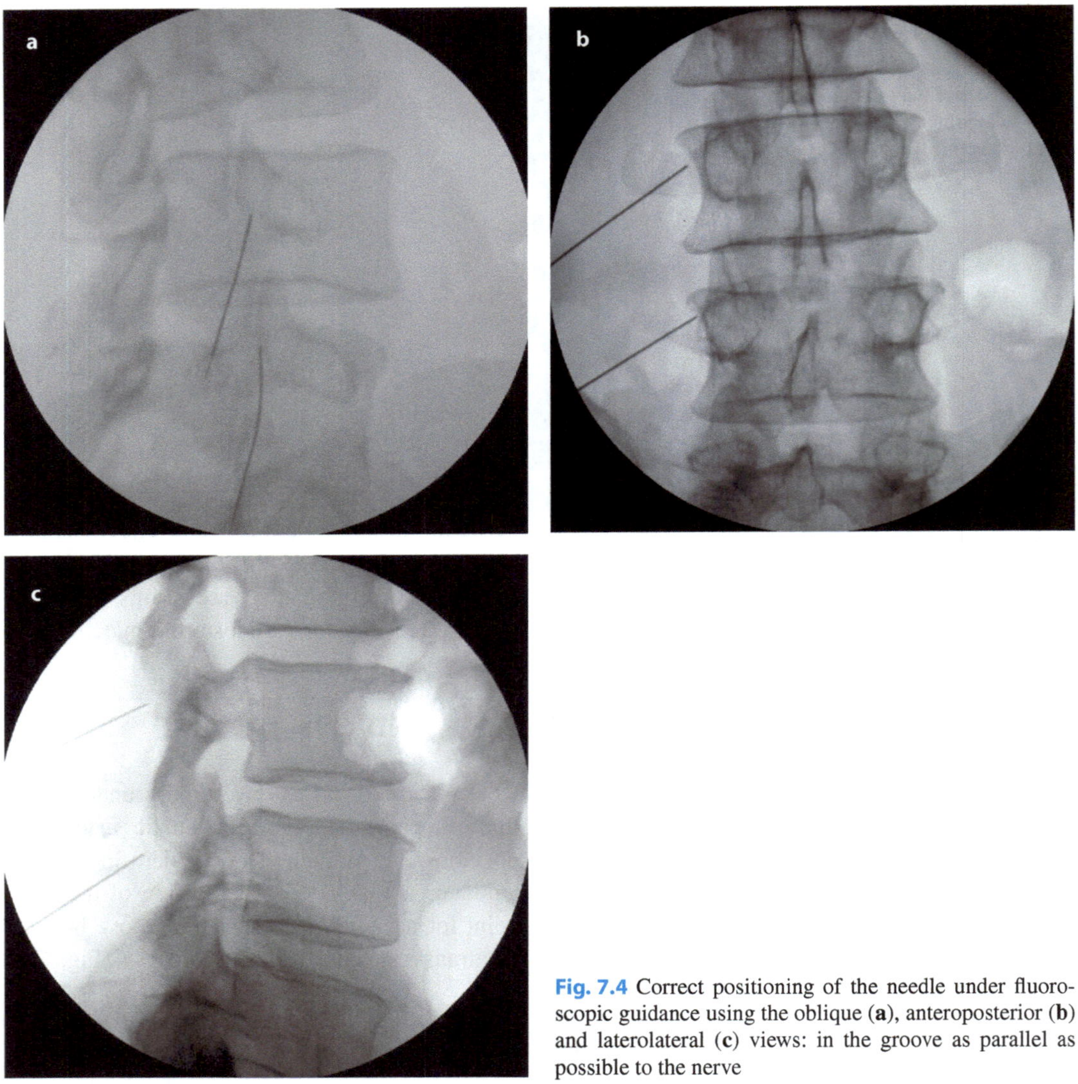

Fig. 7.4 Correct positioning of the needle under fluoroscopic guidance using the oblique (**a**), anteroposterior (**b**) and laterolateral (**c**) views: in the groove as parallel as possible to the nerve

At that site lies the medial arm of the dorsal branch of the spinal nerve before it splits into the two terminal nerves, which allows positioning of the needle parallel to the nerve in the optimal position (Fig. 7.4a–c). Because of anatomical differences, for L5 nerves the dorsal ramus rather than its medial branch is approached on the ala of the sacrum just lateral to the articular process, as discussed above (Fig. 7.5a and b).

One milliliter of lidocaine is administered percutaneously before introduction of a 22-G needle of length 10 cm with a 10-mm exposed tip. When the needle is in the appropriate position (as assessed by anteroposterior and laterolateral views under fluoroscopic guidance) the electrode is introduced. Impedance values of 350–800 Ω suggest correct positioning of the needle. To confirm proximity to the medial branch, sensorial stimulation tests are done (50 Hz and 0.2–0.7 V) to reproduce the typical pain the patient would feel. Motor stimulation tests (2 Hz, 1 V) are also done to avoid motor lesions. Then, without moving the electrode needle, the nerve is ablated by heating to 90°C for 60 s. Thermoablation is then done on the medial branch of the contiguous level according to the neuroanatomy. In the case of two close

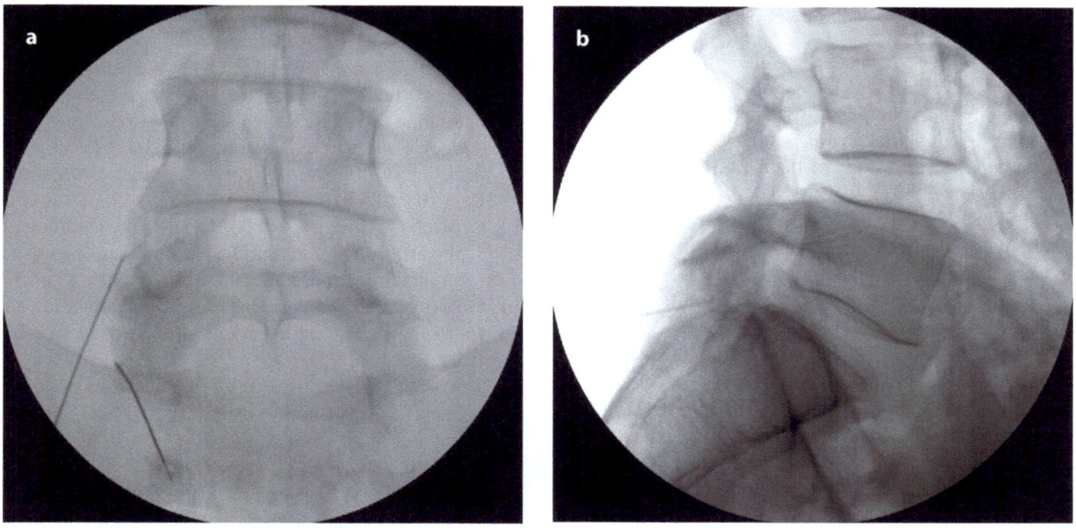

Fig. 7.5 Correct positioning of the electrode needle for the L5 nerve is on the ala of the sacrum, just lateral to the articular process, as showed in AP (**a**) and LL (**b**) view

joints, three levels must be treated. Some newer radiofrequency machines allow simultaneous ablation of four branches. After the procedure, patients are monitored for 2 h in hospital and then discharged.

7.7 Complications

Serious side effects after procedures on facet joints (intra-articular injections, diagnostic blocks, RFD) are extremely rare. Adverse effects to the metabolism and endocrine effects due to corticoteroid depots have not been investigated but are considered to be very rare. Nevertheless, suppression of the hypothalamic–pituitary–adrenal axis must be considered, as must impaired insulin sensitivity causing elevated glucose levels [11]. A possible complication of intra-articular injection is infection. Although very rare, septic arthritis, epidural abscess and meningitis have been reported after injections into facet joints [12, 13]. Anecdotal reports of spinal anesthesia and headache have also been published [14]. Among the possible side effects of RFD, we must consider numbness and/or dysesthesia (although they tend to be transient and self-limiting) [15]. Burning sensations are rare with radiofrequency procedures, and may result from electrical faults or equipment malfunction [16]. The commonest adverse reaction after RFD of facet joints is neuritis, and has a reported prevalence of <5% [17]. Administration of corticosteroid or pentoxifylline has been reported to reduce the occurrence of post-procedure pain [18].

7.8 Follow-up

Corticosteroid injection of the zygapophysial joints is, in general, successful and induces short-term pain relief. This is followed by a relapse of symptoms in an average of 50% of treated patients at 6-month follow-up. Post-procedure beneficial effects have been reported in 60–90% of patients, and long-term effects in 30–50% of treated patients. RFD in patients with a positive response to at least a nerve block test is, in general, followed by a prolonged therapeutic effect as pain relief and function improvement [19, 20]. Nevertheless, data are conflicting and less successful results have also been reported.

References

1. Pedersen HE, Blunck CF, Gardner E (1956) The anatomy of the lumbosacral posterior rami and meningeal branches of spinal nerves (sinuvertebral nerves) with an experimental study of their function. J Bone Joint Surg (Am) 38:377–391
2. Bogduk N (1997) Clinical anatomy of the lumbar spine and sacrum, 3rd edn. Churchill Livingstone, Edinburgh, p 127–144
3. Bogduk N, Wilson AS, Tynan W (1982) The human lumbar dorsal rami. J Anat 134:383–397
4. Bogduk N (1983) The innervation of the lumbar spine. Spine 8:286–293
5. Schwarzer AC, Aprill CN, Derby R, Fortin J, Kine G, Bogduk N (1994) Clinical features of patients with pain stemming from the lumbar zygapophysial joints: is the lumbar facet syndrome a clinical entity? Spine 19:1132–1327
6. Carrino JA (2007) Selective sacroiliac joint and facet joint injections. In: Schweitzer ME, Laredo JD (eds) New techniques in interventional musculoskeletal radiology. Informa Healthcare, London, p 133–149
7. Dreyfuss PH, Dreyer SJ, Herring SA (1995) Lumbar zygapophysial (facet) joint injections. Spine 20:2040–2047
8. Dreyer SJ, Dreyfuss PH (1996) Low back pain and the zygapophysial (facet) joints. Arch Phys Med Rehabil 17:290–300
9. Bogduk N (1997) International Spinal Injection Society guidelines for the per- formance of spinal injection procedures. Part I: zygapophysial joint blocks. Clin J Pain 13:285–302
10. Schwarzer AC, Aprill CN, Derby R, Fortin J, Kine G, Bogduk N (1994) The false-positive rate of uncontrolled diagnostic blocks of the lumbar zygapophysial joints. Pain 58:195–200
11. Ward A, Watson J, Wood P, Dunne C, Kerr D (2002) Glucocorticoid epidural for sciatica: metabolic and endocrine sequelae. Rheumatology 41:68–71
12. Alcock E, Regaard A, Browne J (2003) Facet joint injection: a rare form of epidural abscess formation. Pain 103:209–210
13. Orpen NM, Birch NC (2003) Delayed presentation of septic arthritis of a lumbar facet joint after diagnostic facet joint injection. J Spinal Disord Tech 16:285–287
14. Goldstone JC, Pennant JH (1987) Spinal anaesthesia following facet joint injection: a report of two cases. Anaesthesia 42:754–756
15. Tzaan WC, Tasker RR (2000) Percutaneous radiofrequency facet rhizotomy: experience with 118 procedures and reappraisal of its value. Can J Neurol Sci 27:125–130
16. Shealy CN (1975) Percutaneous radiofrequency denervation of spinal facets: treatment for chronic back pain and sciatica. J Neurosurg 43:448–451
17. Kornick C, Kramarich SS, Lamer TJ, Sitzman BT (2004) Complications of lumbar facet radiofrequency denervation. Spine 29:1352–1354
18. Dobrogowski J, Wrzosek A, Wordliczek J (2005) Radiofrequency denervation with or without addition of pentoxifylline or methylprednisolone for chronic lumbar zygapophysial joint pain. Pharmacol Rep 57:475–480
19. Marcia S, Masala S, Marini S et al (2012) Osteoarthritis of the zygapophysial joints: efficacy of percutaneous radiofrequency neurotomy in the treatment of lumbar facet joint syndrome Clin Exp Rheumatol 30:314
20. Masala S, Nano G, Mamuccari M et al (2012) Medial branch neurotomy in low back pain. Neuroradiology 54:737-44

Epidural and Sacral Spinal Injections

8

Massimo Gallucci and Federico D'Orazio

8.1 Epidural Injections

8.1.1 Anatomy of the Epidural Space

The epidural space is inside the spinal canal and surrounds the dura (which covers the neuraxis, dural sac and root spaces). The epidural space contains adipose tissue, nerve structures and blood vessels (especially veins). It is limited posteriorly by yellow ligaments and structures belonging to the posterior vertebral arches. Laterally, the epidural space opens and continues in the conjugation foramina. Thus, an intraforaminal injection also allows the intracanalar portion of the epidural space to be reached. Each foramen contains a nerve root surrounded by its root sheath and the radicular artery. In one or more levels can be found the radiculomedullary artery, which joins the anterior spinal artery. The epidural space ends at the sacral hiatus, between the coccyx and the posterior aspect of the sacrum.

M. Gallucci (✉)
Neuroradiology Department, San Salvatore Hospital, L'Aquila, Italy
e-mail: massimo.gallucci@cc.univaq.it

8.1.2 Application

An epidural corticosteroid injection can be used to obtain relief from radicular or spinal pain. Spinal pain might be caused by diskopathy, arthrosic degeneration of the spine (thereby causing compression of neural structures) or after unsuccessful spinal surgery for disk herniation (e.g., failed back surgery syndrome (FBSS)). Another application of epidural interventions is the treatment of liquoral hypotension using the "blood patch" method.

8.1.3 Indications and Contraindications to Treatment

Radiculopathy to one or multiple levels caused by diskopathy or degenerative stenosis of the spinal canal is an indication for epidural corticosteroid injections. They can also be useful for back pain secondary to spondylosis with or without significant associated radiculopathy. Precise clinical evaluation is essential; it has been shown that patients with referred axial pain not irradiating to a specific territory, myofascial pain, or neurogenic claudication and severe or worsening neurological deficits respond less well to treatment [1]. One must evaluate if pain might be (even partially) caused by a facet joint syndrome, sacro-iliac dysfunction or coxofemoral disease. A recent CT or MRI is recommended before treatment to exclude other diseases and to confirm the level(s) to treat.

M. Muto (ed.), *Interventional Neuroradiology of the Spine*,
DOI 10.1007/978-88-470-2790-9_8, © Springer-Verlag Italia 2013

Epidural injections can be performed with several technical approaches depending on clinical needs. The most commonly used type of access (especially in anesthesia) is interlaminar posterior access (which can also be carried out in a "blind" fashion). Epidural injections executed under guidance by fluoroscopy or CT are the safest and most precise method [1]. Intraforaminal injections are also used quite often. These must be accompanied by an instrumental guide. Also, selective treatment on a specific nerve root is possible, followed by diffusion of the injected drug into the epidural space. Periradicular injections can be for more selective treatments, and often have a diagnostic role. In fact, one can confirm or exclude if symptoms are caused by the blocked nerve root through an analgesic block. Much less used is the caudal injection. It is carried out to gain access to the sacral hiatus, but is poorly selective [1].

Contraindications include: uncorrectable coagulopathies; thrombocytopenia; use of anticoagulative therapies; local or systemic infections; and known allergies to the drugs to be administered. Furthermore, the corticosteroid injection must be avoided or undertaken with caution in patients with diabetes mellitus or uncontrolled glaucoma, and in the immunossuppressed. Specific pre-procedure preparations are not necessary, but antibiotic prophylaxis might be needed in case the disk is punctured accidentally during the epidural injection [2, 3].

8.1.4 Treatment Techniques

8.1.4.1 Approach to the Epidural Space

Interlaminar injections: The interlaminar approach is a simple and safe way of approaching the epidural space. The metameric level is used for treatment based on accurate clinical evaluation and symptoms [1, 2].

At the lumbar level, the injection can be under guidance by fluoroscopy or CT. Under fluoroscopic guidance, the access site in chosen on the median line in the frontal projection. After anesthesia of the cutaneous, subcutaneous and muscular planes, the needle is advanced to the supras-

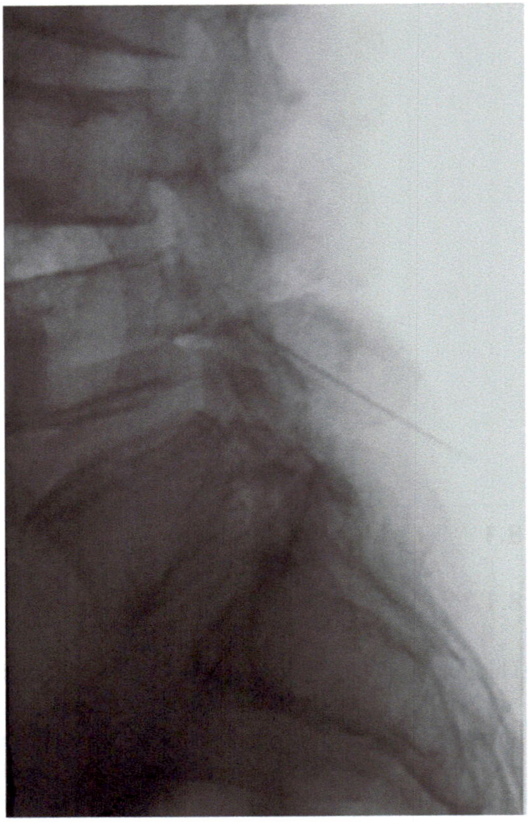

Fig. 8.1 A spinal needle is inserted obliquely through the interlaminar space of spinous process at the L4–L5 level under fluoroscopic guidance (lateral view)

pinous ligament (which is perceived by operator because of an increase in resistance). Once the interspinous ligament is reached, the mandrel is removed and the needle connected to a syringe containing physiological (0.9%) saline. The needle is advanced gently through the interpinous ligament, evaluating the magnitude of resistance felt during the advancement. In this phase, if the procedure is undertaken under fluoroscopic guidance, the C arm is positioned in the lateral view, to confirm the depth of the needle (Fig. 8.1). Immediately after passing through the yellow ligament, an appreciable loss of resistance is felt. At this time, the position of the needle tip must be verified, and must be extra-thecal and extravascular. Thus, in the case of aspiration, neither liquid nor blood should be in the syringe. After confirming this, a mixture of corticosteroids and local anesthetics (triamcinolone acetonide

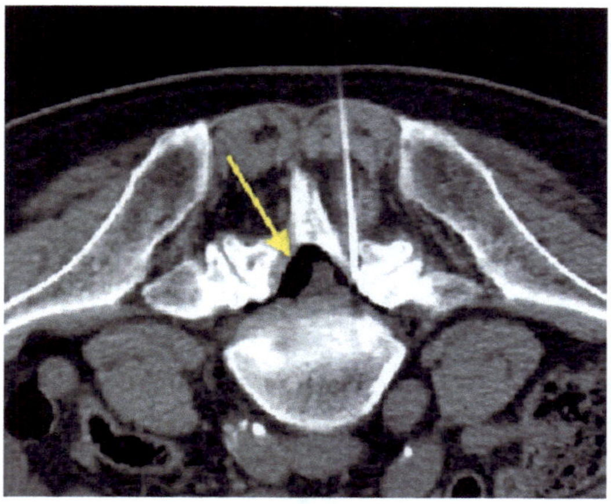

Fig. 8.2 CT showing a spinal needle being inserted through the interlaminar space. Diffusion of ozone inside the epidural space is also shown (*yellow arrow*)

40–80 mg; methylprednisolone acetate 40–80 mg; dexamethasone 4–8 mg; bethamethasone 6–12 mg) diluted with local anesthetic (2–3 mL of ropivacaine 2%) or physiological saline can be injected. The volume injected should be ≤15 mL. The injection is delivered in a similar way under CT guidance. Before injecting drugs, air or ozone can be injected to demonstrate its diffusion in the epidural space [1] (Fig. 8.2).

For interventions at the thoracic level, keeping the needle at a more cranio-caudal tilt is necessary because of the different orientation of the spinous processes [1]. At the cervical level, the procedure is more difficult and involves more risks. Thus, it should be carried out by expert operators in carefully selected patients. The procedure under fluoroscopic guidance is similar to the one described above for lumbar injections except that there are minor differences in terms of the resistance felt by operator when passing through the interpinous ligaments. This is why injection of contrast medium must be carried out before drug administration into the epidural space. The total volume of drugs injected must be ≤4–8 mL, and the injection must be interrupted immediately in case of pain or other disorders [1].

Transforaminal injections: When transforaminal injections are performed under fluoroscopic guidance (Fig. 8.3), the patient is in the prone position and the C arm is placed in the lateral oblique projection so that the "target foramen" is displayed optimally. The needle is into the oblique position so as to follow the same angle of the C arm. One must try to introduce the needle in the posterosuperior aspect of the foramen to obtain better diffusion of injected drugs at periradicular and epidural levels, as well as to reduce the risk of radicular puncture. If the injection is under CT guidance, paravertebral access is used with the patient in the prone position. In this case, the nerve root is displayed clearly. Also, it is eas-

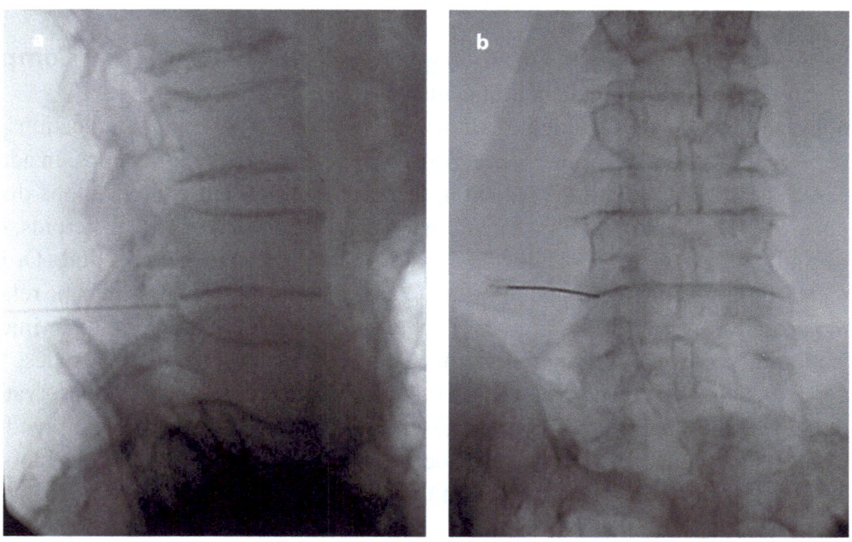

Fig. 8.3 A spinal needle is inserted across the intervertebral foramen to the space between L4 and L5 under fluoroscopic guidance: lateral view (**a**) and anteroposterior view (**b**)

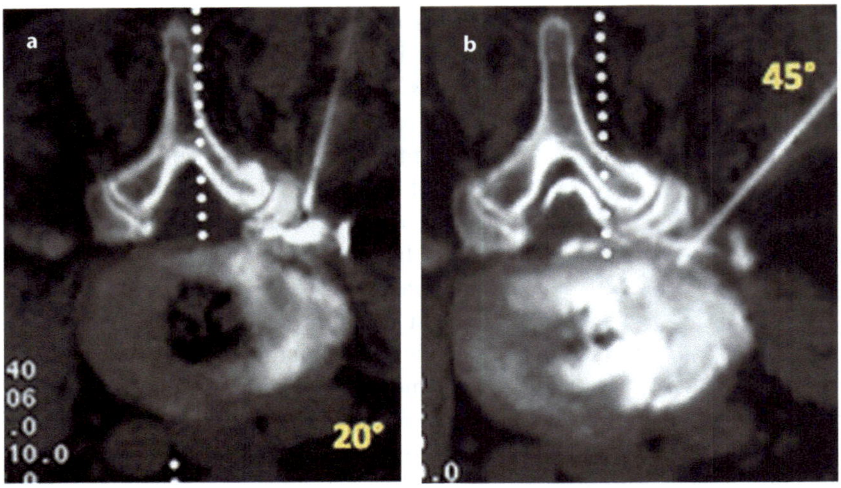

Fig. 8.4 CT showing a spinal needle being inserted at 20° inclination, and the injection is limited to the perigangliar region (**a**). When the angle is increased to 45°, the contrast medium is spread in the peridural space; an amount of contrast enters the intervertebral disk (**b**)

ier to avoid accidental puncture of the nerve root (which is recognizable because of typical radicular pain) [1–3].

Periradicular injections: Lumbar periradicular injections are quite similar to their intraforaminal counterparts, and are often mistakenly confused. Under fluoroscopic guidance in the oblique projection, the needle is directed towards a point 2-mm cranially and 2-mm medially to the inferior-lateral angle of the vertebral body. In this way, drugs tend to be distributed around the nerve root outside the conjugation foramen without entering the epidural space. Usually, a volume of 3–4 mL of anethetics with 1–1.5 mL of corticosteroids is sufficient for each treated level [1, 2] (Fig. 8.4).

At the cervical level, distinguishing between intraforaminal and periradicular injections is less relevant because they coincide. Under fluoroscopy with an oblique projection at 45–50°, access is anterolateral with the patient in the prone position. The neurovascular bundle is spread medially by the operator. Thus, the needle is directed following the obliquation of the C arm to the posterior aspect of the foramen. Frontal projection images may be acquired to check needle depth, which is advanced until the lateral cortical margin of the lateral mass of the chosen layer. Contrast medium (0.5–1 mL) must be injected before drug injection to exclude an intradural or intravascular position of the needle [1].

Caudal injections: Caudal access is a particularly safe type of access to the epidural space. It is found at the level of the sacral hiatus, the upper margin of which is shaped like an inverted "U" when observed in the frontal projection (Fig. 8.5) The needle is inserted at a cranio-caudal angle of 45°. The needle passes through strong resistance produced by the sacro-coccygeal ligament; this resistance disappears when the epidural space is entered. The needel angle is then reduced, and it is advanced for 1 cm. After that, 10–20 mL of a mixture of anesthetics and corticosteroids is injected. This considerable volume is necessary for the mixture to spread widely spread along the sacral and lumbar nerve roots [1].

8.1.5 Potential Complications

Rarely, epidural injections can be the cause of severe complications. In addition to allergic reactions and complications due to the systemic absorption of corticosteroids, there are specific risks linked to the procedure. Orthostatic headache due to dural puncture can be relatively frequent (especially after interlaminar injections) but, given the small size of the needles, it is usually transient or resolved with conservative treatments [1]. If epidural hypotension syndrome persists, placement of an autologous blood patch at the leakage site can be an option. If the intradural position of the needle is not recognized, intrathecal injection

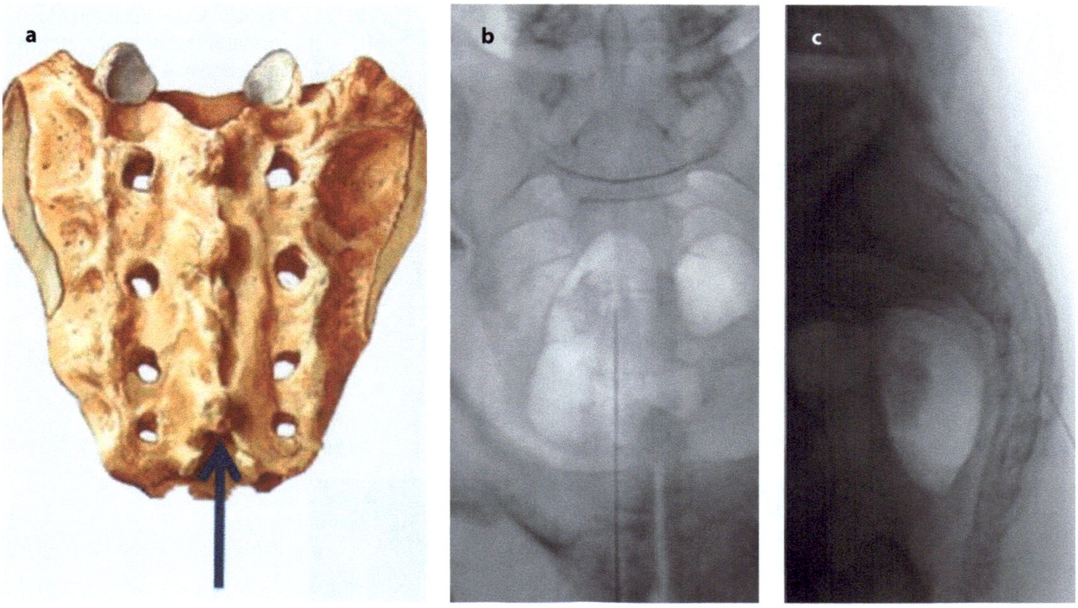

Fig. 8.5 Caudal injection. Sacral hiatus (arrow) (**a**). A spinal needle is inserted at the level of the sacral hiatus under fluoroscopic guidance (anteroposterior view) (**b**). The inclination and depth of the needle is checked during navigation of the needle in the lateral view (**c**)

of corticosteroids and anesthetics may lead to severe complications. Intrathecal injection of corticosteroids does not usually cause damage (even though there have been reports of arachnoiditis after injection of methylprednisolone, which is probably related to the preservatives in the preparation [4]). Intrathecal injection of anesthetics at lumbar or thoracic levels can cause a significant but transient sensory or motor block. At cervical or upper-thoracic levels, uncontrolled injection of anesthetics can cause a complete spinal block (which can lead to respiratory arrest) whereas a sympathetic block can cause severe hypotension. These complications are more frequent after interlaminar rather than transforaminal injections but, even in the latter case, intradural injection can cause direct puncture of the root sheaths [1]. Intramedullary drug injection is very rare. In almost all cases it leads to toxic and ischemic damage to the spinal cord, resulting in severe neurological deficits [1]. Spinal-cord ischemias caused by injection into a radiculomedullary artery are severe complications of epidural injections, and are more likely after transforaminal injections. At the cervical level, injection into the vertebral artery is possible but carries the risk of ischemia in the vertebrobasilar territories of the brain. To avoid these potential complications (which are essentially due to the intra-arterial injection of corticosteroids), injection of a a contrast agent before injection of the drug has been found to be a safe procedure to control the needle position [1]. Nevertheless, corticosteroids with a tendency to form particulates pose a risk and should be avoided in transforaminal injections, and corticosteroids that do not form particulates shoudl be employed [4]. Epidural abscess, meningitis, arachnoiditis, and epidural hematoma are very rare complications but have been described. They can be restricted to minimum with a meticulous technique (Fig. 8.6).

8.1.6 Follow-up

Patients must be followed up to obtain good results and to evaluate if further treatments (even if they are of different types) are needed. If infiltrations are effective, patients typically have significant clinical improvement during the subsequent

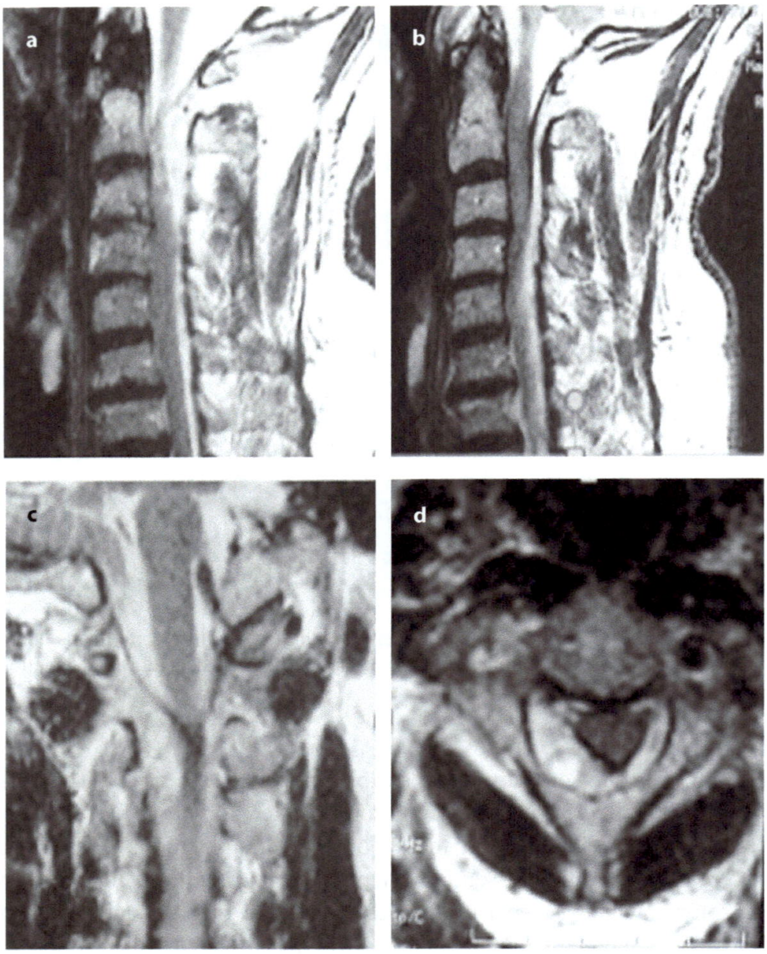

Fig. 8.6 A complication of a peridural injection undertaken at the cervical level without radiological guidance: cervical epidural hematoma (**a**, **b** and **c**). The right vertebral artery is not recognizable; it is dissected and obstructed because of the trauma which presumably caused the hematoma (**d**)

1–3 months. After this period the treatment can be repeated if rehabilitation does not provide sufficient benefit. More than three infiltrations in 6 months should not be repeated because of the relatively high corticosteroid dose employed [1].

8.1.7 Blood Patches

Cerebrospinal fluid (CSF) hypovolemia may result from dural puncture, surgery, trauma, or can be spontaneous. In the case of spontaneous leakage, several mechanisms have been recognized. These include: structural weakness of the dura; collagenopathies (Marfan syndrome, Ehlers–Danlos syndrome); dural dysplasia (neurofibromatosis type 1); as well as periradicular and peridural arachnoid cysts. In general, CSF hypovolemia more commonly affects females aged 40–50 years [1]. When loss of CSF exceeds CSF production, the resultant low CSF pressure may result in traction on the dura, epidural veins, and cranial nerves. Postural headache, nausea and cervicalgia are common presenting symptoms. However, sagging of the brain can lead to more serious complications owing to potential compression of the diencephalon or ischemic traction on the cranial nerves, resulting in permanent neurological deficits. Coma and even death due to spontaneous intracranial hypotension have been reported [5]. In almost 60% of patients, CSF hypovolemia resolves spontaneously. This is because CSF production is a continuous process and because CSF equilibrium may be restored with spontaneous sealing of a dural leak without intervention [6]. However, conservative and in-

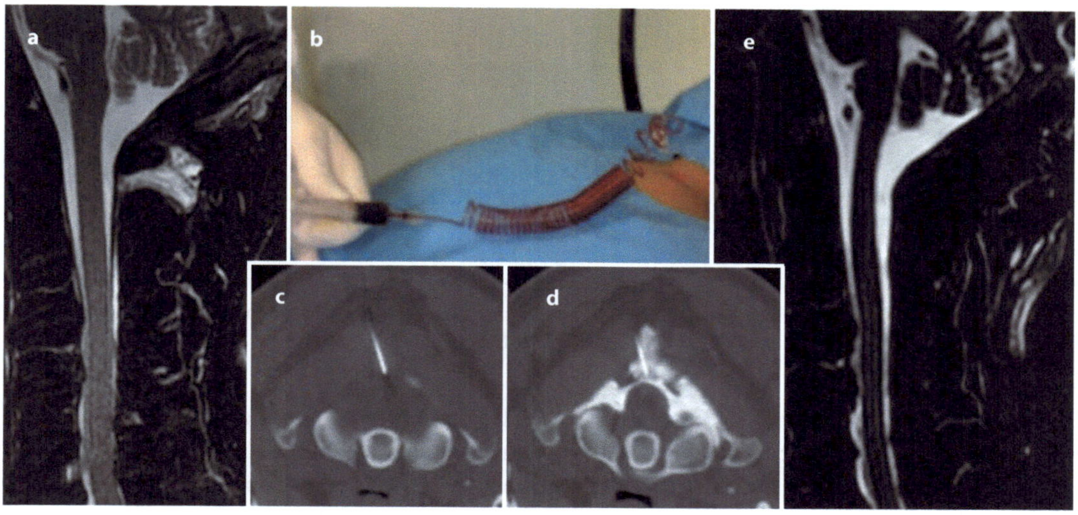

Fig. 8.7 Autologus dural blood patch in a patient with dural fistula at the C1–C2 level. MRI (sagittal plane), T2-weighted fat saturated turbo spin echo: evidence of leakage of cerebrospinal fluid in the posterior wall (**a**). Injection of unclotted blood (**b**). Needle placement under CT control (**c**). CT showing the injection of 10 cm^3 of autologus blood with 1 cm^3 of contrast medium (**d**). MRI (sagittal plane), T2-weighted fat saturated turbo spin echo: control showing complete resolution of the fistula (**e**)

terventional therapies are available for the treatment of symptomatic patients.

The procedure for an epidural blood patch (EBP) is exactly the same as that described for epidural corticosteroid injections, except that autologous unclotted blood is injected. The EBP has been shown to be successful in approximately 75% of cases [7]. The patient's blood (7–20 mL) and 1/10 dilution of myelographic contrast agent with 5,000 IU of sodium heparin should be sufficient for the patch [1]. MRI can be useful to demonstrate the site of CSF leakage (especially if an intervention was not carried out recently). A T2 fat-suppression sequence can be useful to identify the level to treat (Fig. 8.7), and if one is trying to treat CSF leakage in a "non-targeted" fashion (i.e., injecting at the cervico-thoracic passage). This can be equally effective for treating the leakage because of the CSF circulation in the epidural space [1].

When carrying out at EBP, a spinal needle is advanced to the level of the documented CSF leakage towards the epidural space. The loss-of-resistance technique or a syringe containing contrast medium are used for epidurography before injecting blood to document correct placement of the needle. Unclotted blood can then be injected slowly through the needle. A prone position should be maintained immediately for ≥2 h; bed rest for ≥24 h is essential. Image-guidance methods are very important in this intervention. Studies have shown that if the procedure is done "blind", the epidural space cannot be identified in 25% of cases [8].

8.2 Sacral Injections

8.2.1 Painful Sacro-iliac Dysfunction

Low back pain can affect 80–90% of the general population during their lifetime. In ≤47% of cases it can be attributed to painful sacro-iliac dysfunction. If pain is suspected to originate from the sacro-iliac joints (SIJs), several passive joint-mobilization tests (distraction, thigh thrust, Gaenslen, compression, sacral thrust) are available [9]. To understand the concept of sacro-iliac dysfunction one must comprehend the concepts of "form closure" and "force closure", which were expressed first by Snijders, Vleeming and Stoeckhart [10, 11].

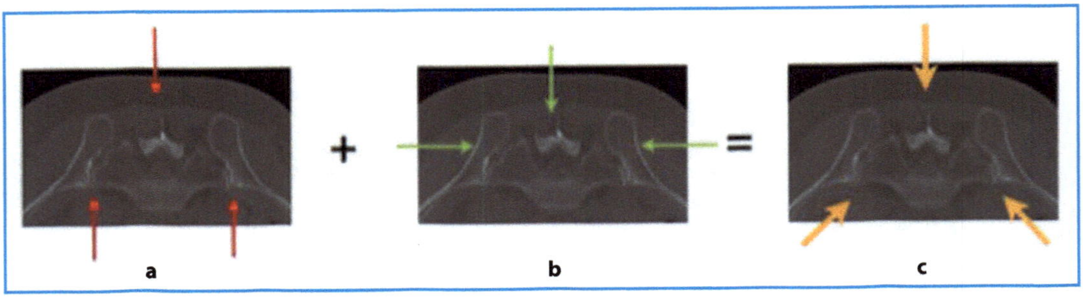

Fig. 8.8 Mechanisms of sacro-iliac joint stabilization; arrows show force lines which are involved in (**a**) form closure, (**b**) force closure, and (**c**) in stabilization produced by the set of form and force closure

Form closure involves stabilizing the joint. This is realized at the sacro-iliac level due to the friction present between the articular surfaces. This is obtained by the effect of:

- perfect complementarity between the ridges (sacral slope) and trenches (pelvic side) facing each other on the articular surface;
- different composition of the opposing surfaces (articular cartilage on the sacral side and fibrocartilage on the iliac);
- almost perfectly vertical spatial orientation of the articular surfaces;
- action of intrinsic and extrinsic ligaments.

Force closure contributes to dynamic stabilization of the joint creating, at this level, an additional force of closure of the articular chain of the pelvis. Three systems participate: (i) passive (capsule, ligaments); (ii) active (stabilizing muscles); and (iii) control (purely neurological) [9]. Figure 8.8 summarizes the concepts of form closure and force closure (panel *a* and *b*, respectively), and provides an overview of the effects of their interaction at the sacro-iliac level.

There are three major frameworks of SIJ dysfunction. They have several etiologies with similar results for each category of dysfunction on joint biomechanics as well as different clinical manifestations. It is possible to distinguish three types of dysfunction, as described below.

Postural dysfunction is due to an alteration in the length or pattern of muscle activation. An example of this type of pathogenetic mechanism is the postural dysfunction of the SIJ observed in cases of disproportion of the lower limbs.

Hypomobility dysfunction arises as a result of microtrauma as well as degenerative or inflammatory processes that cause the stiffness or malpositioning of joints.

Instability dysfunction derives from impairment of one or more elements contributing to determine the form and/or force closure. There is impairment of form closure in the case of the altered morphology of the articular surfaces (sacral, iliac) or the level of the facet joints of the last lumbar vertebrae. Force closure may be compromized by insufficient stabilizing ligaments or ineffective activation of lumbar/pelvic muscles. Moreover, the instability can be defined as "anatomical" (for loss of containment of passive joint-stabilization subsystems in postoperative or fracture outcomes) or "clinical" (for loss of function of neuromuscular stabilization subsystems) [9].

Hendrix (1979) was the first to describe a standardized procedure of intra-articular injection of the SIJs under fluoroscopic guidance. Until then, the origin of back pain was almost invariably attributed to lumbar diskopathy or disease in the facet joints. Recent studies [12] have attributed low back pain to the SIJs in 15–47% of cases. Pain can manifest with a spectrum of intensity and clinical signs that are extremely variable. Rarely, there are associated neurological signs such as paresthesia/dysesthesia, except in cases where contracture of the piriformis muscle (in which the sciatic nerve runs) coexists. Thus, the sacro-iliac origin of bilateral and symmetrical pain is a valid generic distinction which is based on joint overload. The cause of unilateral pain is

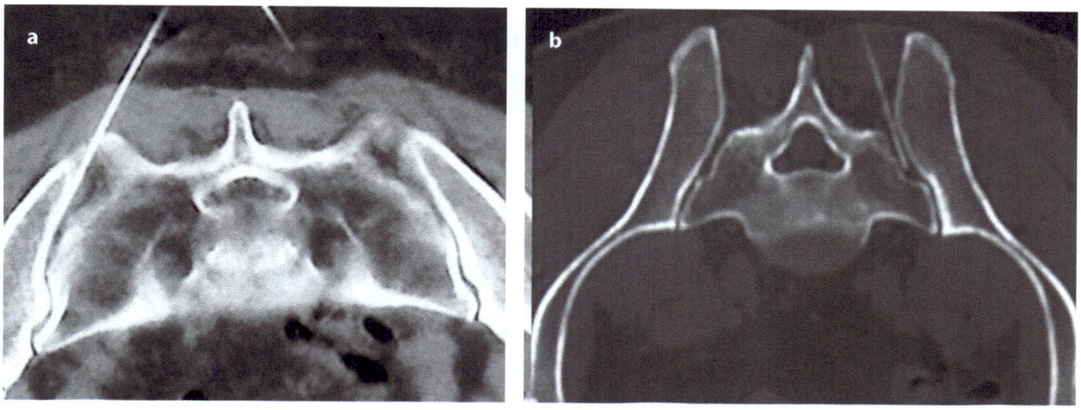

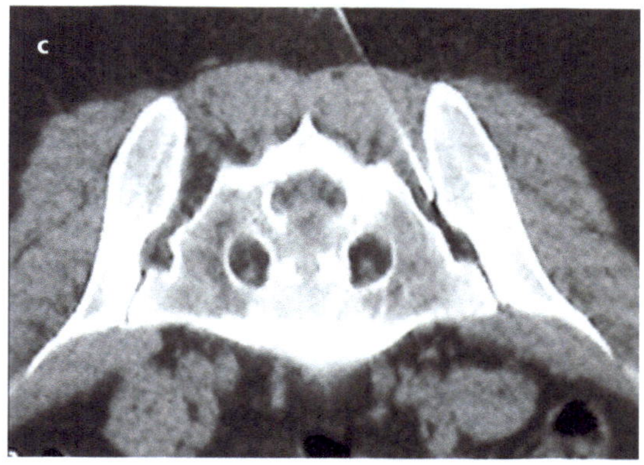

Fig. 8.9 Usefulness of CT guidance when undertaking sacro-iliac injections. The complex anatomy of a sacroiliac joint; nevertheless, the needle is placed correctly within the articular space (**a**). Changing the width and level of the window can simultaneously allow positioning of the needle with respect to bone (**b**) and soft tissues (**c**)

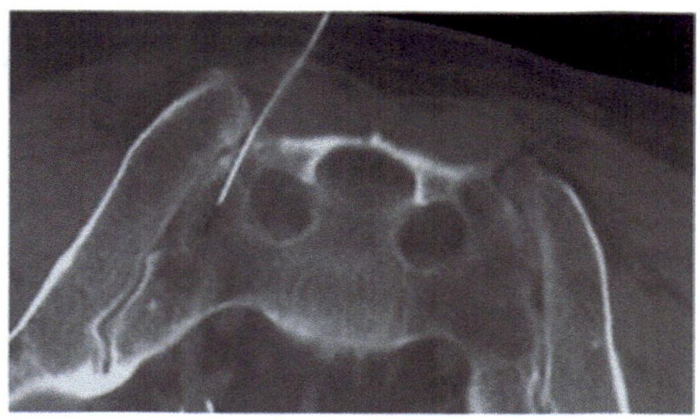

Fig. 8.10 Incorrect placement of a spinal needle as demonstrated by CT in a case in which infiltration was attempted initially without CT guidance

based on post-traumatic arthritis [9]. There are several possible sites of the expression of pain: posterior superior iliac spine; low/high lumbar region; buttocks; groin; medial/front/side/back of thigh; anterior, posterior and lateral leg; or the lower abdomen. The difficulty of obtaining a differential diagnosis between painful sciatica and SIJ dysfunction by clinical evaluation is therefore understandable. However, using the tests of passive joint mobilization described above will aid the differential diagnosis [9].

8.2.2 Sacro-iliac Interventional Therapies

8.2.2.1 Intra-articular Infiltration

Over the years, joint puncture has been carried out using three methods: blind, under fluoroscopic guidance, or under CT guidance [13]. The effectiveness and convenience of conducting blind infiltration of joints has been questioned. In certain cases, the success rate in reducing perceived symptoms (especially when compared with pla-

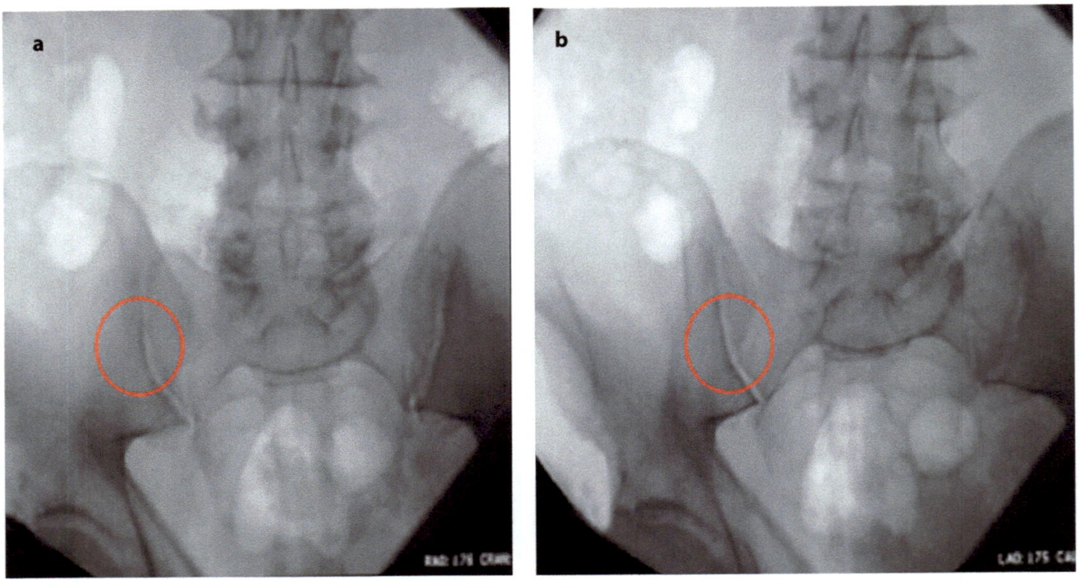

Fig. 8.11 Correct positioning of the C arm to execute a sacro-iliac injection: anteroposterior view (**a**) and oblique anteroposterior view (**b**). After minimal obliquation of the C arm, the two surfaces can be distinguished clearly

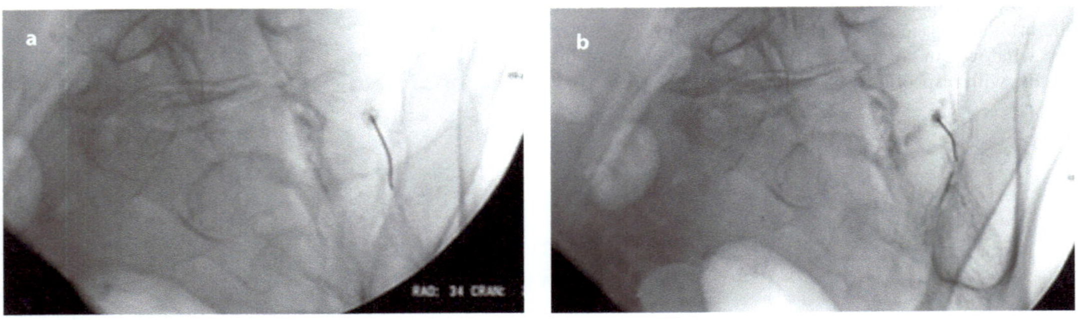

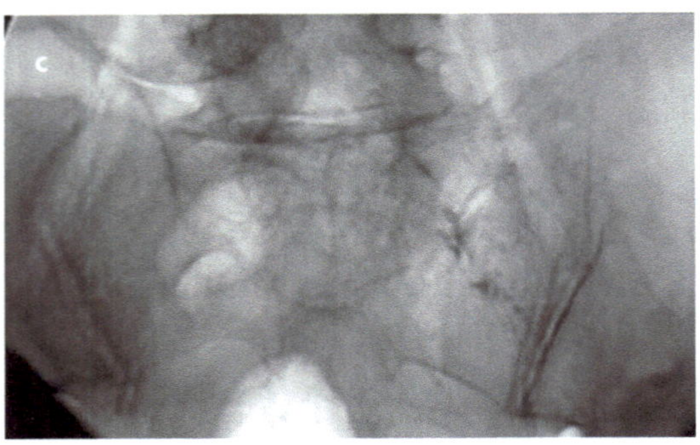

Fig. 8.12 Sacro-iliac injection carried out under CT guidance using an injection of contrast media to demonstrate correct positioning of the needle within the articular space. The needle is first inserted towards the articular space (**a**). A minimum amount of contrast medium in injected through the needle (**b**). Opacification of the articular surfaces demonstrates access to the articular space (**c**)

cebo treatment) was ≤25% of treated patients [14]. Furthermore, it has been estimated that blind infiltration of joints can be used to access the joint cavity in only 22% of cases [14]. This success rate is too low to enable this puncture method to be considered to be an affordable alternative to CT guidance (an established method with success rates close to 100%). We believe

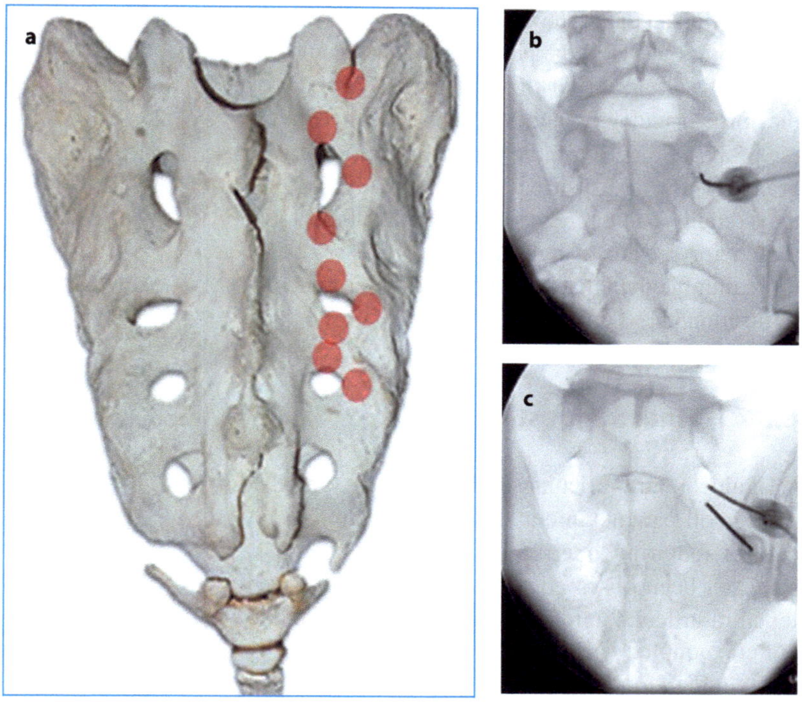

Fig. 8.13 Summary of all the possible sites of needle placement to undertake radiofrequency denervation of the sacro-iliac joint (**a**). A radiofrequency needle is placed at the level of the foramen between S1 and S2 under fluoroscopic guidance (**b**). A second needle is placed in the same patient (**c**)

that the most reliable way to execute infiltration of the SIJs is under CT guidance. In our practice, we have been able to reach the joint space quickly and without risks to patients [1, 15] (Figs. 8.9–8.12).

When injecting into the SIJs, the patient must be in a prone position with a pillow placed under his/her pelvis. A short CT scan is obtained with a low-dose protocol to choose the best entry point for each joint (in case of bilateral treatment). Then, a landmark line can be drawn on the skin to locate the access choosen before undertaking a wide sterile preparation of the soft tissues over the sacrum and buttocks. The overlying soft tissues and skin are infiltrated with local anesthetics, before placing a 22-G spinal needle over the drawn line. Then, navigation of the needle tip towards the joint space can be followed step-by-step by acquiring low-dose, single-slice CT acquisitions each time the operator wants to check its position. Once the joint space is reached, 1 cm^3 of 2% mepivacaine with 1 cm^3 of triamcinolone acetonide (40 mg/mL), followed by about 3 cm^3 of a O_2-O_3 mixture (28 μg/mL), can be injected.

8.2.2.2 Radiofrequency Denervation

Innervation of the SIJs has a high degree of heterogeneity in the population, with many anatomical variants, several of which are considered controversial among clinicians. There is general agreement in attributing multiple innervation to this articulation. For the anterior joint region, the posterior branches of roots are included in the section L1–S2, with possible addition of the secondary sector from the obturator nerve, the gluteal nerve from the top, and from the lumbosacral trunk. For the posterior joint region, the posterior branches of the roots are contained within the tract L4–S3 [9].

A method of denervation through the use of probes capable of emitting a radiofrequency produced by an external transducer enables the insertion of needles that can reach suitable anatomical landmarks for the nerves responsible for articular innervation. By generating local temperatures of around 90°C, a lesion in the branches mentioned above is produced, with consequent denervation of the concerned anatomical part [1] (Fig. 8.13). The main limitation of the method is the anatomical data. The course of the nerves distributed in the SIJ in the population is not homogeneous, and not all of the branches (especially the intra-articular branches) can be reached by the probes. Sometimes, the joint is innervated by branches that are distributed sporadically. This may require re-treatment of the same patient to search for greater analgesia, which tends to be more durable than that observed in intra-articular infiltration [1].

8.3 Final Suggestions

CT-guided intra-articular infiltrations are practised in all patients in our surgical unit. Complications requiring interruption of the procedure have not been observed. The limited benefit after intra-articular infiltration reported in the literature, coupled with the limited effectiveness of re-treatment reported by respondents, suggests that the infiltration should not be repeated if the patient perceives exacerbation of the disease. The use of neurotomy by means of radiofrequencies should be evaluated because of its longer duration of effect. Therefore, the value of CT-guided infiltration of anti-inflammatory drugs and local anesthetics is to identify the origin of the pain that is supposedly arising from the SIJ and to achieve almost immediate benefit to the patient (which could be lower doses of drugs taken by the systemic route). Although this benefit has been demonstrated to be reduced over time, the procedure does not expose patients to the significant risk of major complications. It can therefore be repeated if there is a recurrence of symptoms and alternative strategies are not available. In contrast, radiofrequency neurotomy appears justified only after a positive response to intra-articular infiltration with anesthetics, corticosteroids and ozone. This may allow relief of longer duration, and may be a definitive solution to pain of sacro-iliac origin.

References

1. Gallucci M, Limbucci N, Marcia S, Ricci A (2011) Interventistica articolare del rachide in Caudana. In: Masciocchi G (ed) Radiologia Interventstica Musco-lo-scheletrica. Elsevier-Masson, Milano, p 180–208
2. Johnson BA (2004) Epidural steroid injections and selective nerve blocks. In: Matis JM (ed) Image-guided spine interventions. Springer-Verlag, Heidelberg, p 149–170
3. Delmer O, Dousset V (2006) Foraminal injections of corticosteroids under tomodensitometric control. In: Kastler B (ed) Interventional radiology in pain treatment. Springer-Verlag, Heidelberg, p 49–55
4. Abram SE, O'Connor TC (1996) Complications associated with epidural stroid injections. Reg Anesth 21:149–162
5. Watanabe L (2004) Epidural blood and fibrin patches. In: Matis JM (ed) Image-guided spine interventions. Springer-Verlag, Heidelberg, p 322–333
6. Chung SJ, Kim JS, Lee MC (2000) Syndrome of cerebral spinal fluid hypovolemia: clinical and imaging features and outcome. Neurology 55:1321–1327
7. Safa-Tisseront V, Thormann F, Malassiné P, Henry M, Riou B, Seebacher J (2001) Effectiveness of epidural blood patch in the management of post dural puncture headache. Anesthesiology 95:334–339
8. White AH, Derby R, Wynne G (1980) Epidural injections for the diagnosis and treatment of low back pain. Spine 5:78–86
9. Vanti C, Ferrari S, Ramponi S (2004) Valutazione clinico funzionale. In: Vanti C, Ferrari S, Ramponi S. L'articolazione sacroiliaca. Fisiopatologia, clinica e trattatmento. Masson, Milano, pp. 84-93
10. Vleeming A, Stoeckart R, Volkers AC, Snijders CJ (1990) Relation between form and function in the sacroiliac joint. Part I: clinical anatomical aspects. Spine 15:130–132
11. Vleeming A, Stoeckart R, Volkers AC, Snijders CJ (1990) Relation between form and function in the sacroiliac joint. Part II: biomechanical aspects. Spine 15:133–136
12. Slipman CW, Whyte II WS, Chow DW, Chou L, Lenrow D, Ellen M (2001) Sacroiliac joint syndrome. Pain Physician 4:143–152
13. Rosenberg JM, Quint TJ, de Rosayro AM (2000) Computerized tomographic localization of clinically-guided sacroiliac joint injections. Clin J Pain 16:18–21
14. Laslett M (2008) Evidence-based diagnosis and treatment of the painful sacroiliac joint. J Man Manip Ther 16:142–152
15. Stallmeyer MJB, Zoarski GH (2004) Sacroiliac joint injections. In: Matis JM (ed) Image-guided spine interventions. Springer-Verlag, Heidelberg, p 234–244

Vertebroplasty in Porotic Fractures

9

Mario Muto, Gianluigi Guarnieri, Roberto Izzo
and Alvaro Antonio Diano

9.1 Introduction

Vertebral augmentation methods are minimally invasive and aim to reduce spinal pain in patients with porotic fractures. This is achieved thanks to endovertebral injection of cement that elicits a metameric stabilization effect. Vertebroplasty (VP) and kyphoplasty (KP) are image-guided, percutaneous minimally invasive therapies employed to reduce spinal pain. Each method has a different approach. VP involves metameric injection of cement (polymethylmethacrylate, PMMA) through a needle. KP involves inflation of a small balloon in the vertebral body (VB) to create a void within cancellous bone before the delivery of cement.

The first VP was carried out by Galimbert and Deramond in 1987. These authors treated patients with vertebral hemangioma at the C2 level. The first KP was undertaken in the USA in 1998 in a porotic patient [1–3]. Many patients have been treated worldwide by neuroradiologists, radiologists, orthopedic surgeons, neurosurgeons, anesthesiologists, pain therapists, and rheumatologists using this method. When VP was first employed, the indications adopted by different specialists were not always identical (e.g., type of image guidance). These disparities influenced the results of the treatment and the prevalence of complications between centers.

Osteoporosis is the most accepted indication of VP. Osteoporosis can be related to long-term corticosteroid therapy or be a side effect of therapies for epilepsy, gastrointestinal (GI) disorders and renal dysfunction. The rationale of treatment in osteoporotic fractures is to combine the analgesic and vertebral stabilization effect of VP with or without restoration of the physiological height of the collapsed VB. This strategy can be used to reduce deformity of the VB with resulting normal vertebral biomechanics. Hence, long-term complications in patients with spinal pain can be avoided. Such complications (e.g., cardiorespiratory dysfunction, GI insufficiency, renal insufficiency, psychological problems) can increase the prevalence of mortality by ≤20% [4–6].

In 2009, two randomized clinical trials on porotic vertebral fracture versus sham procedures were published. These studies stimulated discussion, criticism and doubts about the clinical results of VP [7, 8]. However, other randomized controlled clinical trials confirmed the efficacy and safety of balloon KP but also of VP versus medical therapy [9].

The origin of pain in patients with vertebral collapse or fracture (benign or malignant) is related primarily to the stretching of periosteal fibers due to microfractures. However, it can also be due to direct compression of nervous structures with transmission of pain to the paravertebral

M. Muto (✉)
Neuroradiology Department, A. Cardarelli Hospital,
Naples, Italy
e-mail: mutomar2@gmail.com

M. Muto (ed.), *Interventional Neuroradiology of the Spine*,
DOI 10.1007/978-88-470-2790-9_9, © Springer-Verlag Italia 2013

nervous plexus through nerve ganglia and the spinothalamic tract to the parietal cortex (the concept of only one cortical area being responsible for pain is changing with the concept of the "pain matrix") [10–11].

VP is a major indication in porotic patients with spinal pain refractory to conservative medical and physical treatment. That is, if patients are suffering pain with analgesic therapy, they cannot undertake physical therapy, and medical therapy can create side effects such as confusion, excessive sedation and constipation [12–16].

9.2 Mechanism of Action of VP

The mechanism of action of VP in porotic patients is based on the principle that injection of cement (PMMA or another type) within the collapsed soma stabilizes the movements of the trabecular and cortical microfractures that are responsible for the pain. This action is related primarily to the stretching of nerve fibers along the cortical bone. PMMA injection compacts and stabilizes the VB, with a consequent antalgic effect. However, the cement injected into the VB, even though it stabilizes the collapsed soma and elicits an antalgic effect, contributes to biomechanical alterations in the vertebral column:

- restoration of spinal alignment;
- cement injected into the VB has different influences on spinal stiffness based on different properties and features of the cement;
- different distribution of axial loads;
- VP modifies the stiffness and failure strength of functional spinal units (SUs), which could increase the re-fracture rate to adjacent or distant metamers.

9.2.1 Biomechanics

In VP, the cement is injected so that it interdigitates throughout the fractured VB from endplate to endplate. In this way, the loads are transferred from the superior vertebral endplate to the interdigitated cement column and then to the inferior endplate. The weaker cancellous bone is not loaded in series as it is in KP. Kim et al., in an experimental test undertaken to understand differences in the biomechanical behavior of the resultant constructs, did not detect a significant loss of height in VP-treated specimens during repetitive loading [17].

Several biomechanical studies, undertaken on cadaveric spine, have demonstrated that VP with PMMA increases the load on adjacent VBs after surgery, and authors have detailed the possibility of fracture formation because of the rigidity elicited by PMMA [18–19]. According to some authors, in the post-VP spine, there could be an increased prevalence of failure in the adjacent VB to the one that has been augmented; in such studies, the prevalence of failure has been extremely variable [20–22]. This effect also contributes to an increased prevalence of fracture that seems to be due to altered load distributions in which a "pillar of cement" causes an increase in pressure within the nucleus pulposus and an exaggerated deflection of the endplate in the adjacent VB. This phenomenon could also explain the increased risk of new fractures in case of disk leakage (especially if it has a spike shape) [23].

Different cements influence the stiffness and strength of functional SUs to different degrees, resulting in a varying prevalence of re-fracture. All cements are tested to verify resistance to axial and torsional loads, and this capacity is measured in megapascals (MPa). For example, PMMA cement produces a modification of compressive strength of 100 MPa, whereas calcium phosphate cement (CPC) produces one of 80 MPa [26]. Hence, the prevalence of fracture of the adjacent VB after VP using CPC should be lower than that after VP using PMMA. Conversely, the restored strength of VBs augmented with PMMA is significantly higher. VBs augmented with CPC are markedly less stiff than in their original condition, and their strength is not significantly different from their original strength. CPC may be superior to PMMA as a bone-filler material because, although vertebrae augmented with CPC are subject to collapse, they are replaced gradually by new bone and subsequently obtain adequate compressive strength and stiffness. This leads to bone union with a lower risk of inducing new fracture of adjacent VBs than that seen with PMMA.

Using a low-modulus PMMA cement causes less alteration in the stiffness of the augmented vertebrae compared with standard PMMA cement. Numerous studies have explored the biomechanical effect of cement volume on vertebral mechanics. Excessive cement filling is associated with an increased prevalence of complications (e.g., cement embolus, cement leakage), probably due to the high pressures generated within the VB during augmentation. By injecting a conventional bone cement of high elastic modulus into fractured vertebrae, a greater proportion of the load is transferred through the central augmented trabeculae structure than would occur naturally. Abnormal transfer of load arising from the stiffening effect of the cement within the augmented VB causes an accelerated rate of failure of the adjacent vertebrae to an extent that seriously undermines this potentially very effective and easy intervention. Finite element models have suggested a mechanism of failure of adjacent vertebrae. In such models, the cement in the augmented vertebra acts as a "pillar" that prevents endplates from sinking into the VB, thereby increasing pressure in the adjacent nucleus pulposus and subsequently the adjacent vertebrae [23]. Wang et al. undertook a study on 9 fresh, four-level osteoporotic thoracic motion segments from 6 human spinal columns to understand the mechanism of fractures of adjacent and augmented vertebrae after VP by axial loading. In the PMMA-injected vertebral specimens, three steps of fatigue loading (5 Hz for 5 h) were applied incrementally and vertically from 650 N to 950 N to 1,150 N. Specimens of intact, compressively fractured, cement-augmented and post-fatigued loading were imaged by radiography for measurement of deformations of the vertebrae, the canal, and foramen. At the end of fatigue loading, vertebrae were sliced for micro-morphologic analyses. The greatest loss of height after fatigue loading was at the posterior region of the augmented vertebrae. In the augmented vertebrae, fissures were found along the bone–cement interface. These fissures split the cement and the trabeculae, and propagated into the vertebrae and endplates. The compactness ratio of the trabeculae region of the adjacent cranial vertebrae was higher than that for intact and adjacent caudal vertebrae. The authors attributed the fracture of the augmented vertebrae after VP to the initiation of fissures along the cement–bone interface, which, in turn, may be due to uneven deformation of the vertebrae, whereas fracture of the adjacent cranial vertebrae was attributed to collapse of their trabeculae [24].

9.3 General Considerations Regarding VP

The main indications for VP are: spinal pain affected by porotic fractures (Fig. 9.1); metastatic vertebral fractures; vertebral location of multiple myeloma; and a painful or aggressive vertebral hemangioma. The definition of a vertebral compression fracture is reduction of the vertebral height by 20% or 4 mm [25].

Osteoporosis is treated with VP and KP. In Europe, there are approximately 438,750 vertebral collapses per year (which approximates to 117 per 100,000 people) associated with osteoporosis. The natural history of the disease can influence quality of life (QoL), cause psychosocial problems, and influence survival [26]. In women aged >50 years, the incidence of vertebral collapse of an osteoporotic nature has been estimated to be 26% per year with a tendency to increase with age, reaching 40% per year in women aged >80 years [26]. Moreover, there is evidence that women previously affected by a first osteoporotic vertebral collapse have a risk of developing new fractures in the following year of about 19.2% [26–30].

A correct diagnostic approach is very important. Employment of a multidisciplinary team can lead to the best results. Usually spinal pain is focal, non-radicular and increased by digital pressing of the spinous process. The clinical history of a patient affected by an acute porotic fracture usually follows a pattern. That is, the patient presents with acute pain in the thoracic or lumbar spine. After history-taking and clinical evaluation, medical therapy (analgesics and bed rest) and short-term follow-up (usually 2 weeks)

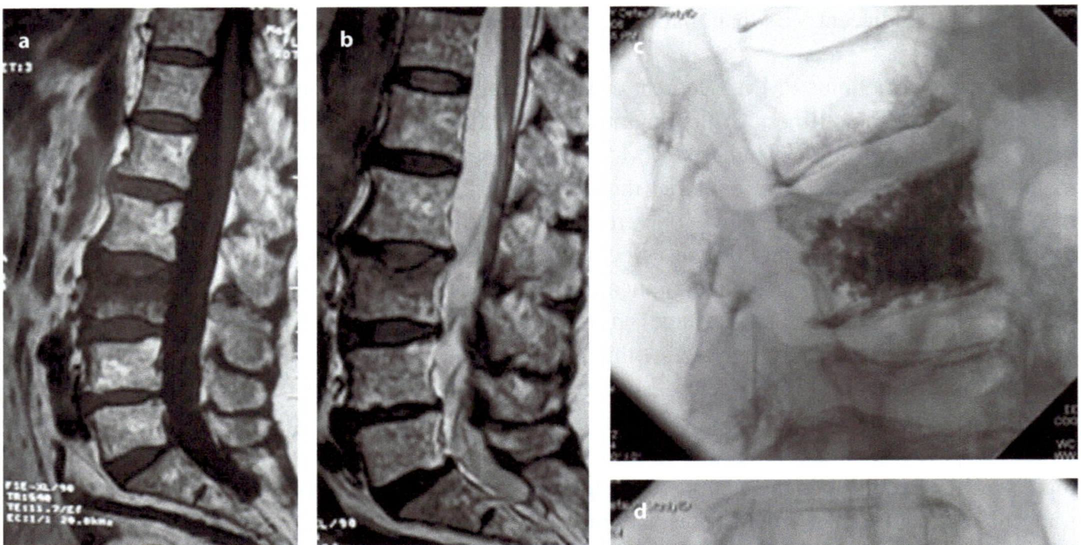

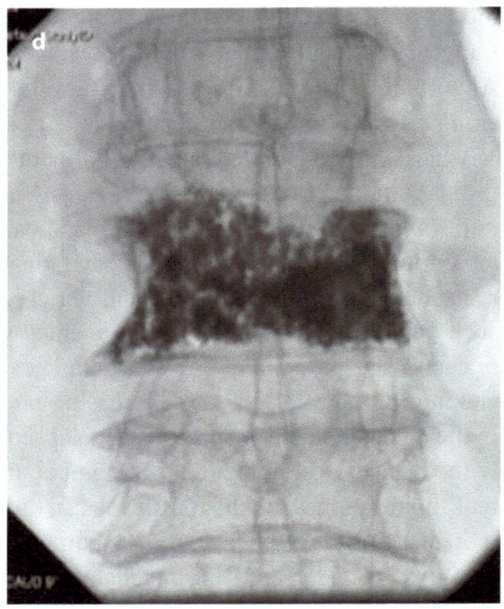

Fig. 9.1 72-year-old female with osteoporosis and acute back pain resistant to medical therapy. Sagittal T1-weighted and T2-weighted MRI show an acute vertebral fracture at the L3 level (**a** and **b**). Left lateral and anteroposterior views under fluoroscopic control after VP at the L3 level show homogeneous distribution of cement into the soma without venous or disk leakage (**c** and **d**)

is recommended. If spinal pain does not lessen within 2 weeks, the second step is radiographic examination of the thoracic and lumbar spine, which can show normal findings or an vertebral abnormality. At this point (usually ≥4–6 weeks after symptom onset), a third step is suggested to patients: examination by magnetic resonance imaging (MRI). Sagittal T2 short-term inversion recovery (STIR) sequences (or any other sequences with T2 fat suppression) are required to decide the treatment and the number of VBs to treat. T2 STIR sequences show hyperintensity in the case of acute fractures or non-healing of fractures and very often can show occult fractures not visible on standard radiographs (Fig. 9.2).

MRI must be carried out close to the date of VP. A delay between the diagnostic examination and VP could result in the treatment of fewer metameric fractures due to the non-identification of occult fractures (not visible on radiographs or CT but visible only with MRI). This could influence the final result of percutaneous treatment.

The radiological patterns used to distinguish between benign and malignant lesions are well known but differential diagnoses can be difficult, especially in vertebral fractures related to multiple myeloma. In such cases, CT is also suggested to better define the lesion, and a biopsy is essential to understand the nature of the lesion. Nevertheless, patients with metastatic disease also

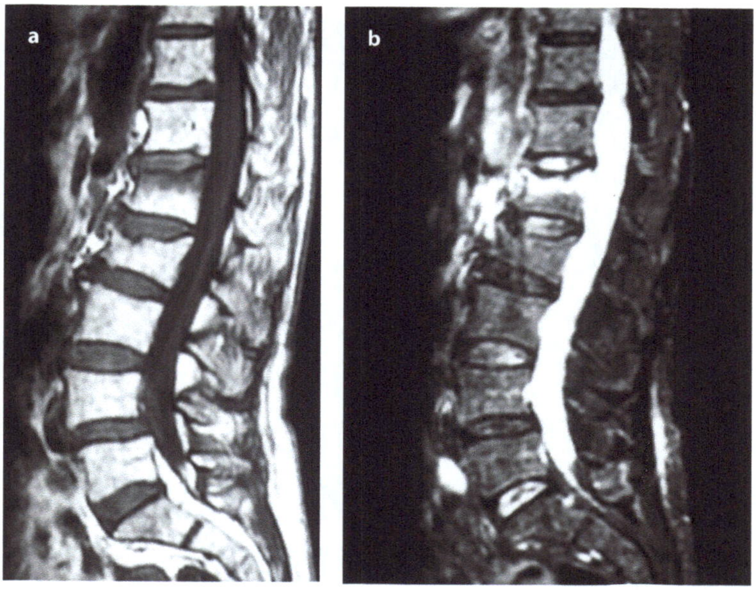

Fig. 9.2 78-year-old female with osteoporosis and acute back pain resistant to medical therapy. Sagittal T1-weighted and T2-STIR MRI show an acute vertebral fracture at the L1 level with a hyperintense signal on T2-STIR (**a** and **b**). The previous VBF presents a normal bone marrow signal (no indication to treatment)

Table 9.1 Absolute and relative contraindications to vertebral cementoplasty

Absolute
Local or systemic infection
Allergy to PMMA
Uncorrectable coagulopathy
Painless vertebral fracture
Relative
Epidural or foraminal extension of soft tissue in a patient with primary or secondary neoplasm associated with a neurological deficit (e.g., radicular or spinal-cord symptoms)
Vertebra plana
Mixed or sclerotic secondary lesions
Disruption of the posterior wall

require CT to better define the type of secondary lesion (lytic, mixed, sclerotic). Bone scintigraphy or positron emission tomography-computed tomography (PET-CT) is also very useful. MRI examination that shows a porotic fracture (hyperintensity in T2 STIR sequences related to bone-marrow edema) in the absence of pain is not an indication for treatment.

The absolute and relative contraindications to VP are shown in Table 9.1 [13, 16, 31]. Vertebra plana is not a typical and unique condition of osteoporosis. It can also be present in patients with other benign or malignant diseases, including aneurysmal bone cysts, giant cell tumors, metastasis or multiple myeloma; biopsy is often essential in these cases. Fragmentation and retropulsion of the posterior wall must also be looked for, and the use of smaller needle is suggested.

Vertebral osteonecrosis with a vacuum cleft inside due to an osteoporotic fracture (Kummel's disease; Fig. 9.3) is a good indication for VP. This cavity can be filled with a greater amount of PMMA cement that usually ≤20 mL for each metamer). A second type of cleft often contains a cystic component which is clearly visible on T2 STIR sequences; the presence of such a cleft is a typical sign of a benign lesion.

To evaluate a "mobile fracture" associated

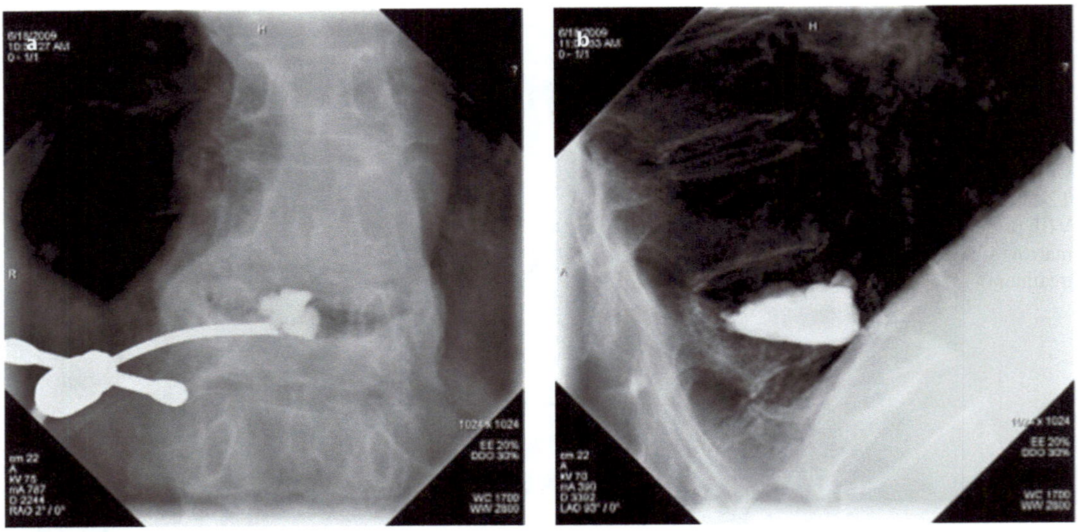

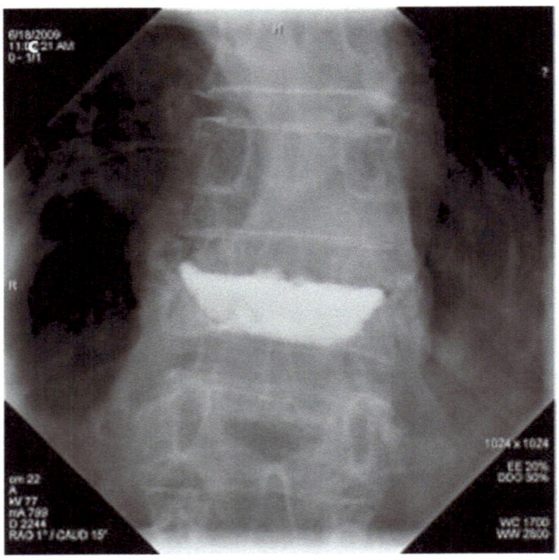

Fig. 9.3 82-year-old male with Kummel's disease and a vertebral fracture at the T11 level with a cleft sign (not shown). Anteroposterior view of fluoroscopic control after VP using a unipedicular approach and initial distribution of cement into a vertebral vacuum (**a**). Left lateral and anteroposterior views under fluoroscopic control after VP at the T11 level show homogeneous distribution of cement into the soma without venous or disk leakage (**b** and **c**)

with a cleft, patients must be asked to inhale and exhale during fluoroscopy in the L–L view to ascertain how the height of the metamer changes during these maneuvers. An appreciable vertebral augmentation effect can be obtained with VP, especially in cases of "vertebral mobile fracture" (Fig. 9.4). Multiple myeloma and spinal metastasis can also be treated with VP [13, 31].

The sacrum is another location for cement injection (sacroplasty). Sacroplasty can be carried out for stress porotic fractures or for neoplastic disease. Stress fractures of the sacrum are painful with low back pain resistant to medical therapy and evidence at STIR T2 sequences of hyperintensity. Sometimes the fracture line can be identified as a "H" shape (Fig. 9.5). Bone scintigraphy can reveal intense uptake of the radionuclide tracer in the sacrum in stress fractures. Clinical and hematological parameters (blood counts, prothrombin time, partial thromboplastin time) should be measured to avoid the risk of complications.

Patients on anticoagulant and anti-platelet therapy must interrupt such treatment for ≥1 week before treatment or they must switch to low-molecular-weight heparin. A bolus of wide-spectrum antibiotics should be infused before and during the treatment to avoid infective complications.

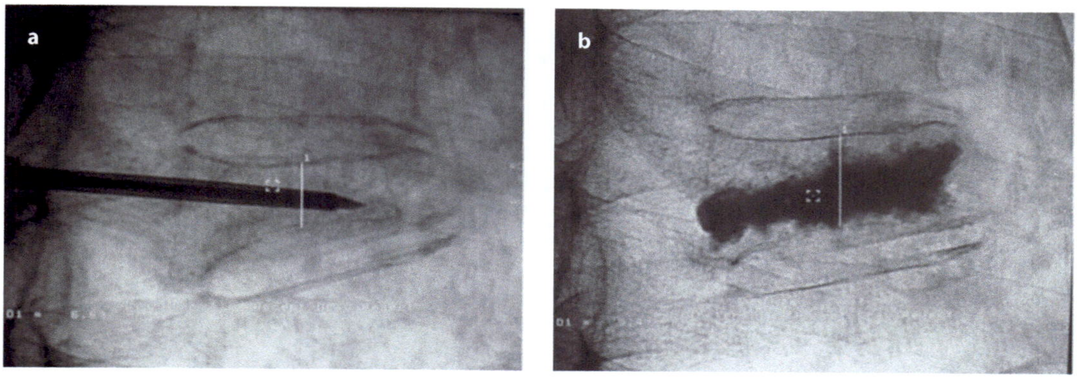

Fig. 9.4 Left lateral view under fluoroscopic control after a unipedicular approach for VP at the L1 level (**a**). Left lateral view under fluoroscopic control after VP shows good distribution of cement without venous or disk leakage as well as good vertebral augmentation (**b**)

There are no absolute rules about the timing of VP. The Percutaneous Vertebroplasty Compared with Optimal Pain Medication Treatment (VERTOS) study showed that patients with vertebral compression fractures treated with VP within a few weeks of the acute onset of symptoms had better results than those who had bed rest and optimal pain medication. However, after 6 months it was still better to undertake VP if the patients were in pain and if MRI showed typical T2 STIR abnormalities. It has been shown that 2/3 of vertebral porotic fractures improve clinically within 6–8 weeks of pain onset, so if pain remains after 8 weeks and abnormal MRI findings are present then VP is indicated [32].

9.4 VP Procedure

A bilateral or unilateral transpedicular approach under fluoroscopic guidance with the patient in the prone position is necessary to obtain good filling of the VB. In the unilateral approach, the needle must reach the VB in the most central position. In the bipedicular approach, the needle can be in a more lateral location. High-quality fluoroscopic guidance is essential for complex and elderly porotic cases to reduce the incidence of side effects and complications related to malpositioning of the needle.

Other common approaches are the trans-somatic, para-pedicular , trans-costo-transversal (for the thoracic level), anterolateral (for the cervical tract) and the trans-oral approach for C2. Different approaches are necessary and are related to the different anatomy of the cervical, thoracic and lumbar tracts (with smaller pedicles in the cervical and thoracic levels compared with the lumbar tract). A combined CT and fluoroscopic approach can be useful for unusual locations such as the lower cervical-upper thoracic spine or for sacral injection. In this way, the needle can be positioned under CT guidance while the injection of the cement can be done under fluoroscopy. It takes longer to carry out KP than to carry out VP.

In general, VP can be done under local anesthesia or minimal neuroleptoanalgesia. Pre-procedure cardiopulmonary evaluation is necessary. Maintaining the prone position is difficult for most patients, so the procedure is usually carried out in the lateral decubitus position. The volume of 2% local anesthesia should be ≤20 mL to avoid side effects such as arrhythmia and vascular disturbances.

The needles employed are usually are quite small (13 G or 15 G). The tips of the needles can be diamond-shaped or beveled without causing significant changes in performance. There are no definitive rules about the numbers of metamer to treat in one session, but usually ≤3–4 are treated. Nevertheless, in selected cases, ≤10–12 metamers can be treated in the same session for vertebral porotic fractures due to long-term cor-

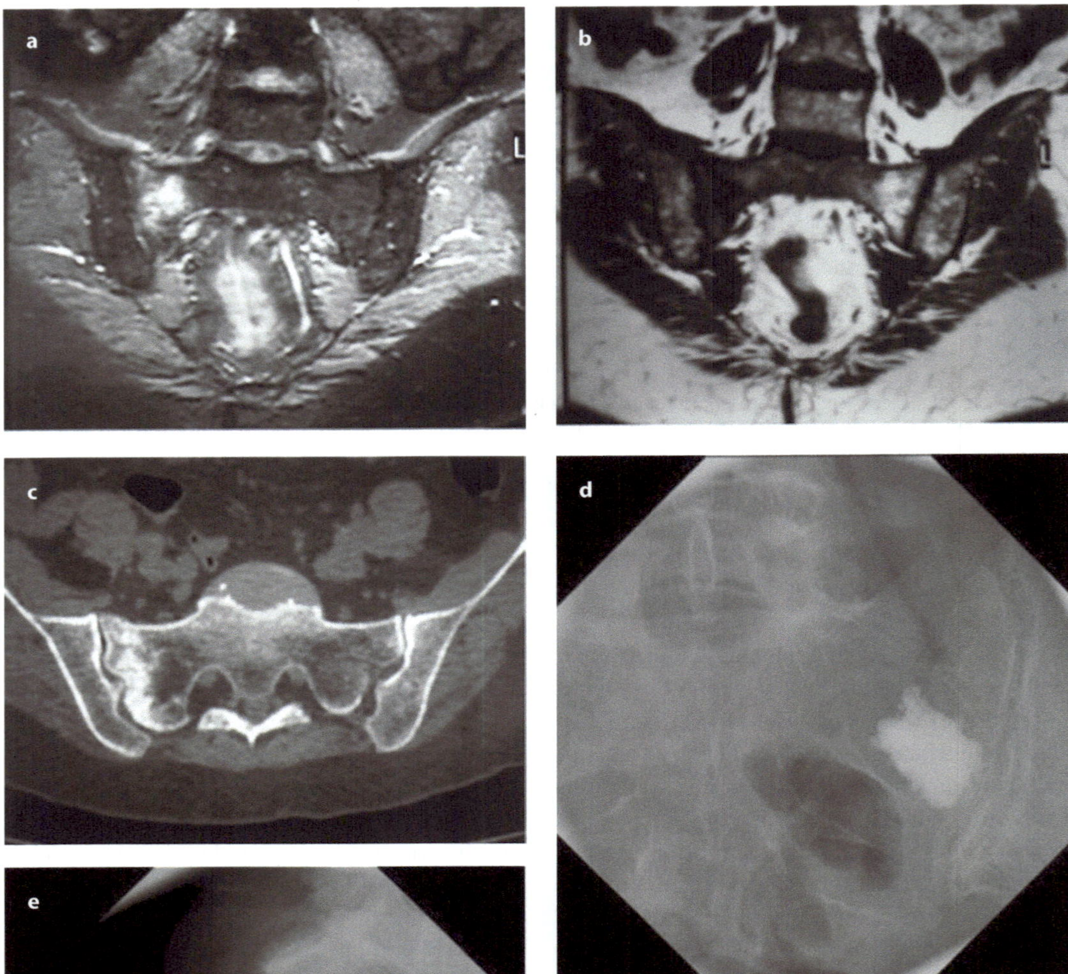

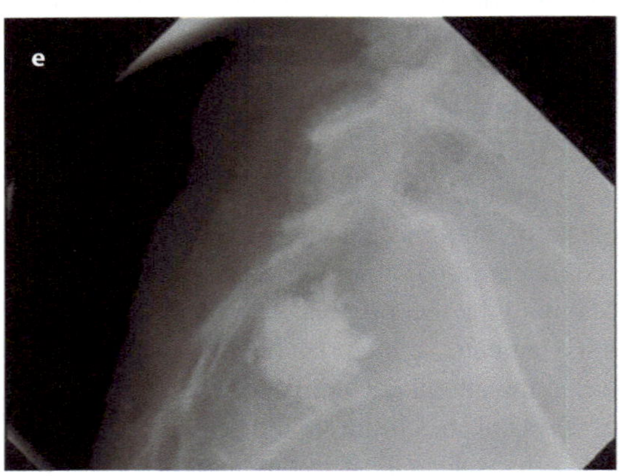

Fig. 9.5 79-year-old female with sacral pain resistant to medical therapy. Coronal T2-STIR MRI shows a hyperintense signal (bone-marrow edema) at the right sacrum: this is a stress porotic fracture (**a**). Coronal T1-weighted MRI shows a hypointense signal at the right sacrum (**b**). Axial multidetector CT shows a right porotic stress fracture at the sacrum with peripheral sclerosis (**c**). Left lateral and anteroposterior views under fluoroscopic control after sacroplasty show good distribution of cement into the fractured sacrum (**d** and **e**)

ticosteroid therapy in patients with collagenopathies, Crohn's disease, epilepsy or allergic rhinitis (Fig. 9.6).

Cutaneous, subcutaneous and periosteal local anesthesia is induced. The needle is positioned in the VB usually through a trans-pedicular approach to reach the posterior wall without going over the medial margin of the peduncle. The medial margin of the peduncle is an absolute anatomical marker to check before going through the posterior wall of the VB to avoid damaging the spinal canal.

The amount of cement injected into the VB can be extremely variable: between 2 mL up to 8–10 mL depending by the metamer to treat (cervical, thoracic or lumbar) and the degree of

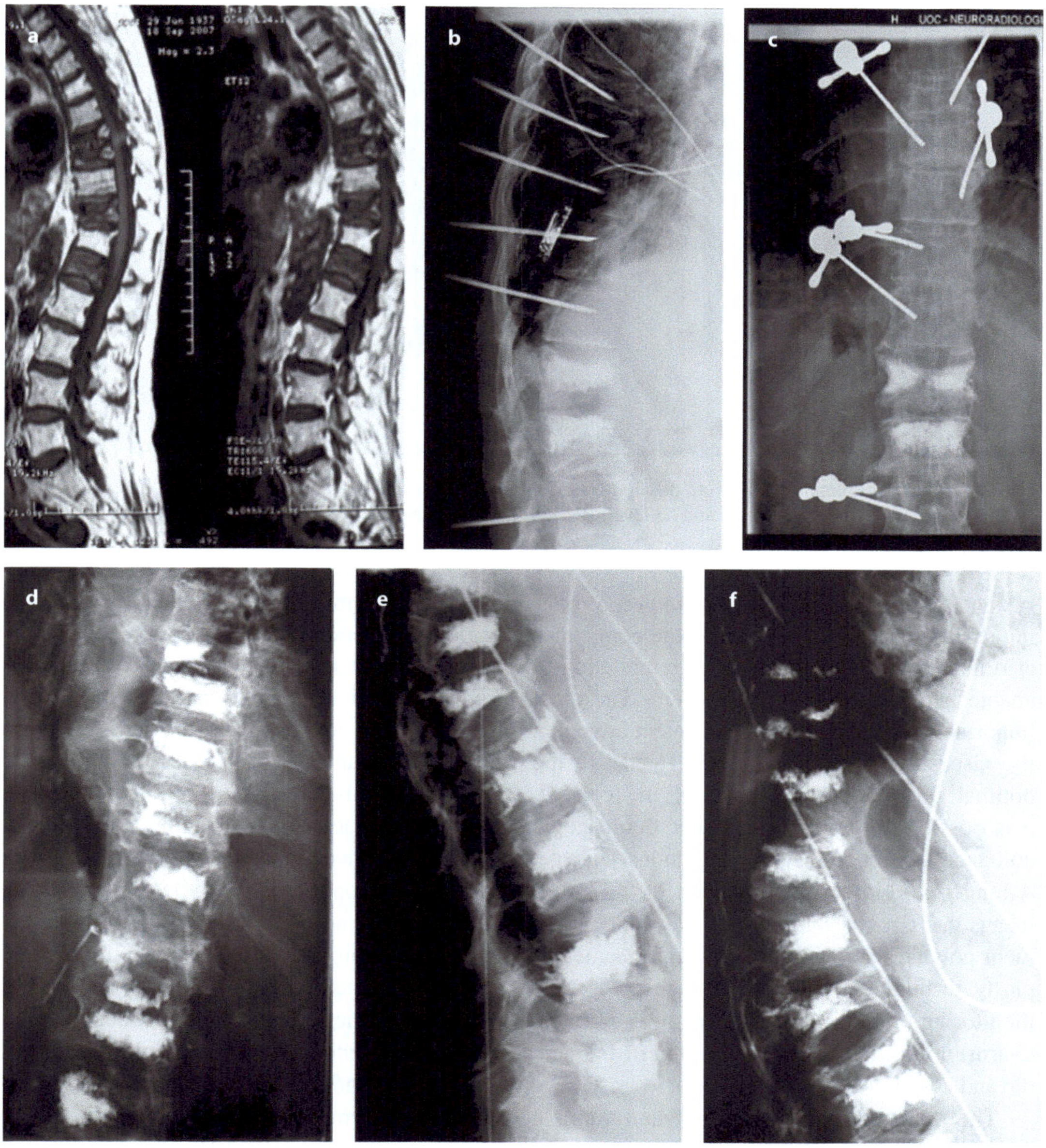

Fig. 9.6 82-year-old female with severe osteoporosis. Sagittal T1-weighted MRI shows multiple vertebral fractures at dorsal and lumbar levels with hypointense signals treated with VP (**a**). Left lateral and anteroposterior views under fluoroscopic control after one session of multilevel VP with a unipedicular approach at dorsal and lumbar levels (**b** and **c**). Left lateral and anteroposterior views under fluoroscopic control after one session of multilevel VP show good distribution of cement without venous or disk leakage (**d–f**)

collapsed vertebrae. There are no absolute rules about the amount of cement to be injected for each vertebra. Cement filling should go from the superior to the inferior endplate by passing through the midline to guarantee the best stabilizing and biomechanical effects. Sometimes this is not possible due to subchondral sclerotic reactions. However, this is not a problem because it represents a point of strength of the ruptured vertebra. Overfilling the metamer to avoid venous and disk leakage is not necessary.

Different VP kits are available with mixing

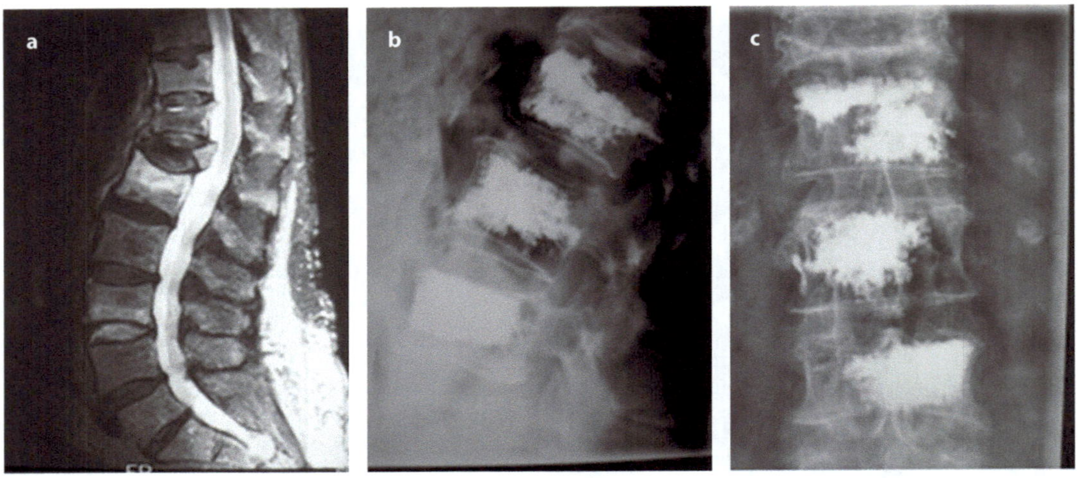

Fig. 9.7 75-year-old female with severe osteoporosis. Sagittal T2-weighted MRI shows complete collapse of the T12 level with hyperintense signals at L1 and L3 levels (**a**). Left lateral and anteroposterior views under fluoroscopic control after VP at L1–L3 levels (**b** and **c**)

systems and cement injections based on a rotating system or a 1-mL syringe. Some companies also have curettes to obtain bony remodeling to enable better distribution of cement. The most important characteristics of the cement are opacity, viscosity and working time. Thanks to the optimal opacity and viscosity of the cement, it is possible to work safely under fluoroscopic guidance to reduce the risk of venous leakage. A longer working time of the cement (≤27 min) means that one does not have to worry about cement polymerization. All the vertebral cementoplasty techniques require constant fluoroscopic monitoring (angiographic equipment or portable C-arm) to ensure correct positioning of the needle and control of cement injection.

The radiation dose is an important variable for patients and physicians alike. Hence, it is important to reduce the fluoroscopy time to protect the patient and operator from over-exposure. Using a system that leads to an increase in the distance between the radiation source and the injection point could be an option.

Preventative VP is not accepted in all centers, and randomized controlled trials proving the efficacy of this type of treatment are lacking. In certain cases, a procedure to prevent new fractures that is related to biomechanics (e.g., preventative treatment of L3 fractures in patients with L2 and L4 fractures ("sandwich fracture") or at the thoracolumbar region in which the kyphotic angle is greater and the axial stress above or below the metamer is higher) (Figs. 9.7 and 9.8) is suggested. This procedure can also be done in patients with collagenopathies (e.g., Takayasu disease, Marfan's syndrome, Crohn's disease). In such patients, the risk of new fractures after the previous fracture is higher compared with patients with conventional osteoporosis [33]. With respect to sacroplasty, 1–4 needles (13–15 G) can be positioned under CT or fluoroscopic guidance. Needle position and cement distribution related to the neural sacral foramina must be checked.

Recently, new types of osteoconductive cements have become available. Bone substitutes (e.g., Cerament™) (Fig. 9.9) and calcium triglyceride (Kryptonite™) (Fig. 9.10) can also be injected within collapsed VBs, thereby inducing the formation of new, normal bone. These bone substitutes comprise 60% alpha-calcium sulfate (α-CaS) and 40% hydroxyapatite (HA). These agents can also stabilize the fracture and elicit an analgesic effect, with a marked improvement in symptoms (>90% of treated patients detail pain relief). However, these materials cannot be used in the presence of metastasis, osteoangiomas or Kummel's disease [34]. Also, these osteoconductive cements are fourfold more expensive than standard PMMA.

In the treatment of osteoporosis, VP stabiliz-

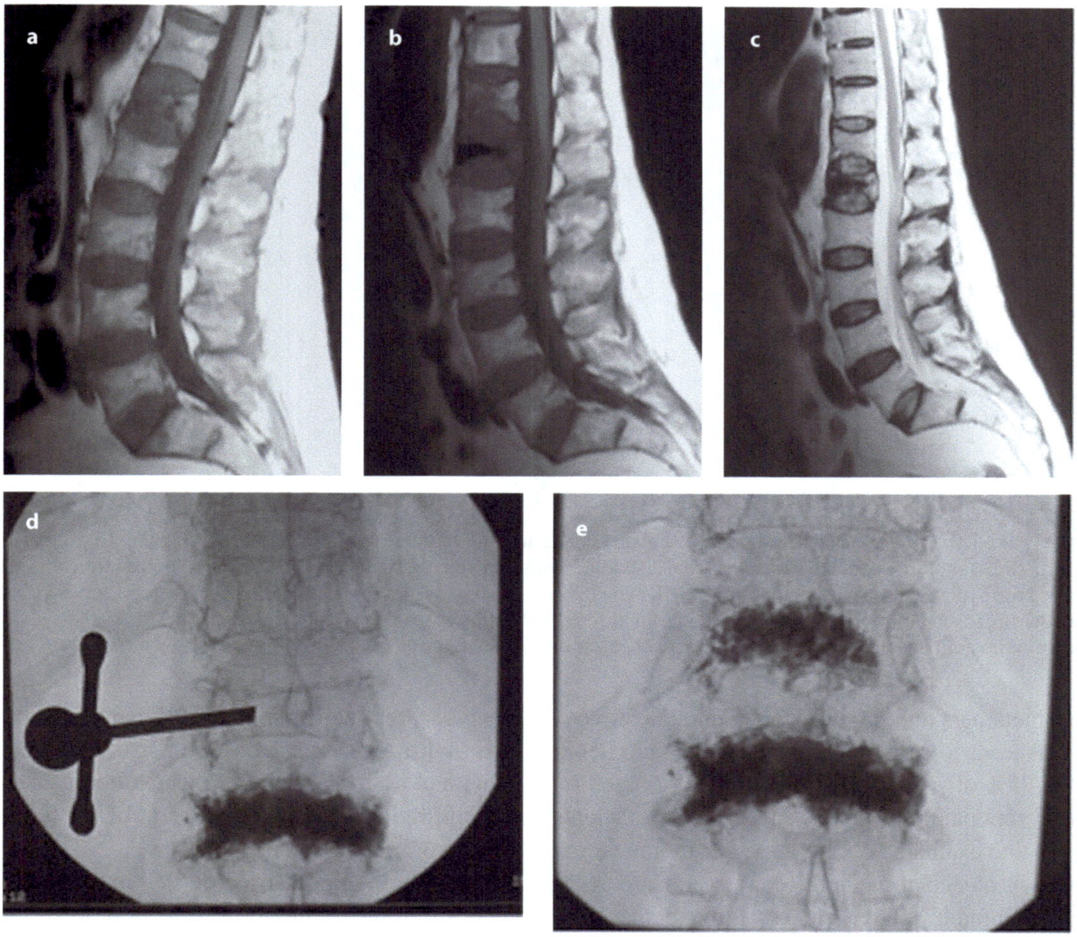

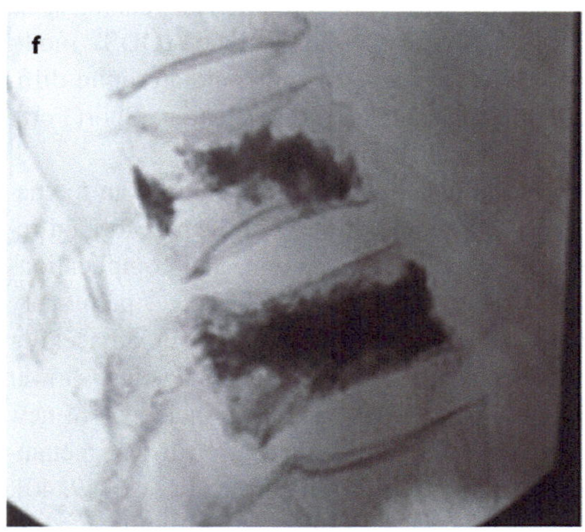

Fig. 9.8 78-year-old female with severe osteoporosis. Sagittal T1-weighted MRI shows acute vertebral fracture at the L1 level with hypointense signals treated with VP (**a**). Sagittal T1-weighted MRI and sagittal T2-weighted MRI control 3 months after VP show a low signal at the L1 level due to PMMA and a hypointense signal on T1-weighted at the T12 level (**b** and **c**). Anteroposterior view under fluoroscopic control after VP at the L1 level with a unipedicular approach at the T12 level (**d**). Anteroposterior and left lateral (**e** and **f**) views under fluoroscopic control after VP at T12 and L1 levels show good distribution of cement without venous or disk leakage (**e** and **f**)

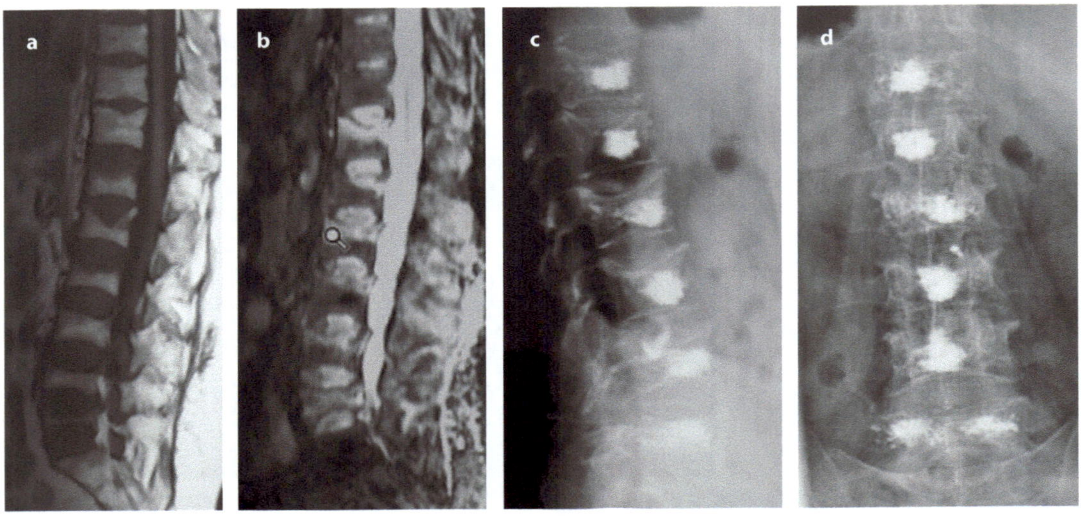

Fig. 9.9 65-year-old female with severe osteoporosis due to long-term corticosteroid therapy. Sagittal T1-weighted MRI shows multiple vertebral fractures from T12 to L5 with hypointense signals (**a**). All vertebral bodies from T12 to L5 show hyperintense signals on T2-STIR MRI due to bone-marrow edema (**b**). Left lateral and anteroposterior views under fluoroscopic control after one session of multilevel VP with a unipedicular approach from T12 to L5 show good distribution of cement (Cerament™) without venous or disk leakage (**c** and **d**)

es metamers and produces good antalgic effects. This leads to early mobilization and pain relief in 80–95% of patients, but these data are based on different pain-evaluation scales [35, 38]. Patients must be evaluated before and after treatment using an objective method. Many scales are available; some of which are easy to understand and complete by the patient (e.g., visual analog scale (VAS), Oswestry Disability Index (ODS), modified MacNab method) and some are quite difficult to understand and complete (e.g., Short Form (SF)36, McGill pain questionnaire).

Several studies have been carried out to analyze the outcome of VP with respect to pain reduction, kyphotic correction, and complications (e.g., cement leakage; disk leakage; pulmonary embolism; new vertebral fractures to adjacent or distant VBs). The risk of cement leakage is lower in KP than in VP, whereas the incidence of new vertebral fractures to adjacent or distant metamers mostly related to the porotic disease [39, 40].

The long-term results are also influenced by appropriate medical therapy after VP. Hence, cooperating with endocrinologists and requesting laboratory examinations are important. Another crucial consideration regarding results in porotic patients is that often we are also dealing with other diseases such as spondylosis and osteocondrosis with degenerative disease also of the facets joints and sacroiliac joints in which corticosteroid infiltration and radiofrequency of the facet joints are suggested [41].

Anselmetti et al. carried out VP in 1,634 patients suffering from painful osteoporotic vertebral compression fractures and followed up over a long time. VP was completed in all patients without recognized clinical complications. They reported a mean VAS score of 7.94 that improved significantly to 1.12; the median ODI values of 82% before treatment decreased significantly to 6%. Before intervention, 1,279 patients wore a brace; after VP, 1,167 (91.2%) patients did not wear a brace. They recorded PMMA leakages in 561 (34.3%) patients. With respect to the prevalence of re-fracture, 1,634 patients had a vertebral fracture secondary to osteoporosis, and 214 (13.1%) had a new painful fracture. Of these patients (13%), a distant fracture occurred in 36.4%, and 63.6% had a new fracture in a contiguous vertebra. Among these patients, 42.7% had a fractured vertebra below the first vertebra treated, whereas 36.0% had a fracture at the level above; 21.3% subsequently had fractures in levels above and below the treated vertebrae [42].

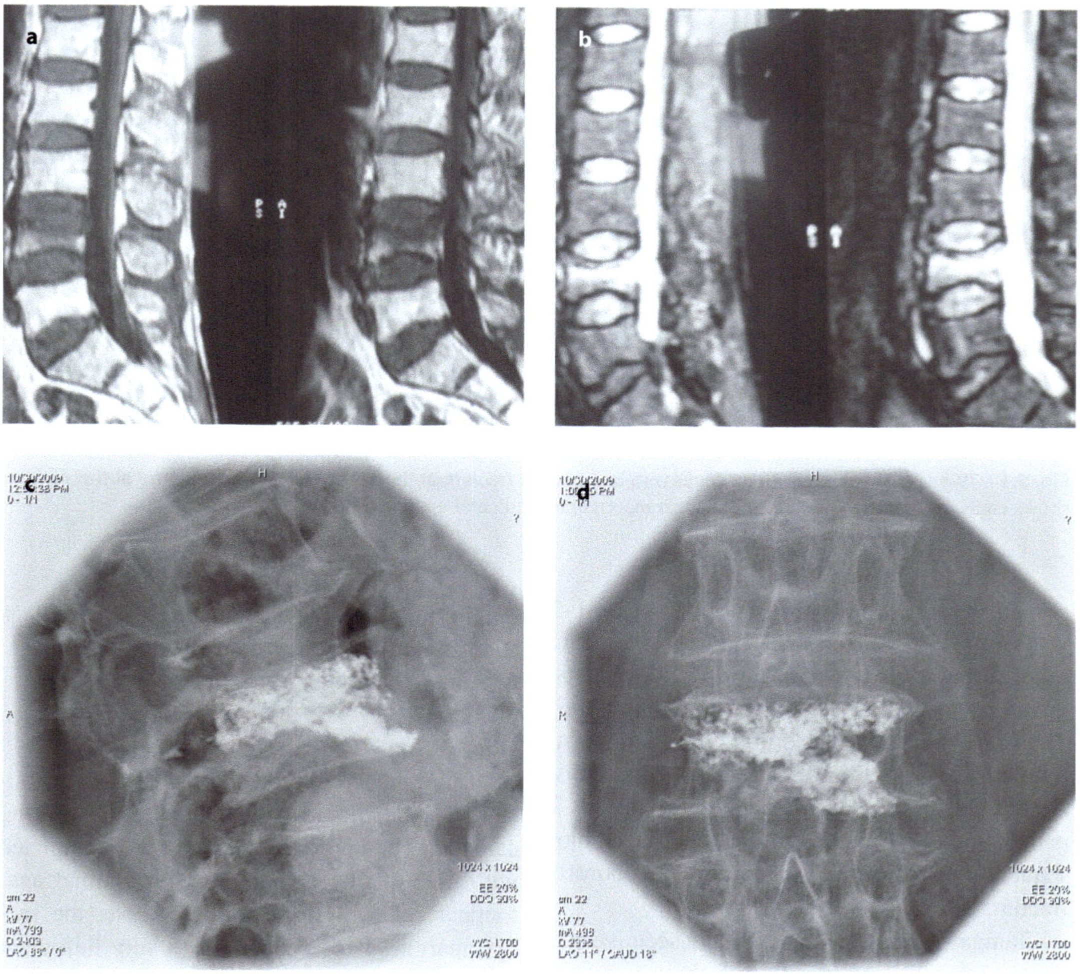

Fig. 9.10 55-year-old male with a vertebral fracture at the L4 level. Sagittal T1-weighted MRI shows a vertebral fracture at the L4 level with hypointense signals (**a**). Sagittal T2-STIR MRI shows the hyperintense signal due to bone-marrow edema (**b**). Left lateral and anteroposterior views under fluoroscopic control after VP of the L4 treated by cement (Kryptonite™) do not show venous or disk leakage (**c** and **d**)

Our research team carried out VP on 805 vertebral bodies in 485 patients affected by osteoporosis (310), metastasis (160) and vertebral hemangioma [16, 43]. In patients treated with VP, the success rates at 24–72 h were 90% for osteoporotic fractures, 100% for vertebral hemangiomas, and 77% for metastatic fractures. Extravertebral vascular or diskal leakage of cement occurred in 39 patients, but only 2 of them reported radicular pain due to epidural involvement. Osteoporotic patients developed new vertebral fractures at adjacent levels in 25 cases and at distal levels in 19 cases.

Kim et al. undertook VP in 159 patients affected by osteoporotic compression fractures with a follow-up for >5 years. They registered pain levels according to the VAS: The VAS score fell by 4.9 from a preoperative mean of 7.0 to the perioperative mean value of 2.1. Forty-six percent of patients reported a score of ≥5 for reduction and maintenance of pain level. Thirty-three cases of newly developed vertebral fracture were reported in the VBs of 22 patients (which signified 32% newly developed vertebral fractures) [44].

Kotwica and Saracen carried out VP in 200 patients suffering from osteoporotic vertebral

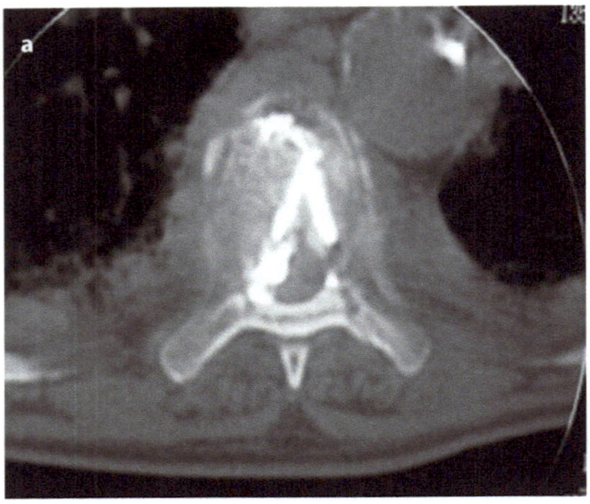

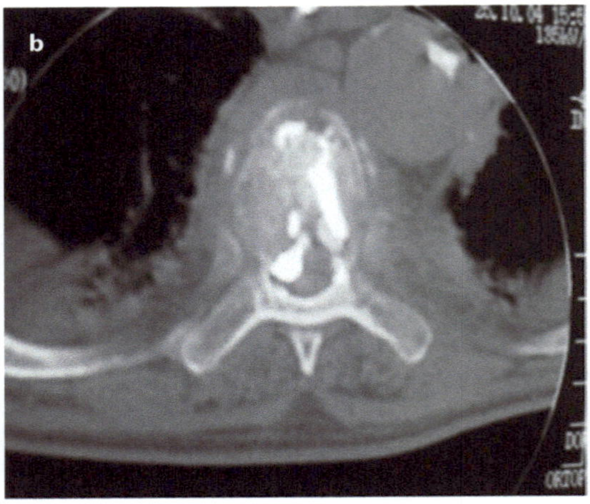

Fig. 9.11 79-year-old female with an acute vertebral porotic fracture at the T8 level. Axial CT control at the T8 level shows endocanal leakage of cement due to an incorrect unipedicular approach (**a** and **b**)

compression fractures with a follow-up of 1–2 years. Twelve hours after VP, very significant relief of pain was observed in 85% of patients; this relief reached 96% on the 7th and 30th day. The same result was noted in 92% of patients at 6 months, and in 90% of patients at 12 months. Among the 80 patients followed up for 2 years, 3 patients reported pain recurrence and were subsequently diagnosed as having new osteoporotic fractures [45].

Tanigawa et al. treated 194 consecutive patients with 500 osteoporotic vertebral compression fractures by VP with a follow of 7 years. The mean VAS score was 7.6 before percutaneous VP. It was 3.1 at 1 day, 2.3 at 1 month, 1.7 at 4 months, 1.5 at 1 year, 1.2 at 2 years, 1.0 at 3 years, 1.1 at 4 years, 0.9 at 5 years, 0.9 at 6 years, and 1.0 at 7 years after VP. They recorded new vertebral compression fractures in 103 vertebrae in 65 patients (33.5%), affecting 65 adjacent vertebrae (63.1%) and 38 non-adjacent vertebrae (36.9%). Cement leakage was seen at 213 levels (42.6%) [46].

9.5 Complications

All procedures must be carried out with the best technology available (digital subtraction angiography or CT–fluoroscopy) to avoid minor and major complications such as endocanal leakage (Fig. 9.11) or venous leakage (Fig. 9.12). Intramuscular paravertebral hematoma is a rare complication (Fig. 9.13). Complications associated with VP and KP are listed in Table 9.2.

The first step in reducing the risk of complications is positioning of the needle and working cannula. These procedures must be completed with high-quality equipment with optimal anatomical control. As mentioned above, the medial margin of the peduncle is a very important anatomical landmark during needle positioning. Complications are associated with abnormal distribution of cement with disk leakage, epidural leakage or vascular leakage but, abnormal leakage is often asymptomatic [13, 31]. Some type of leakages can create only slight radicular pain or compression of the thecal sac, whereas vascular leakage can cause asymptomatic or symptomatic pulmonary emboli, cerebral infarcts or heart/vascular dissection. Disk leakage seems to be related to a higher incidence of fracture to the contiguous VB. To lessen the risk of complications two major practical points must be appreciated: (i) use a dense cement and (ii) inject slowly. A very important anatomical landmark is the posterior wall of the VB, which should never be passed by cement. This is a key point to avoid endocanal cement leakage because it has very dramatic complications: paraplegia or tetraplegia.

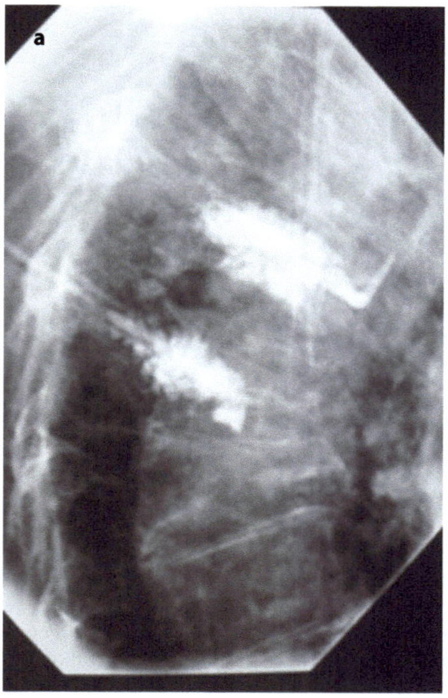

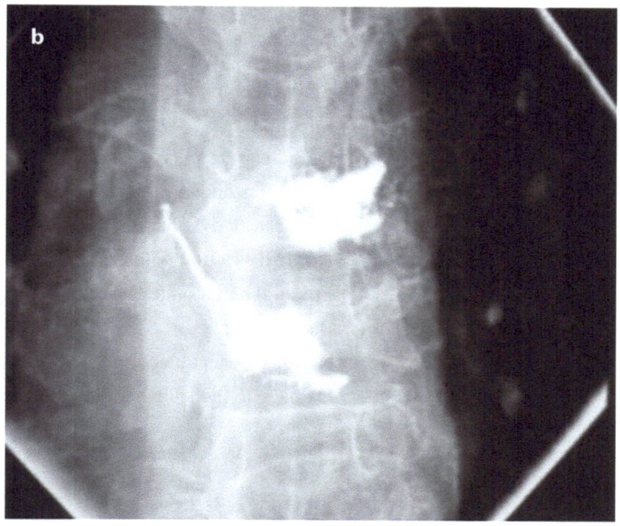

Fig. 9.12 Left lateral and anteroposterior views under fluoroscopic control after VP at two dorsal levels show venous and disk leakages of cement (1 mL) (**a** and **b**)

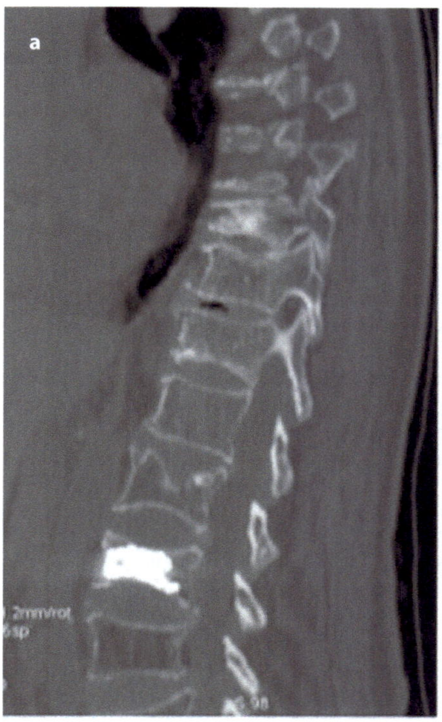

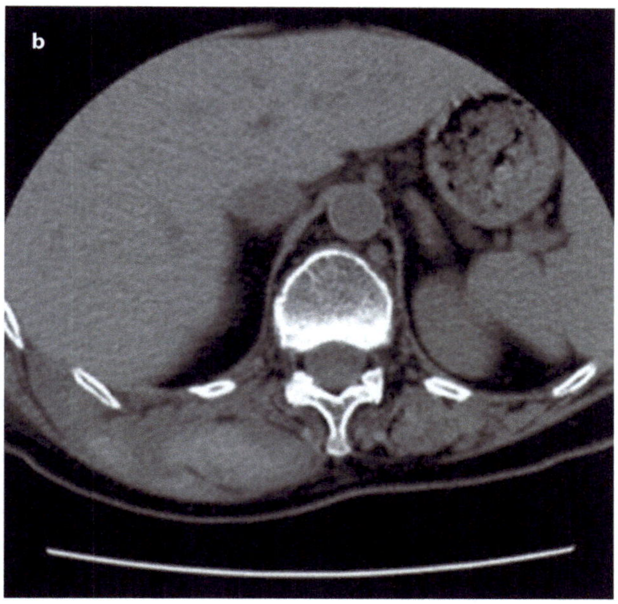

Fig. 9.13 Sagittal multidetector CT after VP at the L4 level (**a**). Axial CT in the thoraco-abdomen shows a complication after VP: right posterior intramuscular hematoma (**b**)

Table 9.2 Complications associated with vertebroplasty and kyphoplasty

Disk and venous leakage
Pulmonary emboli
Cerebral emboli
Infection
Dural tear
Paraplegia and tetraplegia
Respiratory dysfunction
Aortic dissection with arterial emboli
Epidural hematoma
Pneumothorax
Retroperitoneal bleeding
Damage to the spinal cord and compression or rupture of nerve roots
Death

9.6 Conclusions

Vertebral augmentation methods such as VP are safe and effective for the treatment of vertebral compression and primary or secondary spinal tumors with excellent outcomes. VP has some advantages over KP:

- multi-metameric treatment can be completed in one session for certain disorders;
- specific anatomical locations (e.g., cervicothoracic junction, sacrum) can be treated;
- vertebral clefts (cystic or vacuolated) can be treated;
- vertebral hemangiomas can be treated.

The low cost of VP compared with KP and the need of only local anesthesia are also important considerations when deciding which type of vertebral cementoplasty to carry out.

References

1. Wong X, Reiley MA, Garfin S (2000) Vertebroplasty/kyphoplasty. J Women's Imaging 2:117–124
2. Pflugmacher R, Kandziora F, Schroder R et al (2005) Vertebroplasty and kyphoplasty in osteoporotic fractures of vertebral bodies: a prospective 1-year follow-up analysis. RöFo 177:1670–1676
3. Galimbert P, Deramond H, Rosat P et al (1987) Preliminary note on the treatment of vertebral angioma by percutaneous acrylic vertebroplasty. Neurochirurgie 33:166–168
4. Gangi A, Guth S, Imbert JP et al (2003) Percutaneous vertebroplasty: indications, technique, and results. Radiographics 23:10–20
5. Mathis JM, Barr JD, Belkoff SM et al (2001) Percutaneous vertebroplasty: a developing standard of care for vertebral compression fractures. Am J Neuroradiol 22:373–381
6. Muijs SP, van Erkel AR, Dijkstra PD (2011) Treatment of painful osteoporotic vertebral compression fractures: a brief review of the evidence for percutaneous vertebroplasty. J Bone Joint Surg Br 93:1149–1153
7. Kallmes DF, Heagerty PJ, Turner JA et al. (2009) A randomized trial of vertebroplasty for osteoporotic spinal fractures N Engl J Med 361:569–579
8. Buchbinder R, Osborne RH, Murphy B et al (2009) A randomized trial of vertebroplasty for painful osteoporotic vertebral fractures. N Engl J Med 361:557–568
9. Wardlaw D, Cummings SR, van Meirhaeghe J et al (2009). Efficacy and safety of balloon kyphoplasty compared with non-surgical care for vertebral compression fracture (FREE): a randomized controlled trial. Lancet 373:1016–1024
10. Legrain V, Iannetti GD, Plaghki L, Mouraux A (2011) The pain matrix reloaded: a salience detection system for the body. Prog Neurobiol 93:111–124
11. Mouraux A, Diukova A, Lee MC, Wise RG, Iannetti GD (2011) A multisensory investigation of the functional significance of the "pain matrix". Neuroimage 54:2237–2249
12. Guarnieri G, Ambrosanio G, Vassallo P et al (2009) Vertebroplasty as treatment of aggressive and symptomatic vertebral hemangiomas: up to 4 years of follow-up. Neuroradiology 51:471–476
13. Peh WC, Gilula LA (2003) Percutaneous vertebroplasty: indications, contraindications, and technique. Br J Radiol 76:69–75
14. Guglielmi G, Andreula C, Muto M, Gilula L (2005) Percutaneous vertebroplasty: indications, contraindications, technique and complications. Acta Radiol 46:256–268

15. Cotten A, Boutry N, Cortet B et al (1998) Percutaneous vertebroplasty: state of the art. Radiographics 18:311–320
16. Ambrosanio G, Lavanga A,Vassallo P, Izzo R, Diano AA, Muto M. (2005) Vertebroplasty in the treatment of spine Ddisease. Interven Neuroradiol 11: 309–323
17. Kim JM, Lindsey DP, Hannibal M, Alamin TF (2006) Vertebroplasty versus kyphoplasty: biomechanical behavior under repetitive loading conditions. Spine 31:2079–2084
18. Wilke HJ, Mehnert U, Claes LE et al. (2006) Biomechanical evaluation of vertebroplastyand kyphoplasty with polymethyl methacrylate or calcium phosphate cement under cyclic loading. Spine 31:2934–2941
19. Nouda S, Tomita S, Kin A et al. (2007) Adjacent vertebral body fracture following vertebroplasty with polymethylmethacrylate or calcium phosphate cement biomechanical evaluation of the cadaveric spine. Spine 34:2613–2618
20. Uppin AA, Hirsch JA, Centenera LV et al. (2003) Occurrence of new vertebral body fracture after percutaneous vertebroplasty in patients with osteoporosis. Radiology 226:119–24
21. Kim SH, Kang HS, Choi JA et al. (2004) Risk factors of new compression fractures in adjacent vertebrae after percutaneous vertebroplasty. Acta Radiol 45:440–445
22. Trout AT, Kallmes DF, Kaufmann TJ (2006) New fractures after vertebroplasty: adjacent fractures occur significantly sooner. Am J Neuroradiol 27:217–223
23. Furtado N, Oakland RJ, Wilcox RK, Hall RM (2007) A biomechanical investigation of vertebroplasty in osteoporotic compression fractures and in prophylactic vertebral reinforcement. Spine 32:E480–E487
24. Wangn JL, Chiang CK,Yang BD (2012) Mechanism of fractures of adjacentand augmented vertebrae following simulated vertebroplasty. J Biomech [In press]
25. Black DM, Palermo L, Nevitt MC et al; The Study of Osteoporotic Fractures Research Group (1999) Defining incident vertebral deformity: a prospective comparison of several approaches. J Bone Miner Res 14:90–101
26. Anita A, Uppin MD, Joshua A et al (2003) Occurrence of new vertebral body fracture after percutaneous vertebroplasty in patients with osteoporosis. Radiology 226:119–124
27. Bajaj S, Saag KG (2003) Osteoporosis: evaluation and treatment. Curr Womens Health Rep 3:418–124
28. Lindsay R, Silverman SL, Seeman E et al (2001) Risk of new vertebral fracture in the year following a fracture. JAMA 285:320–323
29. Silverman SL (1992) The clinical consequences of vertebral compression fracture. Bone 13: S27–S31
30. Voormolen MH, Lohle PN, Juttmann JR et al (2006) The risk of new osteoporotic vertebral compression fractures in the year after percutaneous vertebroplasty. J Vasc Interv Radiol;17:71–76
31. Guglielmi G, Andreula C, Muto M, Gilula L (2005) Percutaneous vertebroplasty: indications, contraindications, technique and complications. Acta Radiol 46:256–268
32. Jensen ME, McGraw JK, Cardella JF, Hirsch JA; American Society of Interventional and Therapeutic Neuroradiology; Society of Interventional Radiology; American Association of Neurological Surgeons/Congress of Neurological Surgeons; American Society of Spine Radiology (2007) Position statement on percutaneous vertebral augmentation: a consensus statement developed by the American Society of Interventional and Therapeutic Neuroradiology, Society of Interventional Radiology, American Association of Neurological Surgeons/Congress of Neurological Surgeons, and American Society of Spine Radiology. Am J Neuroradiol 28:1439–1443
33. Yen CH, Teng MM, Yuan WH, Sun YC, Chang CY (2012) Preventive vertebroplasty for adjacent vertebral bodies: a good solution to reduce adjacent vertebral fracture after percutaneous vertebroplasty. Am J Neuroradiol 33:826–832
34. Masala S, Nano G, Marcia S, Muto M, Fucci FP, Simonetti G (2012) Osteoporotic vertebral compression fractures augmentation by injectable partly resorbable ceramic bone substitute (Cerament™|Spine Support): a prospective nonrandomized study. Neuroradiology 11 [In press]
35. Maestretti G, Cremer C, Otten P, Jakob RP (2007) Prospective study of standalone balloon kyphoplasty with calcium phosphate cement augmentation in traumatic fractures. Eur Spine J 16:601–610
36. Fuentes S, Metellus P, Fondop J et al (2007) Percutaneous pedicle screwfixation and kyphoplasty for management of thoracolumbar burst fractures. Neurochirurgie 53:272–276
37. Theodoru DJ, Theodorou SJ, Duncan TD et al (2002) Percutaneous balloon kyphoplasty for the correction of spinal deformity in painful vertebral body compression fractures. J Clin Imaging 26:1–5
38. Deramond H, Salioub G, Aveillana M et al (2006) Respective contributions of vertebroplasty and kyphoplasty to the management of osteoporotic vertebral fractures. Joint Bone Spine 73:610–613
39. Teng MM, Wei CJ, Wei LC et al (2003) Kyphosis correction and height restoration effects of percutaneous vertebroplasty. Am J Neuroradiol 24:1893–1190
40. Matthew J, Parker SJ, Wolinsky JP et al (2009) Vertebroplasty and kyphoplasty for the treatment of vertebral compression fractures: an evidenced-based review of the literature Spine J 9:501–508
41. Kamalian S, Bordia R, Ortiz AO (2012) Post-vertebral augmentation back pain: evaluation and management. Am J Neuroradiol 33:370–375
42. Anselmetti GC, Manca A, Hirsch J et al (2011) Percutaneous vertebroplasty in osteoporotic patients: an institutional experience of 1,634 patients with long-term follow-up. J Vasc Interv Radiol 22:1714–1720
43. Muto M, Perrotta V, Guarnieri G et al (2008) Vertebroplasty and kyphoplasty: friends or foes? Radiol Med 113:1171–1184

44. Kim JH, Yoo SH, Kim JH. (2012) Long-term follow-up of percutaneous vertebroplasty in osteoporotic compression fracture: minimum of 5 years follow-up. Asian Spine J 6:6–14
45. Kotwica Z, Saracen A. (2011) Early and long-term outcomes of vertebroplasty for single osteoporotic fractures. Neurol Neurochir Pol 45:431–435
46. Tanigawa N, Kariya S, Komemushi A et al (2011) Percutaneous vertebroplasty for osteoporotic compression fractures: long-term evaluation of the technical and clinical outcomes. Am J Roentgenol 196:1415–1418

Medical Therapy in Porotic Patients

10

Annamaria Colao, Laura Vuolo, Manila Rubino
and Carolina Di Somma

10.1 Introduction

Osteoporosis is a multifactorial skeletal disorder characterized by reduced bone mass and deterioration of the micro-architecture of bone. These features predispose affected subjects to increased susceptibility to fractures. According to the World Health Organization, osteoporosis is diagnosed if the bone mineral density (BMD) is 2.5 standard-deviations below the mean peak value in young adults of the same ethnicity and sex (T-score less than –2.5). The "gold standard" for measuring BMD is dual-energy X-ray absorptiometry (DEXA). Other diagnostic modalities include computed tomography (CT), peripheral quantitative CT, and ultrasonography (which has not been shown to provide additional information about bone quality).

The adult skeleton undergoes a lifelong process of resorption and formation ("bone remodeling") in numerous localized areas called "bone multicellular units" (BMUs). Each BMU has a lifespan of ≈6–9 months, resulting in a turnover of ≈10% of the entire skeleton each year. The cells involved in the highly coordinated process of bone turnover are osteoclasts (bone-resorbing cells), osteoblasts (bone-forming cells), and osteocytes (mechanosensory cells). Osteoclasts are multinucleated cells derived from pluripotential hematopoietic cells. Osteoblasts are mononuclear cells derived from mesenchymal cells. The proliferation, differentiation, and death of cells of both lineages determine the degree of bone remodeling. Bone remodeling is necessary to maintain calcium homeostasis and to remove and prevent the accumulation of bone damage. An imbalance of bone turnover leads to osteoporosis. It can be characterized as "high turnover" or "low turnover". In the former, osteoclastic activity is increased, and resorption lacunae are deeper and more numerous. In low-turnover osteoporosis, osteoblasts fail to form bone during normal turnover of bone.

The most important consequences of osteoporosis are fragility fractures of the spine, hip, and wrist. The impact is considerable: significant pain, long-term disability, and deformity can occur. Degenerative joint alteration distal to the fracture and sympathetic reflex dystrophy can also occur. Medical treatment is recommended to recover an acceptable quality of life (QoL) and functionality, along with certain types of physical or occupational therapy. Hip fractures are less common than vertebral fractures, but account for most of the mortality, morbidity, and costs associated with osteoporosis (hip fractures can lead to long stays in rehabilitation hospitals or nursing homes after acute care). Hip fractures can lead to a 15% increase in mortality within the first year, and >70% of survivors have a significant reduc-

A. Colao (✉)
Department of Molecular and Clinical Endocrinology and Oncology, Federico II University of Naples, Naples, Italy
e-mail: colao@unina.it

M. Muto (ed.), *Interventional Neuroradiology of the Spine*,
DOI 10.1007/978-88-470-2790-9_10, © Springer-Verlag Italia 2013

Table 10.1 Medical options approved for porotic patients

Antiresorptive	Anabolic
Bisphosphonates	PTH 1–34: teriparatide
Selective estrogen receptor modulators	PTH 1–84
Strontium ranelate	Strontium ranelate
Anti-RANKL antibody: denosumab	

RANKL, receptor activator of nuclear factor-kappa B ligand; *PTH*, parathyroid hormone.

Table 10.2 Anti-fracture efficacy of agents

	Vertebral Fractures	Hip Fractures	Non-vertebral Fractures
Alendronate	+	+	+
Risedronate	+	+	+
Ibandronate	+	–	*
Clodronate	+	–	+
Zoledronate	+	+	+
Strontium ranelate	+	*	+
Raloxifene	+	–	–
Denosumab	+	+	+
Teriparatide	+	–	+
PTH 1–84	+	–	–

+ proven efficacy; – no efficacy; * proven efficacy in subsets of patients by post-hoc analyses; *PTH*, parathyroid hormone.

tion in ambulatory capacity, so surgical fixation or hip replacement are usually necessary. Vertebral fractures are also associated with significant morbidity. Although they can be asymptomatic initially, they can result in height loss, kyphotic deformity, long-term pain, as well as impaired ambulation and balance. Once a fracture occurs, the risk of a subsequent fragility fracture at the most common sites is increased regardless of BMD. Multiple vertebral fractures increase the risk of pneumonia and death. Moreover, patients with acquired high disability often develop depression and anxiety.

The goal of therapeutic interventions is to reduce fracture risk in order to preserve the QoL of patients. This aim can be achieved by reducing bone resorption or by enhancing bone formation. The common therapeutic options include anabolic agents and antiresorptive agents. Anabolic agents affect bone formation by increasing the numbers of osteoblast precursors, stimulating the maturation of osteoblasts, and augmenting the function or survival of osteoblasts. Antiresorptive agents affect bone strength by enhancing the programmed cell death (apoptosis) of osteoclasts. Many agents with proven anti-fracture efficacy are available. Bisphosphonates (BPs), hormone replacement therapy (HRT), selective estrogen receptor modulators (SERMs), strontium ranelate (SR) and inhibitors of the receptor activator of nuclear factor-kappa B ligand (RANKL)) are antiresorptive agents. Analogs of parathyroid hormone (PTH) are anabolic agents (Table 10.1). Alendronate, risedronate, zoledronic acid, denosumab and SR reduce the prevalence of vertebral and non-vertebral and hip fractures (Table 10.2).

10.2 Antiresorptive Treatments

10.2.1 Bisphosphonates (BPs)

BPs are the first-line therapy for osteoporosis. BPs are utilized for the treatment of several other metabolic bone diseases characterized by altered osteoclastic function and bone fragility (e.g., Paget's disease of bone, multiple myeloma, bone metastasis, malignancy-related hypercalcemia).

Table 10.3 Formulations of bisphosphonates

Drug	Dosage and Route of Administration				
	Oral			Intramuscular	Intravenous
	Daily	Weekly	Monthly		
Alendronate	10 mg	70 mg			
Risedronate		35 mg	150 mg		
Ibandronate			150 mg		3 mg every 3 months
Clodronate				100 mg weekly or 200 mg every 14 days	
Zoledronate					5 mg every 12 months

Their use has been growing steadily in the last two decades because of the: introduction of simpler dosing regimens; availability of lower-priced generic agents; growing concerns about the safety of long-term treatment with other antiresorptive approaches.

BPs inhibit osteoclastic activity. They are pyrophosphate analogs, and the P-C-P structure acts as a "bone hook" that enables these compounds to bind avidly the hydroxyapatite crystals on the bone surface (particularly at sites of active bone remodeling). Binding potency and antiresorptive efficacy differ among various compounds. The side chains of the structure influence the binding affinity (R1 side chain) and the antiresorptive potency (R2 side chain); modification of these side chains allows for of the development of various agents. The older class of BPs includes non-nitrogen-containing BPs (etidronate, clodronate, tiludronate). They inhibit osteoclastic activity by producing toxic analogs of adenosine triphosphate (ATP), which cause cell death. Second-generation BPs include nitrogen-containing BPs (alendronate, risedronate, ibandronate, pamidronate, neridronate, zoledronate). They inhibit an enzyme called farnesyl pyrophosphate synthase (FPPS). This results in interference with a process called "prenylation" and the accumulation of unprenylated small GTPases (a large family of hydrolase enzymes that can bind and hydrolyze guanosine triphosphate (GTP)) within the osteoclast. This leads to a reduced resorptive activity of osteoclasts and accelerated apoptosis [1].

The clinical potency of nitrogen-containing BPs is dependent upon their binding affinity to hydroxyapatite, their electrical charge ("zeta potential") and their inhibition of FPPS. BPs in common use contain one or more nitrogen molecules in the R2 side chain. The order for binding affinity is zoledronate > alendronate > ibandronate > risedronate. Higher-affinity BPs bind strongly to the bone surface for a long time whereas lower-affinity compounds have a shorter residence time on bone after the withdrawal of treatment. The net result of osteoclast inhibition is a rapid and substantial decrease in the markers of bone turnover in association with an increase in BMD.

Each BP has a unique profile of binding affinity and antiresorptive efficacy that is probably responsible for meaningful differences in clinical characteristics. These include the: speed of onset and offset of effect; degree of reduction of bone turnover; types of anti-fracture effect (vertebral or non-vertebral). They can be administered *via* the oral (daily, weekly, monthly), intramuscular (weekly, monthly) or intravenous (quarterly, yearly) routes (Table 10.3). When taken orally, they must be taken with only water after a prolonged fast (usually in the morning), followed by 30–50 min nil-by-mouth to ensure adequate absorption. Usually, <1% of an orally administered dose of BPs is absorbed; food or anything containing divalent cations completely blocks their absorption. BPs do not have a systemic metabolism and their half-life in plasma is short. Fifty percent of the absorbed dose binds to bone surfaces (mostly avidly at sites of active remodeling); the 50% that does not bind to bone is excreted rapidly by the kidneys. After entering osteoclasts, BPs cause a loss of resorptive function and accelerate apoptosis. BPs may also have effects on osteocytes.

BPs have proven efficacy for the prevention of bone loss due to: aging; estrogen deficiency; glucocorticoid therapy and prevention of fractures in postmenopausal osteoporosis as well as in women and men with glucocorticoid-induced osteoporosis. Head-to-head studies with fracture as the primary outcome are lacking, so a direct comparison of efficacy between several compounds is not possible. However, among all BPs, only three (alendronate, risedronate, zoledronate) showed to reduce the risk of non-vertebral, vertebral and hip fractures [2].

10.2.1.1 Side Effects and Safety Profiles of BPs

BPs offer safe and effective treatment to reduce fracture risk at spinal, hip and non-vertebral sites. They are well-tolerated in most patients with osteoporosis, and the benefits of treatment outweigh the risks. Nevertheless, since their initial introduction in the USA in 1995, some severe adverse events to BPs have been documented even when they have been prescribed and used correctly. The side effects described include esophageal cancer, atrial fibrillation, musculoskeletal pain, atypical fractures and osteonecrosis of the jaw (ONJ); these appear to be rare and may not be caused by BP use [3]. The most common reasons for stopping therapy are gastrointestinal side effects (dyspepsia, esophagitis, esophageal reflux, duodenitis, gastritis, nausea).

Orally administered BPs may irritate the esophagus, and should be avoided in patients who cannot remain upright and in those with active upper gastrointestinal symptoms, including delayed esophageal emptying (achalasia, severe dysmotility). Over the past two decades, some cases of esophageal cancer among patients receiving oral BP therapy have been reported to the Food and Drug Administration (FDA) in the USA. The median time from use to the diagnosis appears to be 1–2 years. These reports lacked details about the risk factors for esophageal cancer in patients and in the control group, which makes the association between esophageal cancer and BPs use quite speculative. The *rationale* for a possible association between esophageal cancer and BP use derives from evidence that this class of medication can cause erosive esophagitis as well as persistent mucosal abnormalities. Further studies investigating the potential risk of carcinogenicity are needed, but current data do not support a cause–effect relationship between oral administration of BPs and esophageal carcinoma.

Approximately 40% of patients receiving their first intravenous dose or monthly oral dose of nitrogen-containing BPs experience an acute phase reaction (APR) with influenza-like illnesses (pyrexia, myalgias, arthralgias, chills): it tends to resolve within 3 days and rarely recurs with repeated administration. Symptomatic management with non-steroidal anti-inflammatory drugs (NSAIDs) and acetaminophen is usually sufficient. The underlying mechanism of an APR comprises increased production of cytokines with a transient, immune-driven response. Ocular inflammations such as conjunctivitis, uveitis, iritis, scleritis and episcleritis have been described (more with intravenous than oral formulations) but are rare. A short course of corticosteroid treatment can resolve ocular inflammation. In cases of scleritis, BP administration must be discontinued. Avoidance of BPs or caution in their use for patients with a history of inflammatory eye disease is recommended. Hypocalcemia may occur, particularly in cases of rapid parenteral administration of BPs (oncology setting) but it is usually mild and not clinically evident in patients treated for osteoporosis.

The only route of elimination for BPs is through the kidney. However, little information on dosing is available in subjects with impaired renal function. BPs appear to be safe and effective in individuals with modestly reduced renal function. However, due to lack of outcome data in such patients the FDA recommend avoidance of these medications in patients with creatinine clearance <30–35 mL/min. Adverse effects on renal function seem to be related primarily to the peak concentration (determined by the dose and infusion rate). The risk of renal toxicity may increase with rapid intravenous administration, and it can be reduced by adequate hydration and prolongation of the infusion rate. Dosage adjustment is not necessary in patients with mild or moderate renal impairment. However, there are inadequate data in patients with more severe chronic kidney disease or end-stage renal failure. Severe pain in bones, joints and muscles are the potential (but rare) adverse effects of BPs that may occur at any point after starting therapy, but which are especially observed during the first weeks of treatment. The underlying mechanism is unknown, and evidence supporting a causal relationship with BPs use is lacking. The FDA recommends that patients inform their physician if such symptoms occur, and in this case the medication should be stopped.

BPs reduce the prevalence of osteoporotic-associated fractures. However, in the past 5 years, several reports have described unusual low-energy subtrochanteric femoral fractures and pelvic-insufficiency fractures, with delayed healing, in patients on long-term BP therapy. This may be due to long-term over-suppression of bone turnover resulting in impaired bone remodeling, accumulation of micro-damage, or increased skeletal fragility. These fractures are typically associated with prodromal pain in the region of the fracture and are frequently bilateral. Characteristic radiographic findings include cortical hypertrophy, a transverse fracture pattern, and medial-cortical spiking. The observed association between long-term BP use and atypical femoral fractures does not prove causality, and additional large-scale studies are needed to elucidate this issue. More definitive data regarding adequate duration of therapy in selected individuals would be critical, but concern about atypical fractures should not lead to the withdrawal of BP therapy in the vast majority of post-menopausal women.

The first suggestion that BPs could elicit an increased incidence in atrial fibrillation (AF) came from the Health Outcomes and Reduced Incidence with Zoledronic Acid Once Yearly-Pivotal Fracture Trial (HORIZON-PVT). In this trial, more patients in the zoledronate group developed arrhythmia compared with those in the placebo group. Reappraisal of the data from the primary licensed trial showed a non-significant trend toward an increase in AF in the alendronate group, but not in the risedronate group, in the Fracture Intervention Trial. There are some data linking previous use of BPs with an increased risk of AF as a serious adverse event but the available information does not confirm a consistent association. The overall evidence does not support a causal relationship. Moreover, there is no convincing mechanism to explain this effect, which appears to be independent of the dose and duration of therapy. The FDA recommends that physicians do not alter their prescribing patterns for BPs while continuing to monitor post-marketing reports of AF.

ONJ is a known complication after radiation therapy in the maxillofacial region for cancer of the head or neck. Recently, cases of ONJ have been reported at an increasing incidence in association with the administration of BPs, especially in patients with multiple myeloma or metastatic bone disease. ONJ related to BP use is defined as exposed necrotic bone in the maxillofacial region that does not heal after 6–8 weeks in patients exposed to BP treatment without a history of craniofacial radiation therapy. Predisposing factors are dental extraction or other invasive dental procedures, poorly fitting dentures or bony exostoses. Possible signs and symptoms include pain, swelling, paresthesias, suppuration, soft-tissue ulceration, intra-oral/extra-oral sinus tracks, and teeth loosening. Epidemiological data suggest an incidence of ONJ in subjects under BP treatment *via* the oral route ranging from 1:10,000 (in Australia and Israel) to 1:250,000 (in Germany) to 1:160,000 worldwide. A higher incidence has been noted in cancer patients exposed to high intravenous doses of BPs at short intervals. The pathophysiology of ONJ is poorly understood. Possible ethiopathogenetic mechanisms include oversuppression of bone turnover due to accumulation of BPs in the jaw bone. This leads to the development of microcracks, osteocyte death and matrix necrosis in association with inhibition of T-cell function and inhibition of angiogenesis. According to the American Dental Association as well as the American Association of Oral and Maxillofacial Surgeons Taskforce on BP-associated ONJ, patients who are starting or taking

BPs should be informed about all the risks of treatment (including a low risk of ONJ). Regular dental visits and maintenance of good oral hygiene are recommended for everyone, as well as encouraging routine dental cleaning and restorative procedures. If dental treatment is needed, it should progress stepwise (if possible). Patients with periodontal disease should receive appropriate non-surgical therapy. Patients starting BPs who need invasive dental procedures should have procedures done and healing should be complete before starting (if possible). Patients already taking a BP may undergo to some time off therapy, even though there is no evidence that this will improve outcomes. However, invasive surgical procedures should be avoided, especially in patients receiving BPs *via* the intravenous route for cancer [4].

10.2.1.2 Duration of BP Treatment and "Drug Holidays"

There has been considerable discussion about the duration of BP treatment. Approval of BPs in USA was based on studies of 3–4-year duration or more, some of which have been extended. BPs bind avidly to bone, so these drugs can accumulate in the skeleton and create a "reservoir", leading to continued release from bone for months or years after treatment has stopped, resulting in a lingering, anti-fracture benefit. Studies with risedronate and alendronate confirmed that, if treatment is stopped after 3–5 years, there is a persistent anti-fracture efficacy of ≥1–2 years. This effect could enable drug holidays (i.e., time-off from BP therapy) for patients after a course of some years, with resumption of therapy if a significant loss of BMD or a new fracture occurs. The duration of treatment and the length of the drug holiday should be tailored to individual circumstances (including the risk of fracture and the binding affinity of each compound used). Although strong evidence is lacking, some time-off treatment should be offered to most patients on long-term BP therapy. Patients at mild risk of fracture could stop treatment after 5 years and remain off therapy as long as BMD is stable and fractures do not occur. Higher-risk patients should be treated for ≈10 years period, followed by a BPs holiday of 1–2 years, and perhaps be on a non-BP treatment during that time [3].

10.2.2 Strontium Ranelate (SR)

SR has been approved for the treatment of post-menopausal osteoporosis in European countries since 2004. This compound consists of two atoms of strontium (inorganic component) and ranelic acid (organic moiety). It exerts its unique effects by substituting calcium ions in the hydroxyapatite crystal. Of all the medical agents used for osteoporosis treatment, SR is the only one with a dual effect: it acts by stimulating bone formation and decreasing bone resorption. *In vitro*, SR has been shown to enhance osteoblastic activity and osteoclastic apoptosis involving the osteoprotegerin/receptor activator of nuclear factor-kappa B ligand (OPG/RANKL) system in favor of OPG.

Clinical trials have demonstrated that SR treatment (2 g/day) over 5 years results in increased BMD at all sites in post-menopausal women with osteoporosis in association with a reduction in vertebral and non-vertebral fractures (including the hip). A recent 5-year, open-label extension of the Spinal Osteoporosis Therapeutic Intervention (SOTI) and Treatment Of Peripheral Osteoporosis (TROPOS) studies supported the maintenance of anti-fracture efficacy over 10 years with SR in post-menopausal osteoporosis, and confirmed sustained increases in BMD over 10 years with a good safety profile [5]. Nevertheless, strontium has a higher atomic number compared with calcium (38 *versus* 20, respectively). Hence, the increased X-ray attenuation may lead to an artificial increase in BMD as measured by DEXA. SR is administered orally (2.0 g daily) with a bioavailability of 27%, and is excreted by the kidneys. Its absorption is reduced by foods such as dairy products, so it should be administered between meals or, preferably, at bedtime.

10.2.2.1 Side Effects and Safety Profile of SR

The most common side effects correlated with the use of SR are nausea, diarrhea, headache and dermatitis. In the SOTI study, 6% of subjects treated with SR showed nausea and diarrhea compared with 3% in the placebo group. Less common effects are: abdominal pains; irritations of oral mucous membranes; muscle pains; fainting; and memory loss. A slight (but significant) increased risk of thromboembolic events was noted from pooled data in phase-III studies, but this result was not supported by a large retrospective observational study. Contraindications to SR administration are renal insufficiency (creatinine clearance <30 mL/min) and an increased risk of venous thromboembolic disease. Moreover, SR should not be associated with drugs such as tetracyclines or chinolones [6]. A few cases (18 reported in Europe, including 2 deaths) of a hypersensitivity reaction (drug rash with eosinophilia and systemic symptoms, DRESS, syndrome) have been described in association with SR treatment. DRESS syndrome is a severe drug reaction characterized by: fever; skin eruptions; hypereosinophilia; lymphocytosis; abnormal liver and renal function; pulmonary and cardiac involvement. The prevalence of mortality is 10%; symptoms usually occur 3–7 weeks after drug consumption. It is hypothesized that DRESS syndrome is triggered by concomitant use of other drugs or concomitant infections. Dress syndrome is an indication for discontinuation of SR treatment, and it can be treated with high doses of corticosteroids [7].

10.2.3 HRT

HRT involves the administration of estrogens alone or in combination with progestins. The indication for post-menopausal osteoporosis is controversial. The Women's Health Initiative (WHI) trial on estrogen replacement therapy was the first large-scale, randomized, controlled study in healthy women aged 50–79 years [8]. This study showed a reduction in the risk of hip and vertebral porotic fractures under estrogen treatment. The positive effects on fractures were offset by long-term side-effects such as vascular events and breast cancer, which limit its widespread use and indication for osteoporosis [9].

10.2.4 SERMs

Selective Estrogen Receptor Modulators (SERMs) are non-steroidal synthetic compounds that bind to estrogen receptors. SERMS induce conformational changes in these receptors, promoting interactions with distinct intranuclear proteins and resulting in estrogen-like and estrogen-antagonistic effects.

Raloxifene is a second-generation SERM. It was the first a second-generation SERM to be approved for the treatment of post-menopausal osteoporosis. It produces agonist effects on bone and the liver as well as antagonistic effects in the breast and genitourinary apparatus. Raloxifene (60 mg per day, p.o.) prevents post-menopausal bone loss, increases BMD, and decreases the risk of vertebral fracture in post-menopausal women with osteoporosis in association with a reduction in the risk of invasive breast cancer. The effectiveness of raloxifene on fractures has been documented in several studies. The Multiple Outcomes of Raloxifene Evaluation (MORE) study demonstrated its effectiveness on vertebral fractures, with no effects on non-vertebral fractures. The MORE study lasted 4 years but was extended for 3 years in the Continuing Outcomes Relevant to Evista (CORE) trial. At the end of these studies, raloxifene therapy showed to lead to an increase of 2.2% and 3% in BMD at the spine and at the total hip, respectively, compared with placebo; the difference in the incidence of non-vertebral fractures was not significant. Other effects of raloxifene were a 58% decrease in the incidence of breast cancer (relative risk (RR) = 0.42; 95% confidence interval (CI), 0.29–0.60) compared with the placebo group. However, non-significant differences were found for the endometrial effects (hyperplasia, cancer, vaginal bleeding) and deep venous thrombosis (DVT) risk with raloxifene compared with the placebo group. The most common unpleasant effects of raloxifene are an increase in menopausal vasomotor phenomena and cramps in the limbs, but the most serious side effects are an increased risk of thromboembolic events and fatal strokes [10].

Bazedoxifene is a third-generation SERM characterized by tissue-selective activities that confer positive effects on the metabolism of bone and lipids without adverse effects on breast or uterine tissues. A 5-year, randomized, placebo-controlled study supported the sustained anti-fracture effects of bazedoxifene on new vertebral fractures in post-menopausal osteoporotic women and on non-vertebral fractures in a higher-risk subgroup of women in association with a significant increase in BMD and reduced bone turnover compared with that seen with placebo. The incidence of hot flushes, leg cramps and venous thromboembolic events after administration of bazedoxifene (20 mg per day, p.o.) is similar to that seen with raloxifene. Bazedoxifene also improves lipid profiles by reducing the serum concentrations of total cholesterol and low-density lipoprotein-cholesterol, with an increase in the serum level of high-density lipoprotein-cholesterol [11].

Lasofoxifene is a third-generation SERM. Its efficacy in post-menopausal osteoporotic women has been demonstrated in an international placebo-controlled trial: Postmenopausal Evaluation and Risk-Reduction with Lasofoxifene (PEARL). After 5 years of treatment, patients who received lasofoxifene (0.5 mg/day) had a 42% and 24% lower RR of vertebral and non-vertebral fractures respectively, compared with the placebo group. Patients in the lasofoxifene treatment group also experienced modest (but significant) increases in BMD at the lumbar spine, femoral neck, and total hip. Similar to other SERMs, lasofoxifene use was associated with a higher incidence of DVT, pulmonary embolism, uterine polyps, and endometrial hypertrophy, but also reduced the risk of breast cancer, coronary heart disease, and stroke. Lasofoxifene is administered via the oral route at 0.5 mg per day [12].

10.2.5 Denosumab

Denosumab has a novel mechanism of action. It exerts proven efficacy in increasing BMD and reducing fracture risk in: post-menopausal women with osteoporosis; men receiving androgen-deprivation therapy for non-metastatic prostate cancer; women receiving adjuvant aromatase inhibitor therapy for breast cancer. Denosumab is a human monoclonal antibody to RANKL. RANKL is a cytokine member of the tumor necrosis factor family expressed by cells of the osteoblast lineage. It has been identified as the principal regulator of osteoclastic bone resorption. When RANKL binds to its receptor (RANK) on the membranes of osteoclasts and pre-osteoclasts, it stimulates their formation, activity, and survival, thereby increasing the rate of bone resorption. OPG is also expressed by osteoblasts. It is a counter-regulatory non-signaling "decoy receptor" for RANKL. The binding of RANKL to OPG reduces the amount of RANKL available for binding to RANK, resulting in a decrease in the formation, activity, and survival of osteoclasts. Thereby, the balance between RANKL and OPG is a key regulator of the rate of bone resorption. Evidence that high levels of RANKL are associated with increased bone resorption and bone loss suggest that inhibition of RANKL might be an effective treatment for skeletal diseases characterized by high bone turnover (including osteoporosis). Denosumab binds with high affinity to RANKL similarly to OPG, preventing interaction of RANKL with its receptor, RANK, which is present on the surface of osteoclasts and their precursors. The inhibition of formation, activity, and survival of osteoclasts obtained decreases bone resorption in trabecular and cortical bone. Denosumab is indicated for the treatment of women with post-menopausal osteoporosis who are at high risk of fracture (defined by the FDA as a history of osteoporotic fracture, multiple risk factors for fracture, or patients resistant or who are intolerant to other available anti-osteoporosis therapy).

10.2.5.1 Efficacy of Denosumab

The rapid, profound, sustained, and reversible decrease in the serum levels of bone turnover markers (BTMs) such as N-telopeptide of collagen type 1 (NTX) and bone-specific alkaline phosphatase (BSAP) observed in a phase-I study of denosumab supported further investigation of the efficacy and safety of this antiresorptive compound as a potential treatment for osteoporosis.

A randomized, placebo-controlled, dose-ranging phase-II study evaluated the effects of denosumab in post-menopausal women with low BMD. It showed that BMD in the lumbar spine increased significantly at 12 months with significant increases at other measured skeletal sites (including total hip and distal third of the radius).

The Fracture Reduction Evaluation of Denosumab in Osteoporosis Every 6 Months (FREEDOM) trial was an international, 3-year, randomized, double-blind, placebo-controlled phase-III trial in 7,868 post-menopausal women with osteoporosis randomized to receive denosumab (60 mg, s.c.) or placebo every 6 months. The primary endpoint of efficacy was new vertebral fractures at 36 months; the secondary endpoints were time to first hip fracture and non-vertebral fracture. Denosumab-treated patients showed, significant (68%) reduction in the risk of new vertebral fractures 40% reduction in the risk of hip fractures, and 20% reduction in the risk of non-vertebral fractures, compared with placebo.

Another phase-III study, Denosumab Fortifies Bone Density (DEFEND) evaluated the efficacy of denosumab for stabilizing or increasing BMD in post-menopausal women with osteopenia. Subjects were randomized to receive denosumab (60 mg, s.c.) or placebo every 6 months, with a primary endpoint of efficacy of percentage change in BMD in the lumbar spine at 24 months compared with placebo. Denosumab significantly increased BMD at the lumbar spine, total hip, distal third of the radius, and total body compared with placebo at 24 months. After drug discontinuation, the increase in BMD was reversed completely. Determining Efficacy: Comparison of Initiating Denosumab Versus Alendronate (DECIDE) was a head-to-head comparison of the effects of denosumab and alendronate (the most commonly prescribed BPs for the treatment of osteoporosis). Subjects were randomized to receive denosumab (60 mg, s.c.) every week plus placebo (p.o.) or alendronate (70 mg, p.o.) weekly plus placebo injections (s.c.) every 6 months. At 12 months, subjects treated with denosumab had a significantly greater BMD increase at the total hip and at all other measured skeletal sites compared with alendronate. Reductions in BTM levels were significantly greater with denosumab than with alendronate. A significant increase in BMD at different skeletal sites was observed with denosumab in women with breast cancer under aromatase-inhibitor treatment. Moreover, increased BMD at all sites in men receiving androgen-deprivation therapy for prostate cancer was described after 24 months in comparison with placebo. In addition, fracture risk was reduced significantly at 36 months. Interestingly, this beneficial effect started after 1 month and was maintained for 3 years [13].

10.2.5.2 Side Effects and Safety Profile of Denosumab

In general, denosumab is well tolerated with total adverse events and serious adverse events similar to those seen with placebo. The benefit of treatment with denosumab is likely to outweigh the risks in women with post-menopausal osteoporosis at high risk for fracture. Denosumab was approved for this indication at 60 mg by subcutaneous injection every 6 months. Safety has been evaluated in all of the denosumab clinical trials and their extensions.

In a report of a phase-I study of denosumab in healthy post-menopausal women, there were no related serious adverse events and no discontinuations from the study due to adverse events. A mild transient hypocalcemia and corresponding increases in serum intact PTH levels has been observed. Infectious adverse events were similar in denosumab (38%) and placebo (33%) groups. Two subjects treated with denosumab showed mild injection-site reactions. There were no changes in the counts for white blood cells, T-cells, B-cells, or natural killer cells, immunoglobulins, or coagulation parameters in association with denosumab treatment.

The four-year data for a phase-II study of denosumab in post-menopausal women with low BMD reported a similar prevalence of all adverse events and all serious adverse events in the placebo, denosumab, and alendronate groups. The prevalence of malignant neoplasms was similar in all treatment groups. The overall prevalence of infections was similar in all treatment groups, but infections requiring hospitalization occurred in 3.2% of denosumab-treated patients and none of those who received placebo or alendronate. All infections were typical community-acquired infections that responded appropriately to standard antibiotic therapy. No patient developed neutralizing antibodies to denosumab.

In the FREEDOM trial, there were no significant differences in the total incidence of side effects between denosumab-treated patients and those receiving placebo. The overall risk of death, malignancies, infections, cardiovascular events, atrial fibrillation, stroke and hypocalcemia were similar between the two groups. There were no cases of ONJ. There was a theoretical safety concern that over-suppression of bone remodeling might increase fracture risk or impair fracture healing. There was, however, no evidence of adverse clinical consequences due to suppression of bone turnover observed with denosumab. Significant differences were seen with several skin-related conditions. Eczema was reported in 3.0% of denosumab-treated patients compared with 1.7% in the placebo group. Cellulitis as a serious adverse event was more common with denosumab (0.3%) than placebo; cellulitis as an adverse event was similar in both groups. The prevalence of falling and concussion was probaly less common with denosumab than with placebo. Hence, the tolerability of denosumab is excellent and the long dosing interval of 6 months is likely to be attractive to patients with poor compliance to the more frequent requirements for other antiresorptive compounds. It has ben reported that adherence (defined as meeting the study criteria for compliance and persistence) was significantly greater with denosumab than with alendronate [14].

10.3 Anabolic Treatment

10.3.1 PTH Analogs

The evidence of striking clinical benefits of intermittent, low-dose administration of PTH in osteoporosis introduced a new era for the medical treatment of osteoporosis: the era of skeletal anabolic agents. The use of PTH as a skeletal anabolic agent in the treatment of post-menopausal osteoporosis is relatively recent. Only two forms of PTH are licensed for this purpose: teriparatide (a recombinant formulation of endogenous PTH containing a 34-amino-acid sequence which is identical to the N-terminal portion of the human hormone (rhPTH 1–34)) and a full-length PTH (PTH 1–84) manufactured using a strain of *Escherichia coli* modified by recombinant DNA technology. In Europe, both are available for the treatment of osteoporosis in post-menopausal women at the highest risk for fracture, whereas in the USA only teriparatide is approved for treatment of post-menopausal osteoporosis. Teriparatide has also been approved for primary or hypogonadal osteoporosis in men at high fracture risk as well as glucocorticoid-induced osteoporosis (GIOP) in men and women. Teriparatide and PTH 1–84 are given as a subcutaneous injection once daily into the thigh or abdominal wall at 20 μg and 100 μg, respectively. They are not approved for use >24 months. Their high cost (more than the other anti-porotic drugs) limits their selection for high-risk osteoporotic patients such as those with previous fragility fractures, severe osteoporosis, and lack of efficacy or intolerance to BPs. The exclusion of metabolic bone diseases other than osteoporosis is crucial before initiating therapy because PTH analogs are not indicated for metabolic bone disease other than osteoporosis.

The anabolic effect of PTH in cancellous bone in primary hyperparathyroidism was suspected as long as 20 years ago. When considering the significant bone loss that occurs with hyperparathyroidism, the use of PTH analogs as anabolic agents may initially seem counterintuitive because it is well known that PTH acts directly through the PTH receptor type 1 (PTHR1) on osteoblasts. It then stimulates bone formation and also indirectly stimulates the differentiation and development of osteoclast cells, leading to active bone resorption by increasing the RANKL/OPG gene-expression ratio. Continuously high levels of PTH stimulate generalized bone turnover to mobilize calcium from the bone and accelerate bone loss. However, pulsatile exposure to lower doses (which occurs with once-daily dosing with PTH analogs) enhances bone formation (possibly due to the inhibition of osteoblast apoptosis or the transformation of bone-lining cells back to functional osteoblasts), resulting in increased BMD and bone mass. Moreover, independently from growth hormone (GH) activity, PTH induces the synthesis of insulin-like growth factor 1 (IGF-1; a strong bone anabolic factor) in bone tissue. Simultaneously, PTH blocks the expression of the osteocyte-derived SOST protein sclerostine, which inhibits the activity of the Wnt–β-catenin pathway responsible for the promotion of many transcription processes, leading to the increased proliferation and activity of osteoblasts. All of these effects are reflected in bone-marker behavior with PTH-analog therapy. Levels of bone-formation markers rise more rapidly and peak within the first 3 months of therapy as compared with bone-resorption markers (which peak at 6 months). This overriding of bone formation *versus* bone resorption is referred to as the "anabolic window of PTH." Administration of PTH analogs also increases bone strength and the micro-architecture; skeletal improvements are more rapid and evident in areas of cancellous bone (lumbar spine) than in sites of cortical bone (radius and femoral neck).

10.3.2 Efficacy of PTH Analogs

The effects of teriparatide therapy on the risk of osteoporotic, vertebral and non-vertebral fractures in post-menopausal women were evaluated in the Fracture Prevention Trial (which involved 1,637 women with a diagnosis of post-menopausal osteoporosis). After 18 months of therapy with daily subcutaneous injections of teriparatide in 20-mg doses, a significant reduction in new fractures (vertebral by 65% and non-vertebral by 54% *versus* placebo) was demonstrated. Moreover, treatment with teriparatide resulted in significant, dose-dependent BMD increases in the lumbar spine, hip and whole skeleton compared with the control group.

The Treatment of Osteoporosis with PTH (TOP) study, with its Open Label Extension Study (OLES), and the PTH and Alendronate for Osteoporosis (PaTH) clinical trial, provided most of the data on the efficacy and safety of PTH (1–84), leading to its use in the treatment of post-menopausal osteoporosis. Similarly to teriparatide, a significant reduction in the prevalence of vertebral fractures, and a non-significant decrease in the prevalence of non-vertebral fractures has been observed in high-risk patients under treatment with PTH (1–84). In the PTH (1–84)-treated group, a significant increases in BMD in the lumbar spine, total hip and femoral neck has been observed, while at distal radius BMD decreased.

Multiple scenarios can occur when considering therapy with PTH analogs. They can be employed: after other prior therapies (sequential therapy); in those treated with other agents (combination therapy); in previously untreated patients ("treatment-naïve patients"). The reasons to consider switching therapy to teriparatide or PTH 1–84 may be a new fragility fracture or loss of BMD on current therapy, and/or drug intolerance. Regarding combination therapy, there are concerns about potential over-suppression of bone. The official viewpoint of the National Osteoporosis Foundation in the USA is that the added cost, unknown efficacy and potential side effects of combination therapy should be weighed against potential gains. Conversely, sequential therapy (use of PTH analogs after BPs or other antiresorptive compounds) is a common approach to porotic patients. Indeed, PTH analogs appear to retain their anabolic effect in post-menopausal women with osteoporosis previously treated with BPs for a long time. However, the benefits of sequential therapy are probably less than those seen in treatment-naïve patients, with fewer relative increases in BMD and markers of bone formation.

Finally, when comparing teriparatide with alendronate in naïve-post-menopausal osteoporotic women, teriparatide showed to increase BMD at all skeletal sites to a greater degree than alendronate (except for BMD at the distal third of the radius). The prevalence of non-vertebral fractures was significantly lower in the teriparatide-treated group than in the alendronate group. However, not many direct comparisons of fracture reduction can be made compared with other antiresorptive agents due to a lack of head-to-head studies focusing on fracture outcomes. In women and men with GIOP, teriparatide led to a greater increases in BMD in the lumbar spine as well as a favorable profile in preventing vertebral fractures when compared with alendronate therapy.

10.3.3 Side Effects and Safety Profile of PTH Analogs

In general, PTH analogs are well tolerated. Transient orthostatic hypotension may occur within 4 h of administration but it is usually limited to the first several doses. Dosing at bedtime helps to minimize this occurrence. Hypercalcemia and hypercalciuria are frequent (but transient) consequences of PTH treatment, and are usually well-controlled by reducing supplementation with calcium and vitamin D. Serum and urinary levels of calcium require only periodic assessment. Nausea, dizziness, headache, limb pain, and hyperuricemia can occur, but these are usually not sufficiently severe to require discontinuation of therapy. Post-marketing case reports of acute dyspnea, allergic reactions, facial and/or oral edema, hypercalcemia, injection-site reactions (bruising, pain, swelling), muscle spasm, and urticaria have also been documented. Compliance with treatment with PTH analogs can be limited by daily subcutaneous injection route of administration.

Few data are available about the use of these medications in patients with cardiovascular, hepatic, or liver disease, so caution should be applied in those with severe renal and hepatic impairment. Although it has not bee studied specifically, the clearance of PTH analogs is presumed to be identical to that of endogenous PTH, with metabolism mainly in the liver with excretion by the kidneys. Dosage adjustment is not required with renal insufficiency (though bioavailability and half-life may increase if creatinine clearance <30 mL/min). PTH analogs should also be used with caution in patients with active or recent urolithiasis, and in those under digitalis treatment. PTH analogs are contraindicated in case of hypercalcemia and hyperparathyroidism.

The pivotal registration trial for teriparatide was stopped due to the appearance of osteogenic sarcoma in all of the Fischer strains of rats receiving lifelong, high-dose teriparatide. This risk was related to the dose and duration of the medication. However, a limitation of these rat studies derived from very high doses were used in the short lifecycle of rats. The rats were also treated with relatively supra-therapeutic doses for their size. Subsequently, a repeat study was done by the same research team looking at osteosarcoma risks because it was related to age at treatment as well as dose range (3- and 60-times higher than that approved for human use). They found that, if doses more compatible with human use were used, an increased risk of osteosarcoma was not documented. Osteogenic sarcoma was also observed in PTH 1–84 preclinical data in rats, with a dose-responsive increased incidence.

Hence, it seems that there is no real concern about the carcinogenic action of PTH with dose and treatment duration approved in humans, but continuous monitoring is ongoing. As a result, use of PTH analogs should be avoided in patients with an increased baseline risk of osteosarcoma. This includes subjects with Paget's disease of bone, previous radiation therapy, unexplained elevations in levels of alkaline phosphatase, or in young adults with open epiphyses. Similarly, it should not be used in pregnant women. A theoretical potential exists for teriparatide to accelerate local tumor extension if non-primary bone tumors are unknowingly present in bone because anabolic therapy enhances bone remodeling. All of these findings has led to a hesitancy to use teriparatide in patients with active or recent non-osteosarcoma cancers that have a likelihood to metastasize to bone (e.g., breast, prostate, lung, thyroid, kidney) [15–18].

10.4 New Perspectives

Although many compounds are available, considerable emphasis is being placed in the development of new agents for the treatment of osteoporosis to obtain a better efficacy, tolerability, and simplicity of administration. Hence, new treatment modalities of osteoporosis (including

Table 10.4 New perspectives for medical treatment of porotic patients

Antiresorptive	Anabolic
Cathepsin K inhibitors: odanacatib	New delivery systems for parathyroid hormone
Src kinase inhibitors: saracatinib	Modulation of calcium-sensing receptor: ronacaleret
	Antibodies to sclerostin (Wnt antagonist)

novel antiresorptive and anabolic agents) are at various stages of development.

Novel antiresorptive agents include cathepsin K (CTSK) inhibitors such as odanacatib and Src kinase inhibitors such as saracatinib. Cathepsin K is a lysosomal cysteine protease that degrades type-I collagen, which is preferentially expressed by osteoclasts. *Ctsk* null mice exhibit increased trabecular and cortical bone volume. However, studies of the biomechanical properties of *Ctsk* null mice have been controversial. Src kinase is a non-receptor tyrosine kinase that has a role in the survival and activity of osteoclasts. In *Src* null mutants, osteoclasts do not form a "ruffled" border and do not resorb bone. Saracatinib is a novel, orally available competitive inhibitor of Src kinase that inhibits bone resorption *in vitro*.

Novel anabolic therapies involve the use of factors with anabolic properties for bone or the neutralization of antagonists of growth factors. The limitation of current PTH anabolic therapy is the need for daily subcutaneous administration. Thus, alternative delivery systems of PTH (e.g., oral, transdermal, intranasal) have been tested. Another approach consists in the stimulation of endogenous PTH secretion by oral agents (e.g., ronacaleret) that interfere with the calcium-sensing receptor on the parathyroid cell. A novel target for anabolic treatment of osteoporosis is the Wnt signaling pathway. The Wnt–β-catenin signaling pathway induces osteoblastogenesis and bone formation, and suppresses osteoclastogenesis and bone resorption. Antibodies to Wnt antagonists (e.g., sclerostin) are under study but non-specific Wnt activation could result in adverse effects, including increases in carcinogenesis in non-skeletal tissues [19]. The success of all of these compounds will be dependent upon their long-term effectiveness and safety profile (Table 10.4).

10.4.1 Supplementation with Vitamin D and Calcium

Adequate mineral nutrition, including daily supplementation with calcium and vitamin D, is a crucial prerequisite for successful treatment of porotic patients. Lack of calcium and/or vitamin D is a very common cause of a poor response to osteoporosis drug therapy and is associated with an increased risk of osteoporosis and fragility fractures *per se*. The mean daily intake of calcium in the general population is often insufficient (especially in the elderly) and hypovitaminosis D is very common. Calcium supplementation should be commensurate to the degree of nutritional deficiency (in general, 500–1,000 mg/day) and is contraindicated in the presence of increased risk of hypercalcemia and/or nephrolithiasis.

Recently, increases in the prevalence of cardiovascular events (particularly myocardial infarction) have been reported in women allocated calcium supplements. These data justify reassessment of the use of calcium supplements in older people. With regard to analogs of vitamin D, supplementation with 800–1,000 IU/day of cholecalciferol is recommended, with higher doses in the elderly and during winter, in order to obtain serum levels of 25-hydroxyvitamin D >75 nmol/L (30 ng/mL). Cholecalciferol can also be administered weekly (4,000–14,000 IU); monthly (25,000–50,000 IU); quarterly (50,000–300,000 IU); every 6 months or yearly (≥600,000). Active metabolites of vitamin D such as calcidiol or calcitriol are not indicated for the prevention of hypovitaminosis D because they enhance the risk of hypercalcemia and hypercalciuria. However, active metabolite represent the best option in selected cases (severe renal or hepatic dysfunction, severe intestinal malabsorption, hypoparathyroidism) [20].

10.5 Conclusions

Lifestyle factors (physical activity, sun exposure, avoidance of consumption of alcohol and tobacco) and ensuring adequate intake of calcium and vitamin D represent the baseline approaches for preventing and treating osteoporosis. Pharmacological treatments are recommended for subjects: with fragility fractures, with a T-score of BMD ≤2.5, currently taking high-dose corticosteroids for a long time.

Several antiresorptive and anabolic compounds are available. BPs are first-line therapy for established osteoporosis. Anabolic agents have a place in the management of severe osteoporosis and in specific forms characterized by the decreased formation and remodeling of bone (e.g., glucocorticoid-induced osteoporosis). Drug selection is guided by sex, menopausal status, medical and fracture history, patient preference and, in certain countries, eligibility for government subsidy. Osteoporosis is under-diagnosed and under-treated; compliance and persistence to treatment are often poor, resulting in a higher risk of fracture and greater healthcare costs. More effective communication between physicians and patients may enhance patient awareness of the balance of benefits and risks, and may improve adherence to therapy. Patient compliance is a critical factor to be considered when choosing agents. On a long-term basis, optimal anti-fracture effects can be obtained by using a tailored therapy, with an orchestrated sequence of anti-catabolic and bone-forming agents.

References

1. Russell RGG, Watts NB, Ebetino FH, Rogers MJ (2008) Mechanisms of action of bisphosphonates: similarities and differences and their potential influence on clinical efficacy. Osteoporos Int 19:733–759
2. Pazianas M, Epstein S, Zaidi M (2009) Evaluating the antifracture efficacy of bisphosphonates. Rev Recent Clin Trials 2:122–130
3. Watts NB, Diab DL (2010) Long-term use of bisphosphonates in osteoporosis. J Clin Endocrinol Metab 4:1555–1565
4. Shannon J, Shannon J, Modelevsky S, Grippo AA (2011) Bisphosphonates and osteonecrosis of the jaw. J Am Geriatr Soc 12:2350–2355
5. Reginster JY, Kaufman JM, Goemaere S et al (2012) Maintenance of antifracture efficacy over 10 years with strontium ranelate in postmenopausal osteoporosis. Osteoporos Int 3:1115–1122
6. Cesareo R, Napolitano C, Iozzino M (2010) Strontium ranelate in postmenopausal osteoporosis treatment: a critical appraisal. Int J Women's Health 2:1–6
7. Kinyó Á, Belso N, Nagy N et al (2011) Strontium ranelate-induced DRESS syndrome with persistent autoimmunehepatitis. Acta Derm Venereol 2:205–206.
8. Rossouw JE, Anderson GL, Prentice RL et al (2002) Risks and benefits of estrogen plus progestin in healthy postmenopausal women: principal results from the Women's Health Initiative randomized Controlled Trial. JAMA 288:321–333
9. Holloway D (2010) Clinical update on hormone replacement therapy. Br J Nurs 8:496, 498–504
10. Deal CL, Draper MW (2006) Raloxifene: a selective estrogen-receptor modulator for postmenopausal osteoporosis – a clinical update on efficacy and safety. Women's Health (Lond) 2:199–210
11. Silverman SL, Chines AA, Kendler DL et al; Bazedoxifene Study Group (2012) Sustained efficacy and safety of bazedoxifene in preventing fractures in postmenopausal women with osteoporosis: results of a 5-year, randomized, placebo-controlled study. Osteoporos Int 23:351–363
12. Cummings SR, Ensrud K, Delmas PD et al; PEARL Study Investigators (2010) Lasofoxifene in postmenopausal women with osteoporosis. N Engl J Med 362:686–696
13. Tsourdi E, Rachner TD, Rauner M, Hamann C, Hofbauer LC (2011) Denosumab for bone diseases: translating bone biology into targeted therapy. Eur J Endocrinol 6:833–840
14. Lewiecki EM (2011) Safety and tolerability of denosumab for the treatment of postmenopausal osteoporosis. Drug Healthc Patient Saf 3:79–91
15. Han SL, Wan SL (2012) Effect of teriparatide on bone mineral density and fracture in postmenopausal osteoporosis: meta-analysis of randomised controlled trials. Int J Clin Pract 2:199–209
16. Pietrogrande L (2010) Update on the efficacy, safety, and adherence to treatment of full length parathyroid hormone, PTH (1-84), in the treatment of postmenopausal osteoporosis. Int J Women's Health 1:193–203
17. Carpinteri R, Porcelli T, Mejia C, Patelli I, Bilezikian JP, Canalis E, Angeli A, Giustina A, Mazziotti G (2010) Glucocorticoid-induced osteoporosis and parathyroid hormone. J Endocrinol Invest 33 (7 Suppl):16–21
18. Sikon A, Batur P (2010) Profile of teriparatide in the management of postmenopausal osteoporosis. Int J Women's Health 2:37–44
19. Canalis E (2010) New treatment modalities in osteoporosis. Endocr Pract 5:855–863
20. Adami S, Bertoldo F, Brandi ML et al; Società Italiana dell'Osteoporosi, del Metabolismo Minerale e delle Malattie dello Scheletro (2009) Guidelines for the diagnosis, prevention and treatment of osteoporosis. Reumatismo 4:260–284

Vertebroplasty and Spinal Tumors

11

Luigi Manfrè, Gianluigi Guarnieri
and Mario Muto

11.1 Introduction

The spine can be affected by several primary or secondary tumors, with progressive osteolysis of each part of the vertebra (i.e., posterior arch, pedicles, body), causing unsustainable local pain and motor impairment secondary to vertebral collapse [1]. In the last decade, prolongation of life expectancy in patients affected by neoplastic disease has been responsible for an increase in vertebral metastases, particularly in the case of cancer of the breast, lung, kidney and prostate cancer [2]. Approximately 70% of patients with secondary lesions have at least one vertebral lesion [3] (Table 11.1). Moreover, because of the improvement in survival related to implementation of cancer treatment, most methods (including vertebroplasty) have changed from being end-of-life palliative care to become part of management of chronic disease [4].

Pain is the main symptom related to vertebral tumors, not only related to bony weakness of the vertebra, but also to the local periosteum and paravertebral tissues. In general, the pain is: drug-resistant; unrelated to mechanical distress; present even in the resting position. It usually precedes extravertebral spread of the tumor as well as radicular and spinal cord syndrome related to compression fracture.

11.2 Diagnosis

Symptoms of spinal metastases are the initial presentation of the disease in ≥20% of patients affected by neoplastic disease [5]. Despite care-

Table 11.1 Classification of spinal tumors

Benign	Malignant
Hemangioma	Solitary
Osteoid osteoma	Chordoma
Aneurysmal bone cyst (ABC)	Chondrosarcoma
Osteochondroma	Ewing's sarcoma
Osteoblastoma	Plasmacytoma
Eosinophilic granuloma	Multiple
Hemangiopericitoma	Multiple myeloma
Giant cell tumor	Lymphoma
	Leukemia

M. Muto (✉)
Neuroradiology Department, A. Cardarelli Hospital,
Naples, Italy
e-mail: mutomar2@gmail.com

M. Muto (ed.), *Interventional Neuroradiology of the Spine*,
DOI 10.1007/978-88-470-2790-9_11, © Springer-Verlag Italia 2013

ful evaluation of clinical findings such as motor and sensory impairment, abnormal reflexes and pain can be useful if one suspects neoplastic involvement in the spine [6]. The correct diagnosis is usually achieved using conventional computed tomography (CT) and magnetic resonance imaging (MRI), particularly in patients with a known history of cancer, with vertebral bone biopsy being undertaken in case of solitary lesions with equivocal radiological findings. Detailed history-taking, physical examination, bone scintigraphy and total-body CT enables the primary disease to be identified in 85% of cases; additional bone biopsy can bring this figure up to 93% [7]. Thanks to more precise selection of the targeted area required for analyses, CT-guided biopsy enables the correct histological diagnosis to be reached in 93% of cases [8]. Plain radiographs are not considered appropriate for the diagnosis because lesions are detected in only 30% of cases [9]. CT, despite excellent accuracy in the detection of bony abnormalities, shows moderate sensitivity (about 66%) [10], but remains fundamental for planning vertebroplasty. In fact, the size and location of lytic lesions is important to assess the risk of vertebral collapse in patients with vertebral disease. Hence, careful evaluation in multiple planes of the vertebra affected by the tumor is fundamental for CT studies, if augmentation with polymethylmethacrylate (PMMA) is being considered. According to Taneichi and coworkers, the risk of sudden collapse of a vertebra at the thoracic level is higher in the case of vertebral body (VB) involvement (>60%) and in the case of 30% destruction of the VB if there is involvement of the costovertebral joint. In patients with lumbar involvement, lesions involving 35–40% of the VB, and those with only 20–25% VB destruction associated with involvement of the posterior arch and/or pedicle are considered to be at high risk rate for vertebra collapse [11]. MRI is the ideal method for demonstrating neoplastic involvement of the spine, with a sensitivity and specificity of 98.5% and 98.9%, respectively [11]. Hence, study of the entire spine, including T1-weighted spin echo (SE) and T2-weighted short T1 inversion recovery (STIR), is preferred in cases of suspected neoplastic disease [6], with enhanced imaging to be added if extravertebral tumor spread is suspected.

11.3 Conventional Treatment

Management of spinal tumors includes medical therapy (corticosteroids, chemotherapy), radiotherapy and surgical treatment. Therapy is according to the histological type as well as the location and size of the tumor. Even though pain relief can be achieved in ≤71% of treated patients [12], chemo-radiotherapy has delayed efficacy [13] and surgery is not always possible. Moreover, despite the high prevalence of success in reduction/resolution of tumor size with chemotherapy and/or radiotherapy, the immediate risk of vertebral fracture remains. Despite being palliative in the case of metastatic disease, surgical management of spinal tumors is proposed for compression of the spinal cord (laminectomy, corpectomy, *en bloc* resection), spinal instability and severe pain [14].

11.4 Augmentation Treatment

Vertebral augmentation has been validated as an excellent procedure for increasing spinal stability if spine osteolysis occurs. The pain resolution observed with vertebral augmentation is almost immediate. With respect to the safety, feasibility and efficacy of vertebroplasty, it should be considered to be part of conventional analgesic treatment [15], thereby reducing narcotic use for all stages of the disease [16]. With regard to surgery, augmentation procedures should be carried out before chemo-radiotherapy [17] to reduce tumor size and to allow the patient to better tolerate anti-tumor therapies [4]. Pain relief after vertebroplasty has been reported to 84–92% [18], with asymptomatic paravertebral leakage accounting for 4–9.2% [19, 20].

Augmentation in the case of an osteolytic vertebral tumor has two aims: mechanical stabilization of the vertebra (preventing creep deformation of the VB and complications related to neural compression) and resolution of the focal

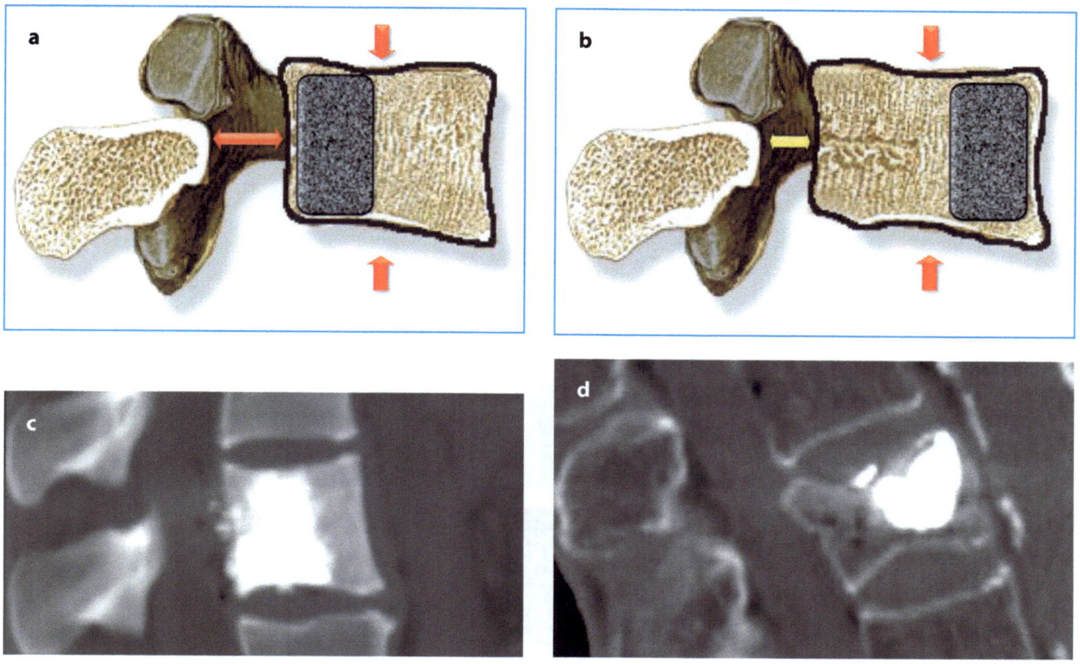

Fig. 11.1 Best position to obtain vertebral stability. When PMMA is introduced into the posterior-third of the vertebral body (**a** and **c**), the variation of the spinal canal under compression is minimal in comparison with augmentation undertaken in the anterior-third (**b** and **d**)

pain related to the disease. According to recent biomechanical studies on metastatic spinal tumors, mild-to-moderate reduction in size of the spinal canal (with a consequent risk of increasing compression of the spinal cord) has been demonstrated in the case of compression of a vertebra augmented in the anterior-third only. Hence, the best position for PMMA injection for reaching vertebral stability is the posterior-third of a neoplastic VB [21] (Fig. 11.1).

Different mechanisms (i.e., thermal ablation of the vertebral nerve plexus or neurolytic actions of the monomer used) have been advocated for the explanation of pain relief [22], but mechanical stabilization seems to be the main mechanism. Recently, increasing interest in biological-bioactive cements has become evient in the literature [23]. Osteoconductive material as an association between alpha-calcium sulfate and hydroxyapatite [24] has been proposed in the attempt to obtain bone regrowth in focal osteolytic areas, with the original tumor being removed by conventional chemo-radiotherapy (Fig. 11.2).

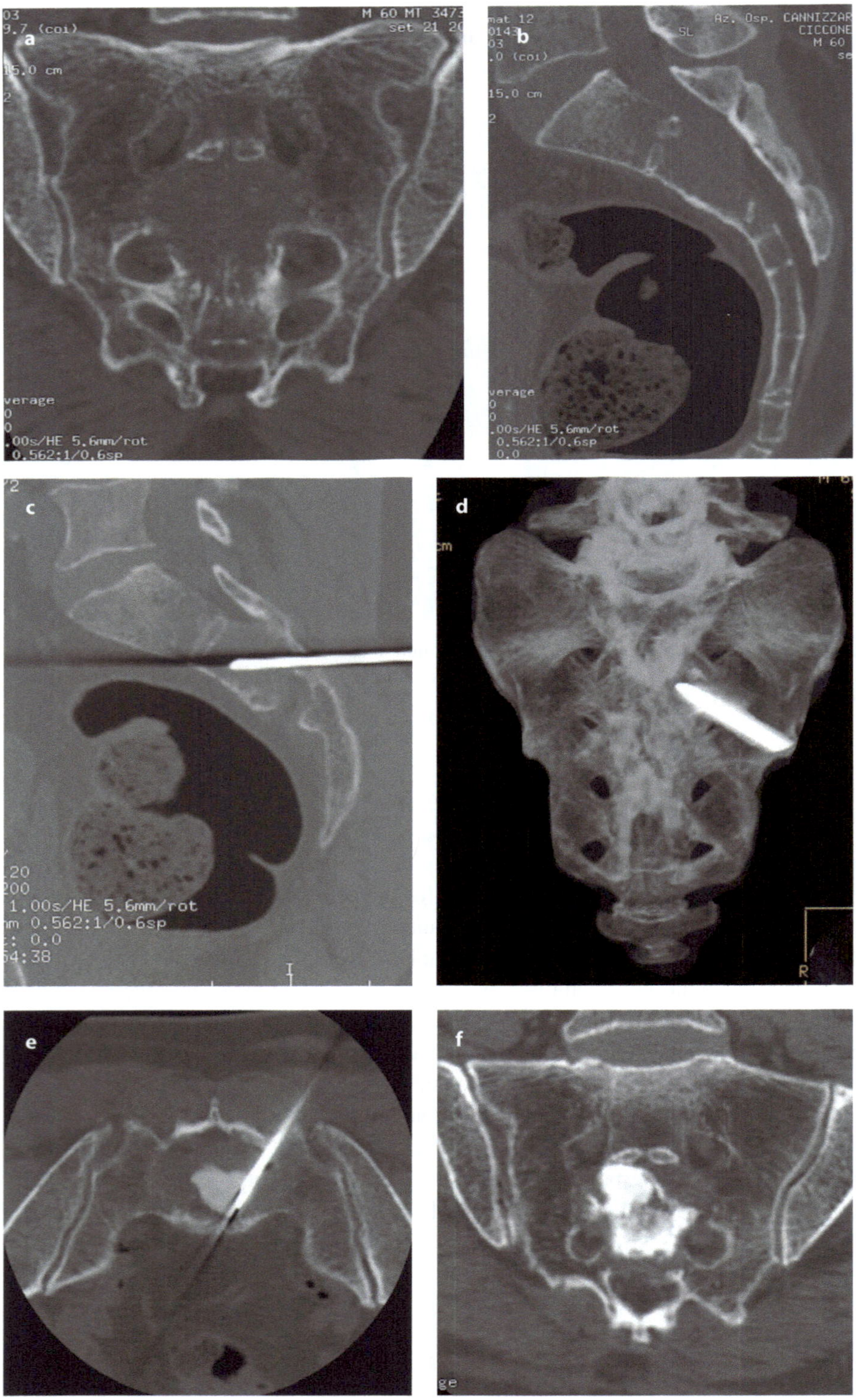

Fig. 11.2 Osteoconductive augmentation of the sacrum. A large sacral defect into the S2 body is observed in a patient previously affected by multiple myeloma (**a** and **b**). A 11-G needle is placed into the sacrum (**c** and **d**) and a small amount of osteoconductive material introduced using a X-ray–CT-guided technique (**e**). After 45 days, regrowth of new bone into the sacrum is observed (**f**)

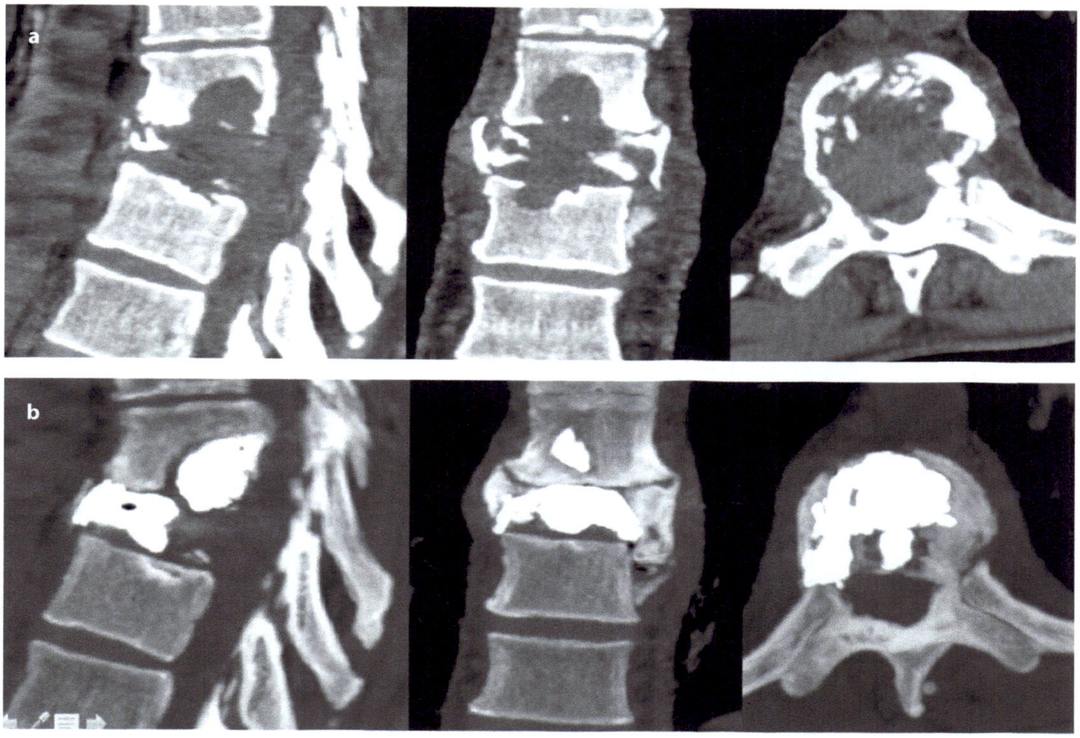

Fig. 11.3 Vertebral augmentation using radiofrequency-applicable PMMA. Severe T7 vertebral collapse with erosion of the posterior wall is observed in a 56-year-old male with by multiple myeloma (**a**). After slow injection of very dense PMMA, reduction of kyphosis related to vertebral augmentation with partial restoration of vertebral height, and respecting the posterior wall profile, is observed (**b**)

11.5 Vertebroplasty and the Posterior Wall

If vertebroplasty is planned in the case of neoplastic vertebral erosion, discontinuity of the posterior somatic wall and/or epidural tumor involvement has been referred as severe contraindications to the procedure [25] because of the presumed risk of dislocation of tumor tissue into the spinal canal [26]. Some authors suggest that pre-vertebroplasty treatment (chemo-radiotherapy or embolization-radioablation of the tumor [27–29]) should be carried out to reduce the size of the tumor, and to carry out PMMA augmentation with concurrent myelography to monitor epidural changes during kyphoplasty/vertebroplasty [30]. Recently however, new trends related to technical considerations have been reported. First, according to a biomechanical study by Pollintine et al. on PMMA spreading into a VB [31], cement distribution is strongly influenced by the physical property of material injected and hardening behavior. Hence, the use of polymers with radiofrequency-controlled hardening could be useful in augmentation of tumor VBs with defects in the posterior wall [32, 33] (Fig. 11.3). Moreover, stress distribution in the VBs can be normalized using repeated injections of small volumes of PMMA (Fig. 11.4) to reduce the risk of epidural leakage [34–38]. Hence, despite not being indicated for epidural compression [39, 40], augmentation procedures can be undertaken cautiously even in patients with severe erosion of the posterior wall (Fig. 11.5) and/or epidural extension of the tumor [41]. This is because worsening neurological symptoms after vertebroplasty have not been described in patients with symptomatic epidural compression 42 (Figs 11.6 and 11.7).

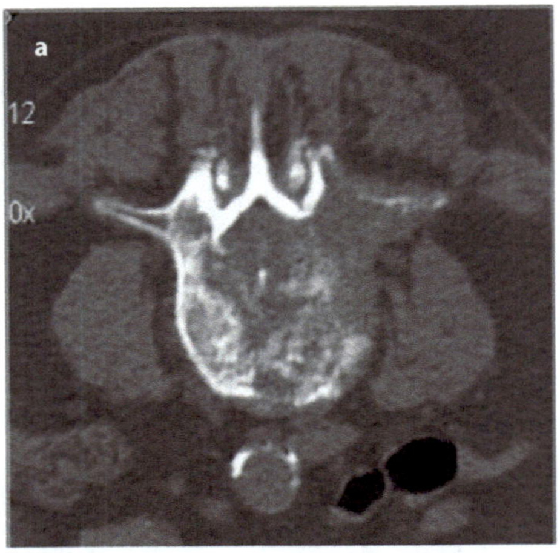

Fig. 11.4 Small-volume injections of PMMA in pedicle reconstruction in a patient with severe osteolysis secondary to a breast lesion of the right pedicle (**a**). Using multiple injections of small amounts of PMMA, careful reconstruction of the pedicle and tranverse process is achieved (**b**)

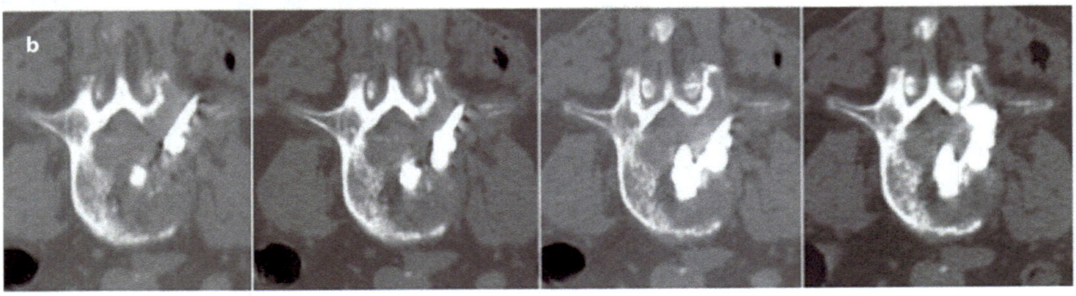

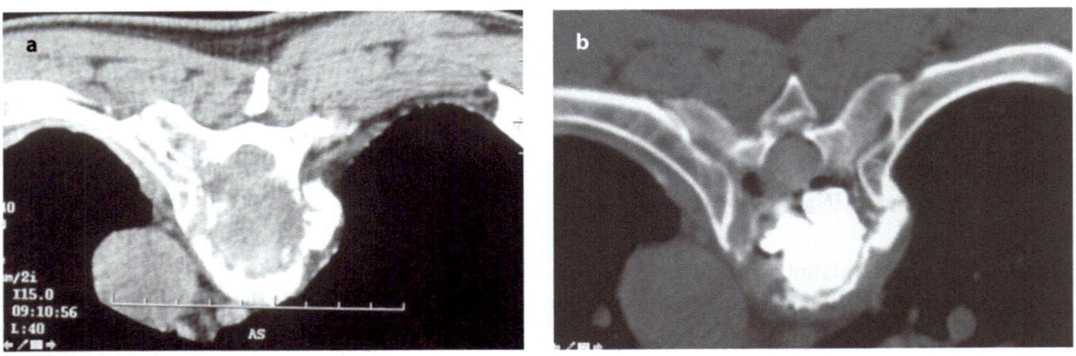

Fig. 11.5 Vertebroplasty in a patient with erosion of the posterior wall secondary to metastases due to primary lung carcinoma. Before treatment, a large defect at the level of the posterior wall of T9 can be seen (**a**). After treatment, subtotal augmentation of the vertebral body without epidural leakage can be achieved (**b**)

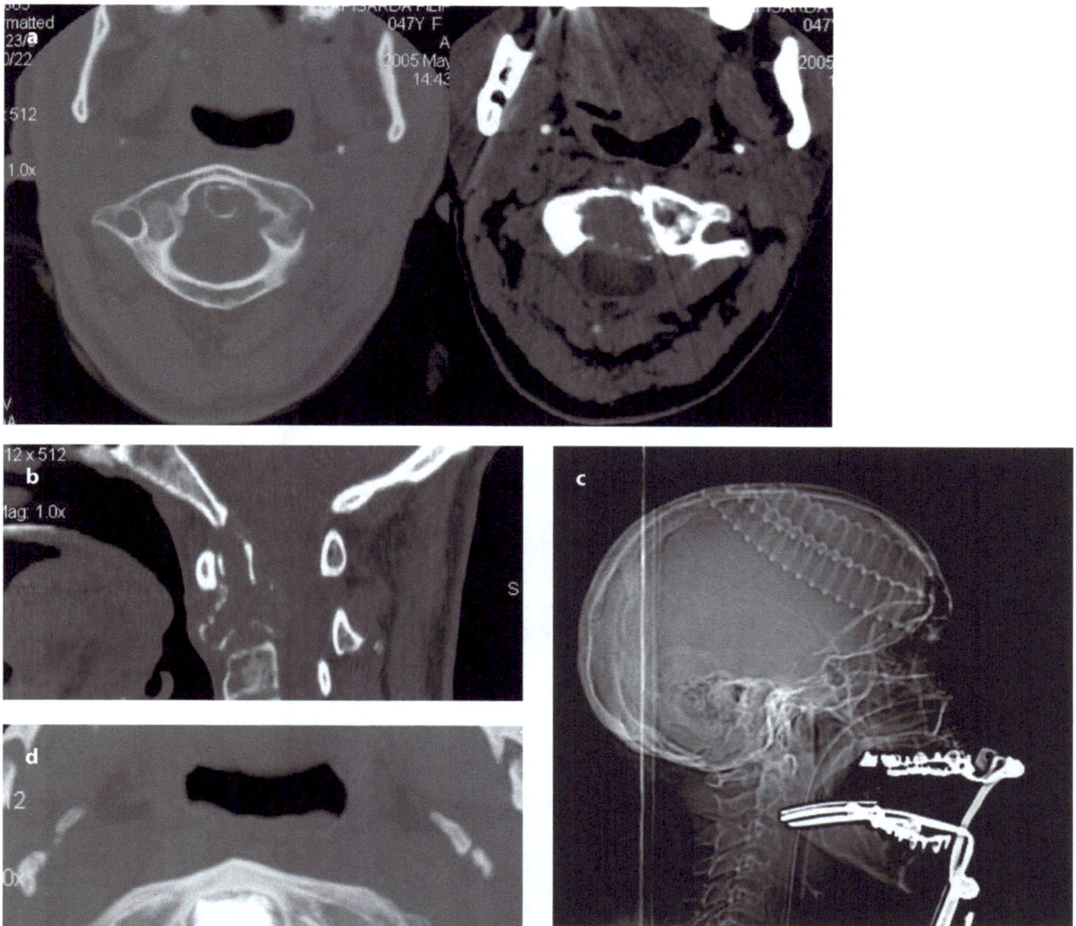

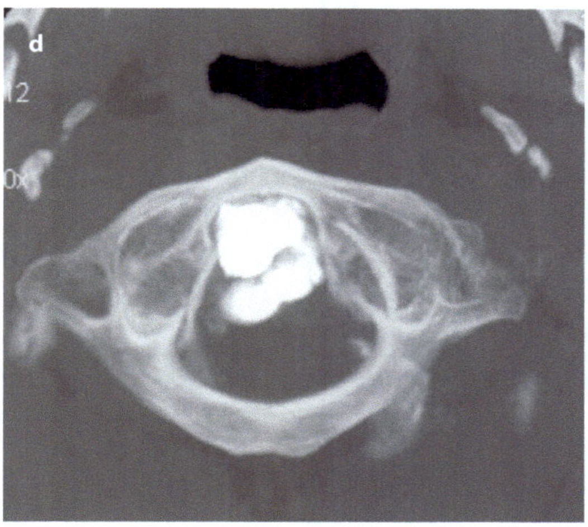

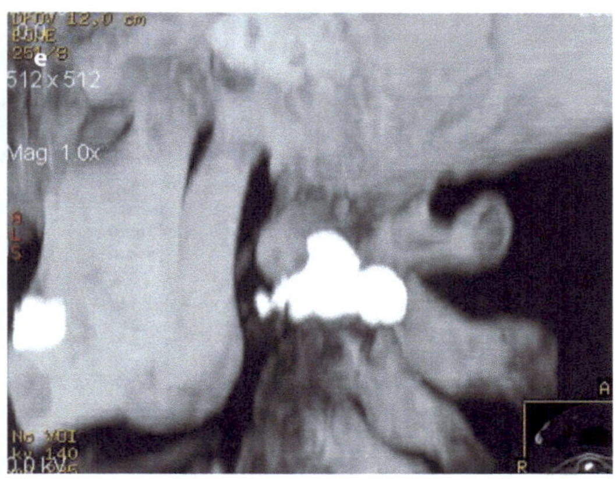

Fig. 11.6 Odontoid reconstruction using CT-guided PMMA augmentation. A large odontoid defect can be observed in a patient with lymphoma (**a** and **b**). The patient is placed in the supine position, under general anesthesia, and the mouth remains open usinf distractors (**c**). After PMMA injection, total remodeling of the odontoid process recreating the C1–C2 articulation is demonstrated (**d** and **e**)

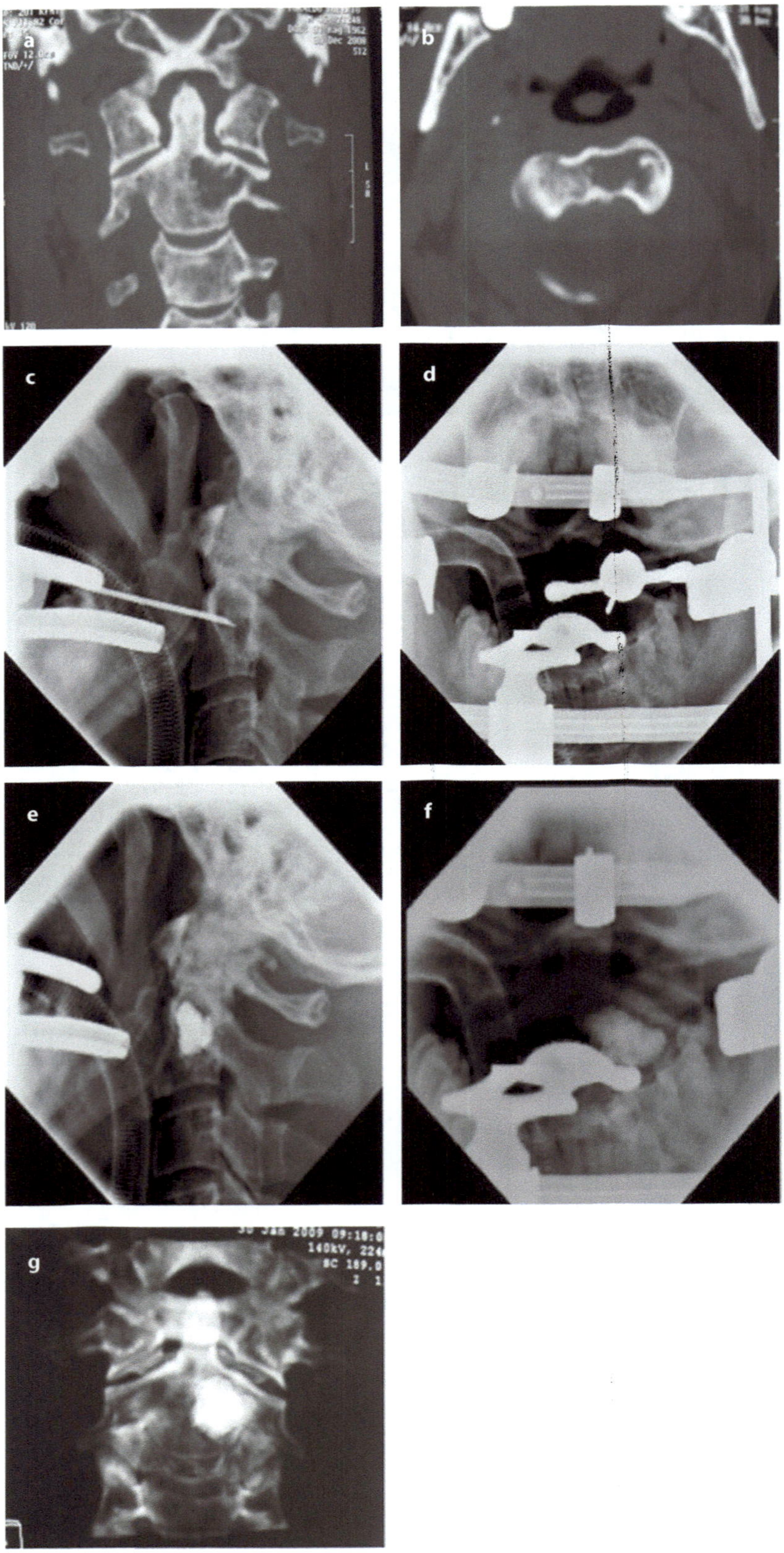

Fig. 11.7 C2 vertebroplasty. Multidetector-row computed tomography (MDCT) coronal and axial MP reconstruction at the cervical level show a multiple myeloma lesion at C2 (**a** and **b**). The patient is placed in the supine position under general anesthesia. The mouth remains open by the use of distractors (**c** and **d**). Left lateral and anteroposterior views under fluoroscopic control after PMMA injection show good distribution of cement into the lesion without leakage (**e** and **f**). Three-dimensional volume-rendered MDCT shows good distribution of the PMMA (**g**)

11.6 Vertebroplasty and Extravertebral Tumors

Another point to consider is whether conventional vertebroplasty can be carried out in cases of a neoplastic vertebra with an extravertebral soft-tissue tumor. Previously, an extravertebral tumor was considered to be a contraindication for vertebroplasty (especially in cases of severe epidural extension). Even though severe compressive myelopathy remains an indication for conventional open surgery to decompress the spinal cord, an increasing number of studies focusing on the "emboligenous" effect of injected PMMA has been published [43–45], and the procedure has become used widely (even in cases of epidural involvement of the disease) with very low prevalence of complications [15]. Ischemic changes of paravertebral tissue immediately after vertebral augmentation can be demonstrated by contrast-enhanced CT or MRI, and persistent regression of the tumor can be documented in follow-up studies (Figs 11.8–11.10). Even though the cause of spontaneous regression of extravertebral extension of metastatic disease after vertebroplasty remains unknown, several mechanisms have been proposed. Deramond et al. suggested that the thermal effect related to PMMA could be responsible for the observed cytolytic effects [46], but this does not seem probable considering the low-temperature hardening PMMA that is commonly used. Kayamura et al. suggested that the regression could be related to the activation of messenger ribonucleic acid (mRNA) by PMMA, with new synthesis of tumor necrosis factor (TNF) [47]. However, considering the size reduction detected a few days after augmentation, this mechanism do not seems feasible. Considering the embolic effect of PMMA injection demonstrated in the literature [44], ischemic changes could be considered to be the main cause of immediate reduction in tumor size after vertebroplasty [45].

11.7 Vertebroplasty and the Neoplastic Posterior Arch

The pedicle and posterior arch are crucial for spinal stability. At the thoracic level, ≥60% involvement of the VB is considered to suggest the risk of vertebral collapse. However, if the pedicle/posterior arch is involved, 25% erosion of the VB is sufficient to cause vertebral creeping [48]. Moreover, the entire posterior arch is considered to be a very sensitive area for local pain. Several authors have demonstrated neoplastic involvement of elements of the posterior arch to be associated with severe local pain, and local infiltration in case of persistent pain after vertebroplasty has been suggested [49, 50].

Previously, neoplastic involvement of the posterior arch was considered to be a contraindication to vertebroplasty. This was mainly because of the difficulty in visualizing PMMA distribution during injection into the pedicle using the C-arm assisted procedure, as well as the consequent risk of PMMA leakage into the spinal canal. However, if a CT-guided technique is employed, use of a small-gauge needle (13–15 G) and multiple mini-injections of PMMA can be used to reconstruct almost every part of the posterior arch, thereby sparing the spinal canal (Figs 11.11–11.15).

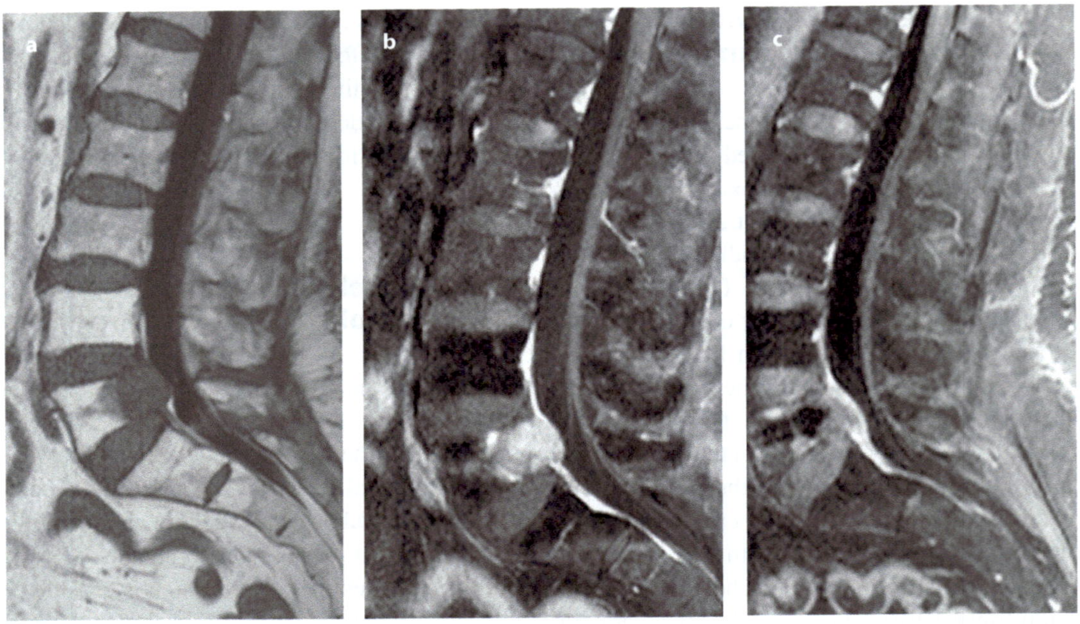

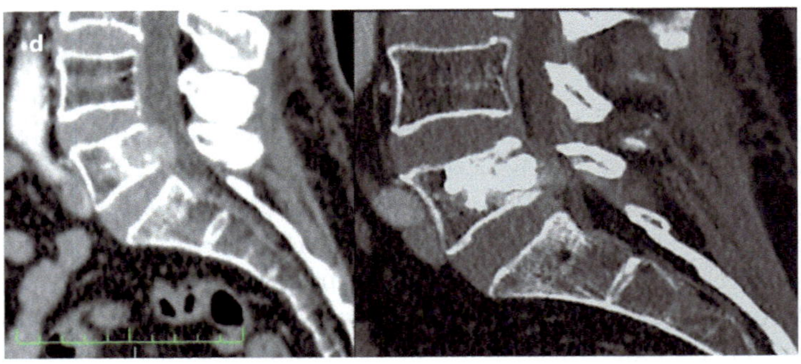

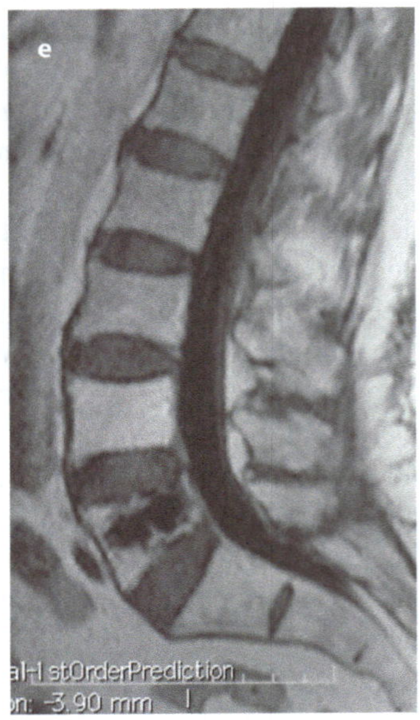

Fig. 11.8 Spontaneous regression of a tumor after PMMA injection in a patient with a gastric cancer metastatic lesion of the posterior-third of L5 with intra-canal extension of the tumor. The preoperative T1-weighted image shows a large hypointense mass bulging into the spinal canal (**a**) with extensive enhancement of contrast after intravenous injection of GdDTP (**b**). Immediately after vertebroplasty, the posterior location of the PMMA can be observed on MRI (**c**) and CT image reconstruction (**d**). Follow-up MRI after 4 weeks shows regression of the epidural mass without other chemo- or radiotherapeutic treatment (**e**)

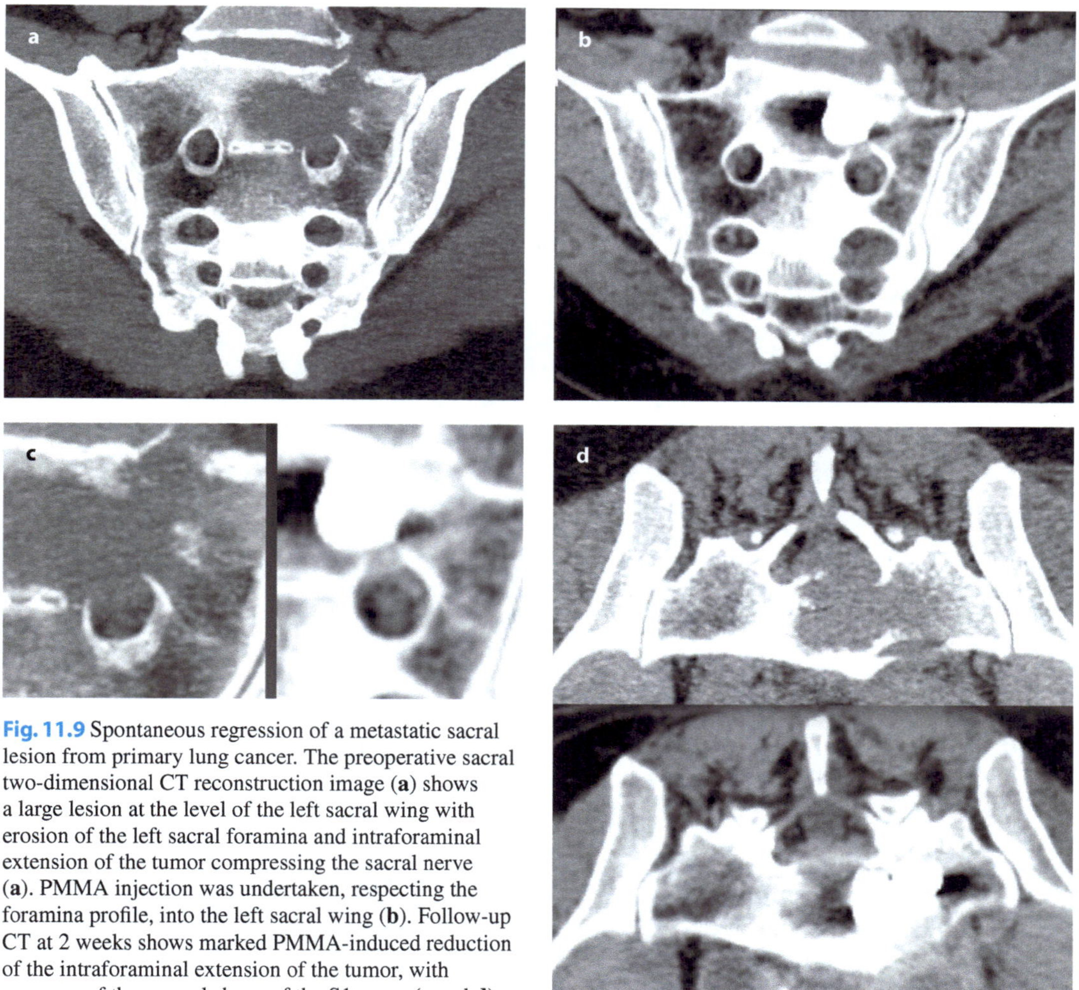

Fig. 11.9 Spontaneous regression of a metastatic sacral lesion from primary lung cancer. The preoperative sacral two-dimensional CT reconstruction image (**a**) shows a large lesion at the level of the left sacral wing with erosion of the left sacral foramina and intraforaminal extension of the tumor compressing the sacral nerve (**a**). PMMA injection was undertaken, respecting the foramina profile, into the left sacral wing (**b**). Follow-up CT at 2 weeks shows marked PMMA-induced reduction of the intraforaminal extension of the tumor, with recovery of the normal shape of the S1 nerve (**c** and **d**)

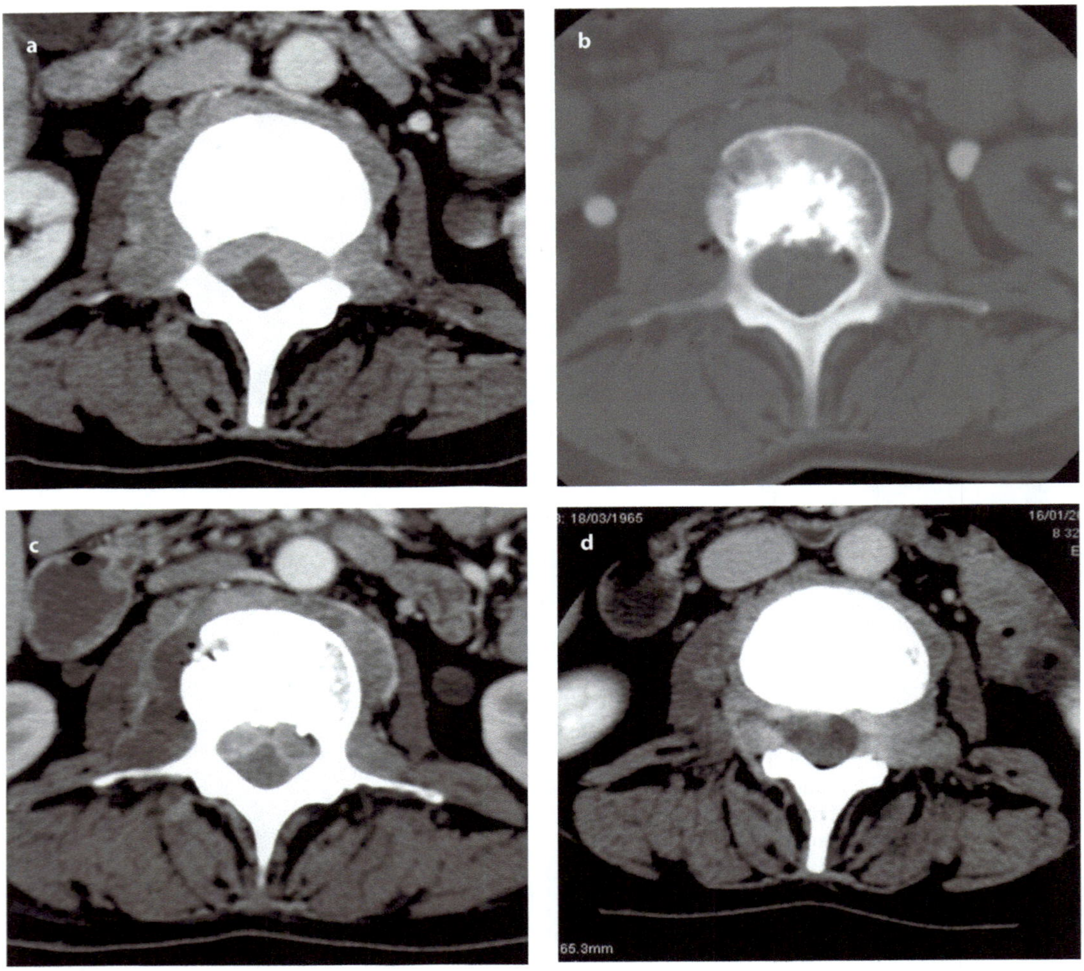

Fig. 11.10 Spontaneous regression of epidural tumor extension in a female with T11 involvement due to breast cancer metastasis and paraparesis. The preoperative contrast-enhanced CT study shows tumor extension into the perivertebral space and spinal canal with spinal-cord compression (**a**). PMMA augmentation is undertaken involving mainly the posterior-third of the vertebral body of T11 (**b**). Upon immediate contrast-enhanced follow-up, no enhancement of the epidural intrathecal lesion and paravertebral lesion on the right side can be seen, which is probably related to ischemic chances induced by PMMA augmentation (**c**). At 4-week follow-up, the paraparesis has resolved and no recurrence of the tumor can be seen in the spinal canal (**d**)

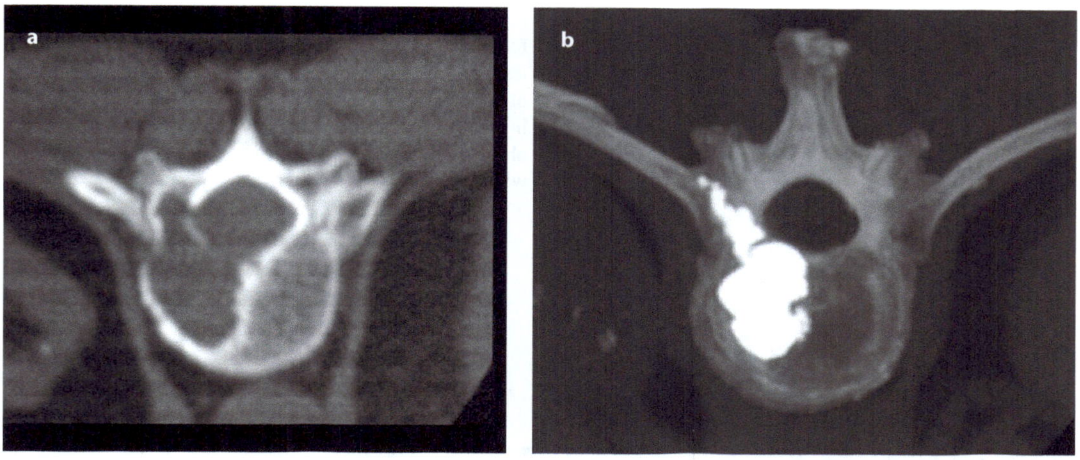

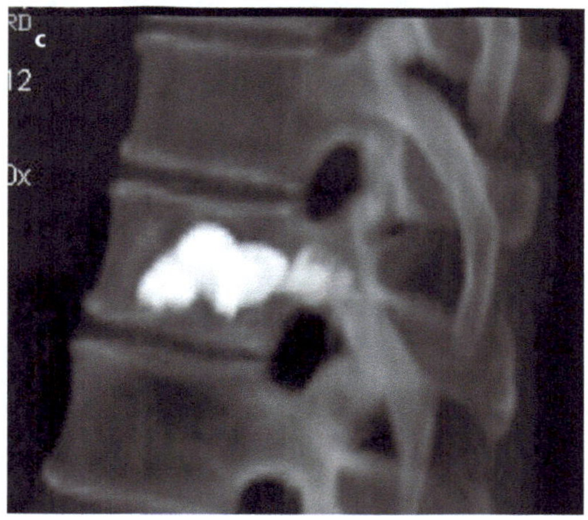

Fig. 11.11 Pedicle reconstruction in a patient with multiple myeloma. The preoperative image shows a large defect of the body as well as the pedicle and rib processes of a T10 vertebra on the left side (**a**). After PMMA augmentation, subtotal filling of the lytic lesion occurs (**b** and **c**), thereby resolving the original costovertebral pain

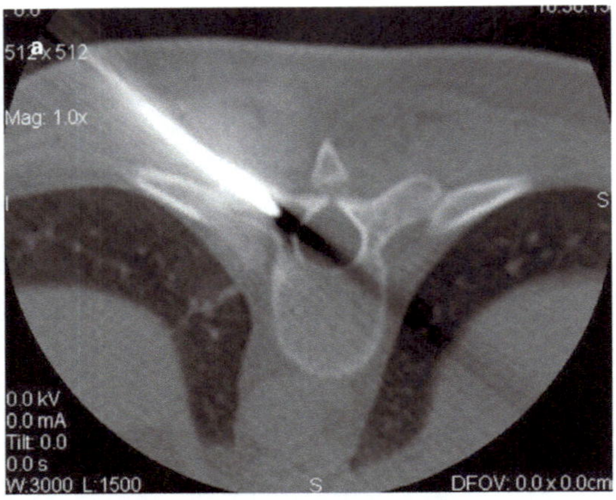

Fig. 11.12 Pedicle augmentation in a female with painful focal left pain at the T6 level. Before augmentation, a lytic lesion of the left transverse process related to localization of breast cancer metastases can be seen (**a**). After PMMA injection, total filling of the left transverse process can be observed on axial, sagittal and coronal CT reconstruction, with resolution of the pain (**b**)

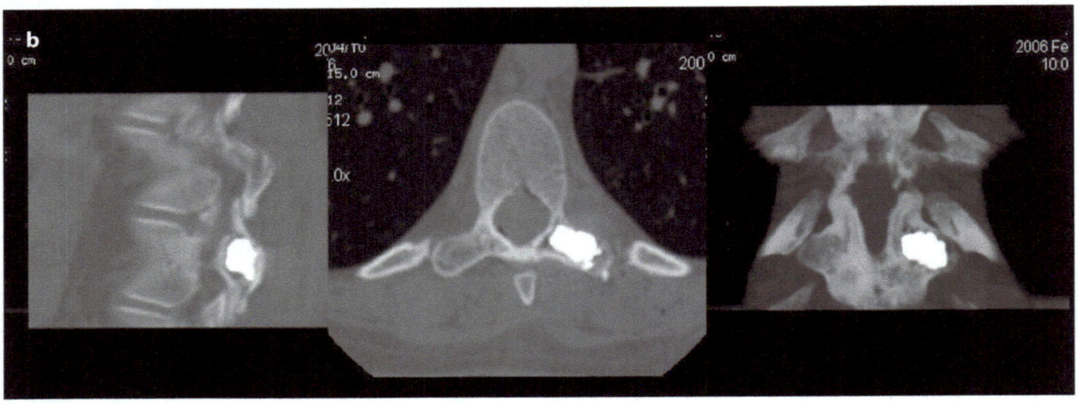

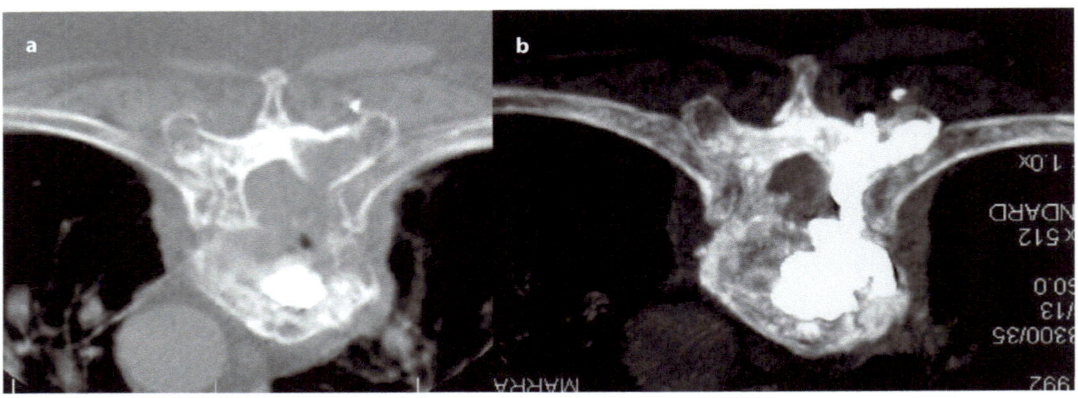

Fig. 11.13 Reconstruction of the body, pedicle and transverse process in a patient with T12 lung cancer metastases. Before PMMA injection, a large painful osteolitic lesion can be seen involving the left pedicle and transverse process of the T12 vertebra (**a**). After PMMA injection, full remodeling of the vertebra can be seen, recreating the missing left pedicle and articular process (**b**)

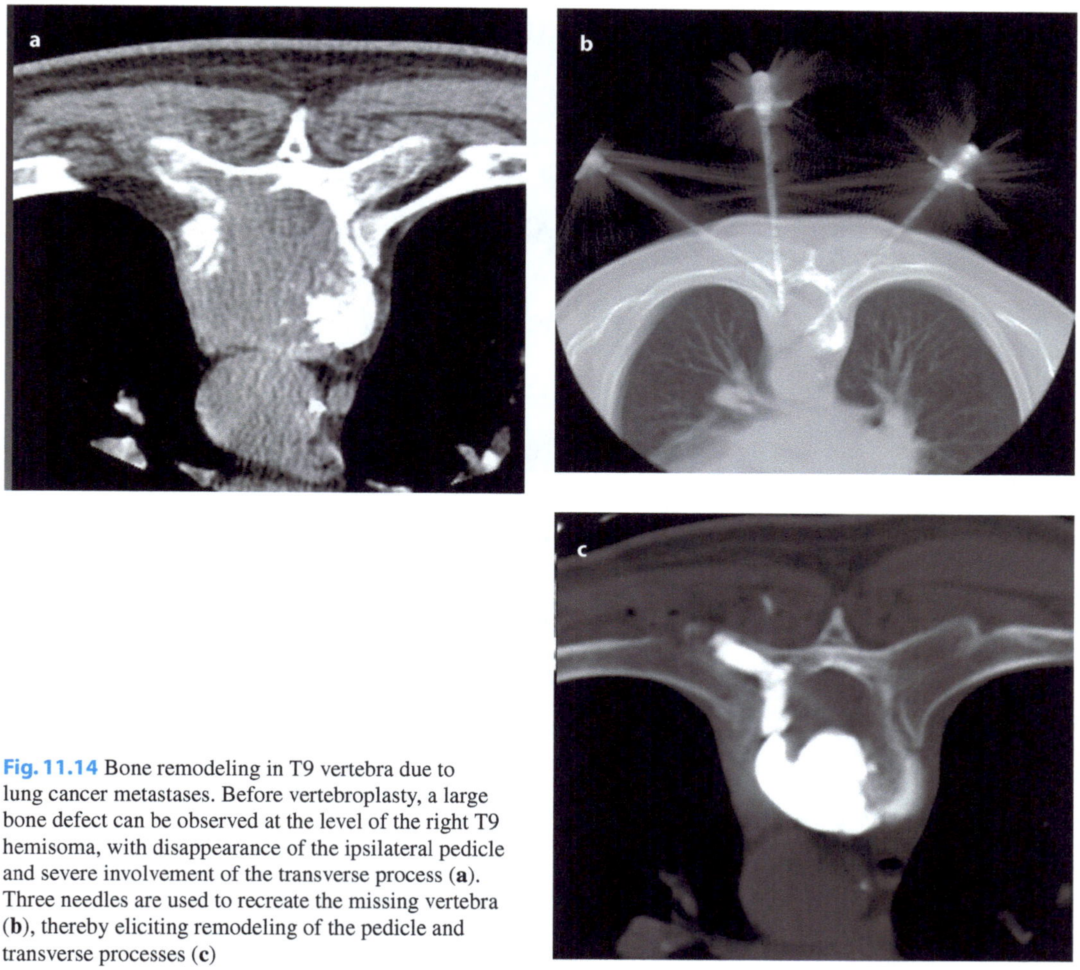

Fig. 11.14 Bone remodeling in T9 vertebra due to lung cancer metastases. Before vertebroplasty, a large bone defect can be observed at the level of the right T9 hemisoma, with disappearance of the ipsilateral pedicle and severe involvement of the transverse process (**a**). Three needles are used to recreate the missing vertebra (**b**), thereby eliciting remodeling of the pedicle and transverse processes (**c**)

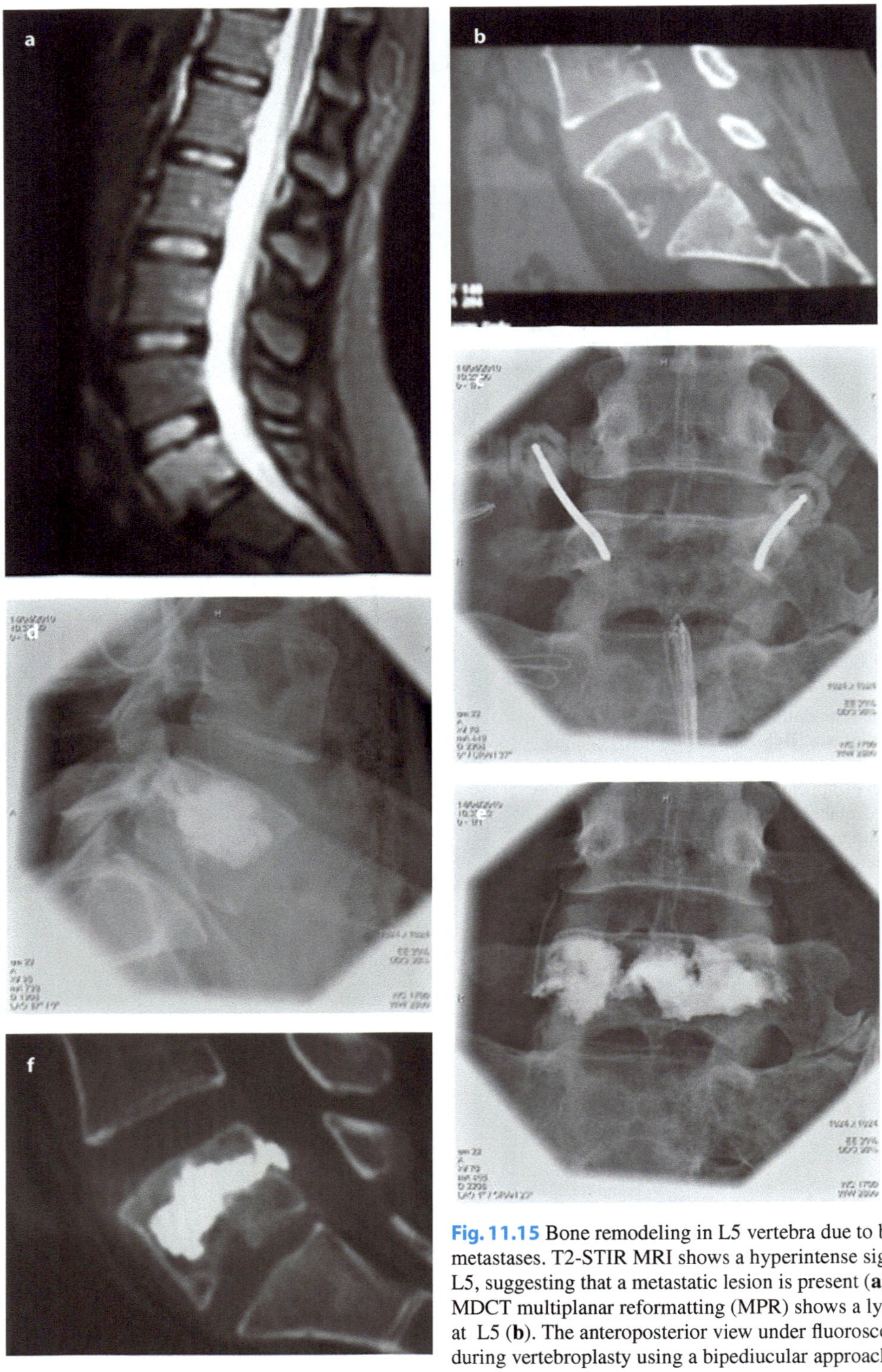

Fig. 11.15 Bone remodeling in L5 vertebra due to breast cancer metastases. T2-STIR MRI shows a hyperintense signal at L5, suggesting that a metastatic lesion is present (**a**). Sagittal MDCT multiplanar reformatting (MPR) shows a lytic lesion at L5 (**b**). The anteroposterior view under fluoroscopic control during vertebroplasty using a bipediucular approach shows good positioning of the needles (**c**). Left lateral and anteroposterior views under fluoroscopic control post-vertebroplasty show PMMA remodeling of the lesion without cement leakage (**d** and **e**). Sagittal MDCT MPR shows the remodeling effect due to PMMA (**f**)

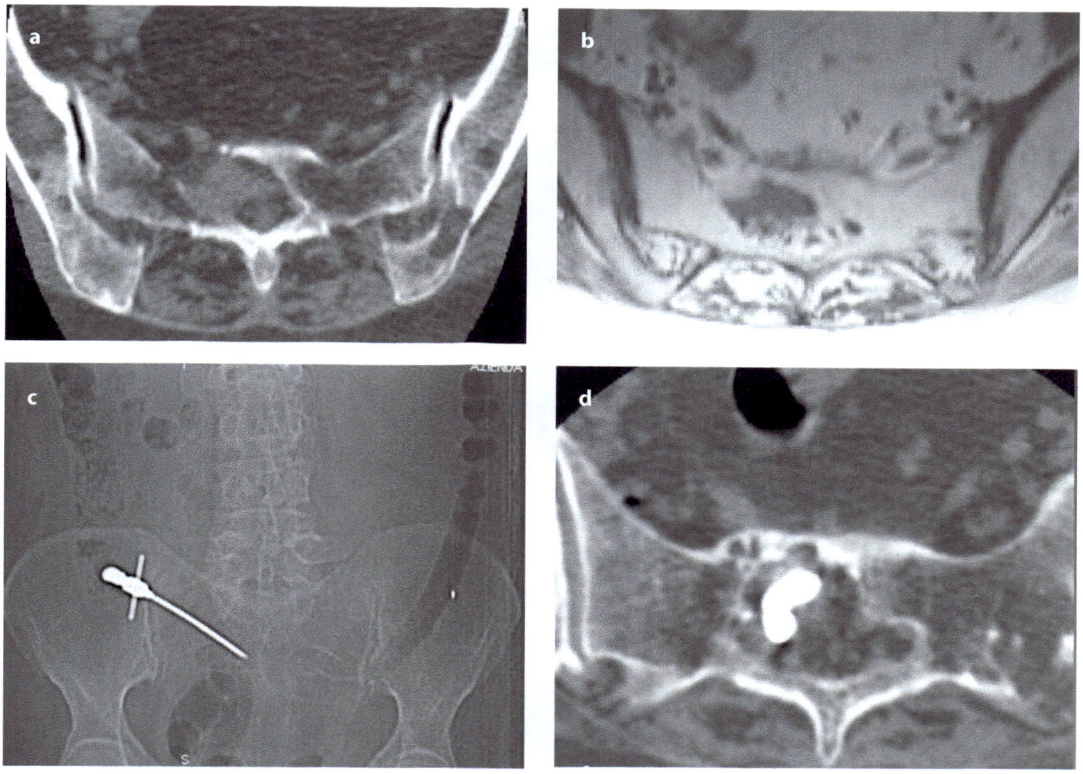

Fig. 11.16 Small sacral lesion and targeted PMMA injection in a patient with multiple myeloma. On CT (**a**) and T1-weighted MRI (**b**), a small lesion can be observed at the body-to-wing line of the sacrum. A 11-G needle is placed carefully into the lesion *via* a CT-guided transalar approach (**c**) and the lesion filled with PMMA, resulting in pain resolution (**d**)

11.8 Vertebroplasty and the Neoplastic Sacrum

Neoplastic involvement of the sacrum can be part of secondary disease. It can be responsible for severe local pain, preventing the patient from sitting or standing up. Pain control is based on radiotherapy and/or drug use. More recently, percutaneous interstitial laser photocoagulation (ILP) of vertebral bone tumors such as osteoid osteomas under CT or MRI guidance has been used to obtain thermal destruction of the nidus tumor with low-power laser energy. ILP is a minimally invasive method that can be an alternative to conventional surgical treatment (i.e., percutaneous laser photocoagulation of spinal osteoid osteomas under CT or MRI guidance [51–54]. Sacroplasty using intra-tumor injection of cement is a powerful tool for pain relief, even for very small sacral lesions (Fig. 11.16). From a technical viewpoint, if C-arm fluoroscopy is adopted to introduce a needle, the overlapping bony pelvis usually obscures sacral visualization to a considerable extent. This complicates assessment of whether the injected cement is contained within the sacrum or has leaked outside the sacral boundaries (i.e., into the sacral foramina) [55]. Garant et al. [56] attempted to overcome this problem by placing several 15 cm-long, 20-G Chiba needles in the sacral foramina to identify their location during PMMA injection. However, lateral-view C-arm fluoroscopy is frequently insufficient for safe depiction of the sacral foramina and sacral boundaries.

CT guidance during sacroplasty and adoption of manual PMMA micro-injection with small syringes (i.e., 1.5–2.0 cm^3 by time) appears to be the best choice to reduce the risk of extrasacral leakage

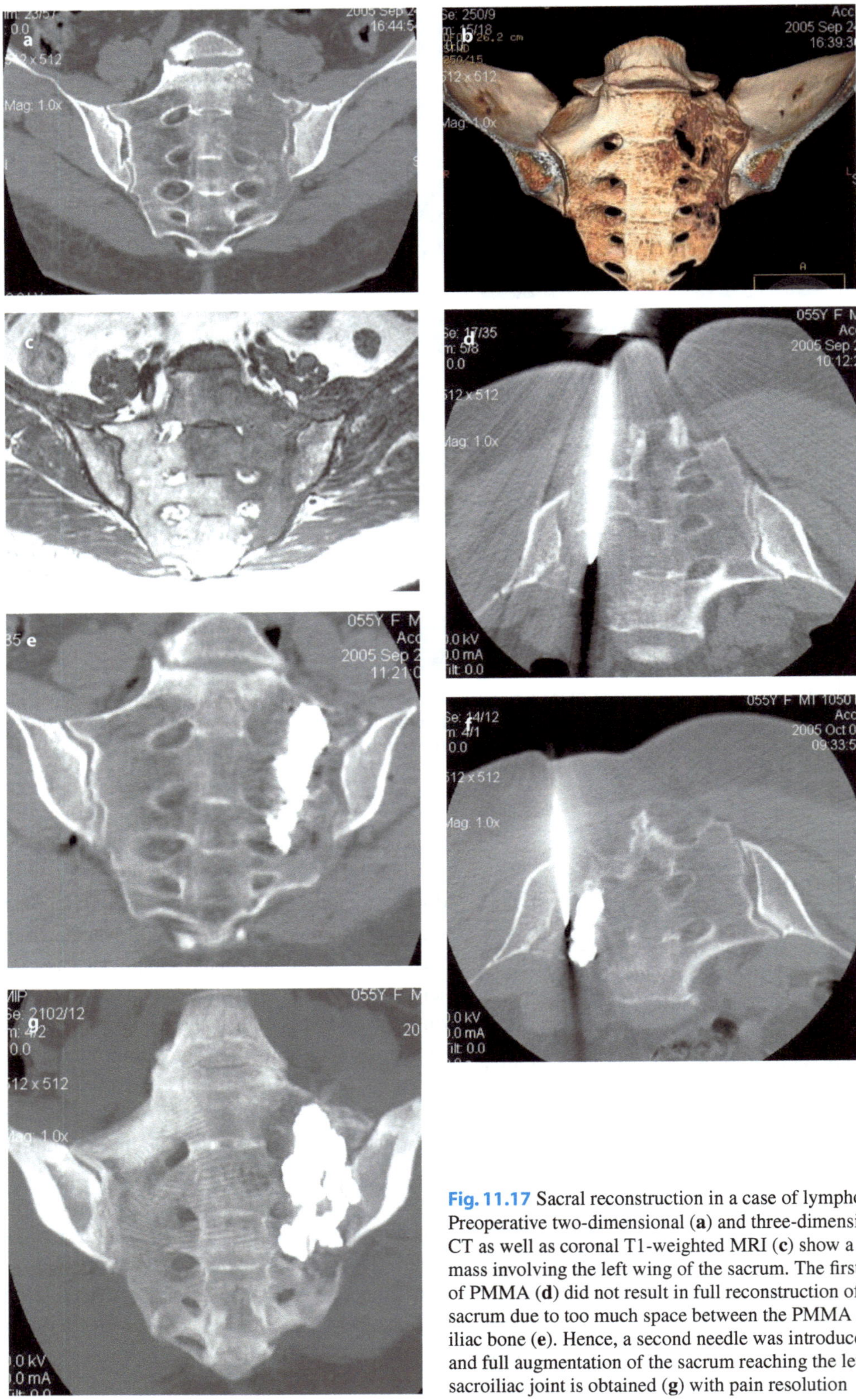

Fig. 11.17 Sacral reconstruction in a case of lymphoma. Preoperative two-dimensional (**a**) and three-dimensional (**b**) CT as well as coronal T1-weighted MRI (**c**) show a large mass involving the left wing of the sacrum. The first injection of PMMA (**d**) did not result in full reconstruction of the sacrum due to too much space between the PMMA and the iliac bone (**e**). Hence, a second needle was introduced (**f**) and full augmentation of the sacrum reaching the level of the sacroiliac joint is obtained (**g**) with pain resolution

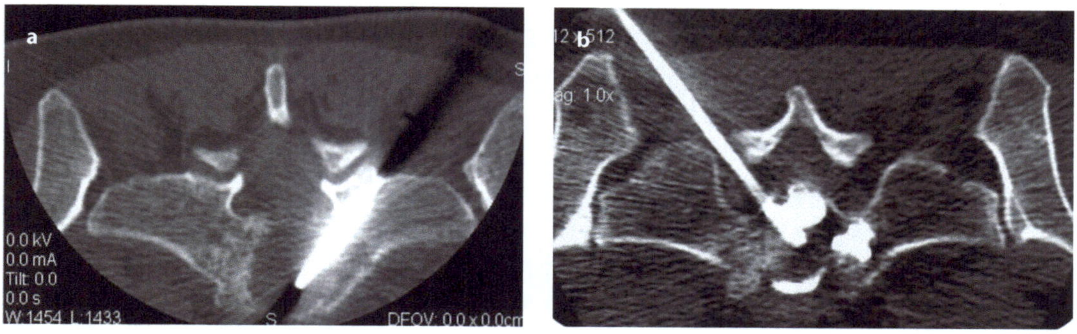

Fig. 11.18 A different approach to carrying out a sacroplasty. The Jamshidi needle can be introduced through the sacral wing (**a**) or directly into the sacral body *via* the posterior sacral foramina (**b**), paying sparing attention to sparing the sacral nerve

for two main reasons. First, one can immediately appreciate the initial intraforaminal leakage. The procedure can be stopped and the needle moved away from the foramen to prevent intraforaminal extravasations (Fig. 11.17). Second, the best orientation of the needle can be chosen easily. The vertebroplasty needle should be oriented to cover the entire extension of the sacral fracture according to the shape of the sacrum and the distribution of the sacral tumor osteolysis. New access routes different to the traditional transpedicular approach (e.g., parapedicular route, transdiskal access) have been adopted by several authors [57] to reach the VB. One of the advantages of a combination of a C-arm-assisted procedure and CT-guided procedure [58] is the abilty to choose the best route to reach the target because markers (i.e., pedicles) are not needed. In general, the transalar and transforaminal approaches can be adopted to minimize the risk of complications (Fig. 11.18). Moreover, in patients with anarchic osteolysis related to malignancies, the chance to see the true PMMA distribution inside the sacrum permits consolidation of all the area occupied by the disease. This allows sacral remodeling to be undertaken in the case of extensive osteolytic disease (Fig. 11.19). Finally, as demonstrated by several authors, CT-guided spinal interventional methods significantly reduce radiation exposure to the patient and the operator. Recently, Perisinakis et al. demonstrated that fluoroscopic-guided vertebroplasty and kyphoplasty exposed patients to significant radiation doses: 10 min of fluoroscopic exposure equated to a mean value of 173 mGy for vertebroplasty and 233 mGy for kyphoplasty. Histological analyses of skin specimens of patients who underwent 10 min of kyphoplasty demonstrated cellular injuries [59, 60].

11.9 Aneurysmal Bone Cysts (ABCs)

ABCs are expansive osteolytic lesions with thin walls containing blood-filled cystic cavities. Although benign, ABCs can be aggressive and can cause extensive weakening of the bony structure and impinge on surrounding tissues. Malignant transformation is extremely rare [61]. ABCs predominantly affect individuals aged <20 years, with a female preponderance [62–64]. The cause of ABCs is not known [65]. The tibia and femur are affected in 24.7% and 17.3% of all cases, respectively, followed by the upper extremities (10%) and pelvis (9%). About 14% of all ABCs are encountered in the spine, with those in the cervical spine making up only 2% [66]. The expansive nature of the lesions can cause pain, swelling, deformity, disruption of growth plates, neurological symptoms (depending on their location), and pathologic fractures [66–67]. ABCs can be asymptomatic, but usually produce pain that is resistant to medication. Occasionally, ABCs can be found incidentally or cause acute onset with spinal cord syndrome.

The treatment of spinal ABCs is controversial. For vertebral lesions, the choice of treatment must

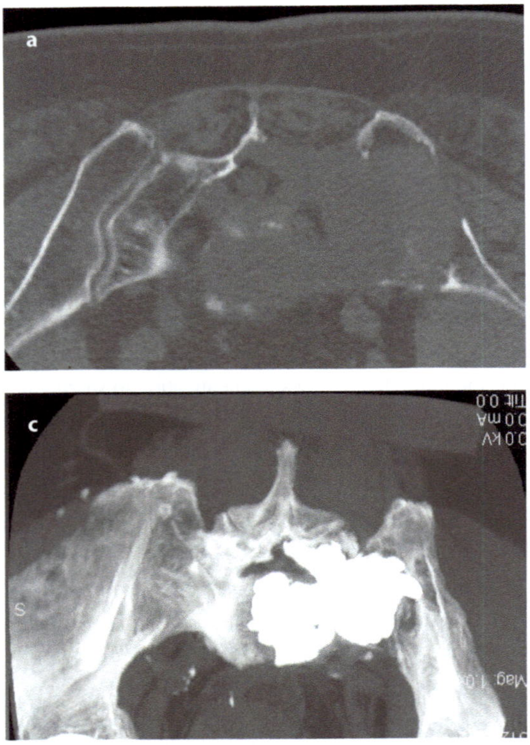

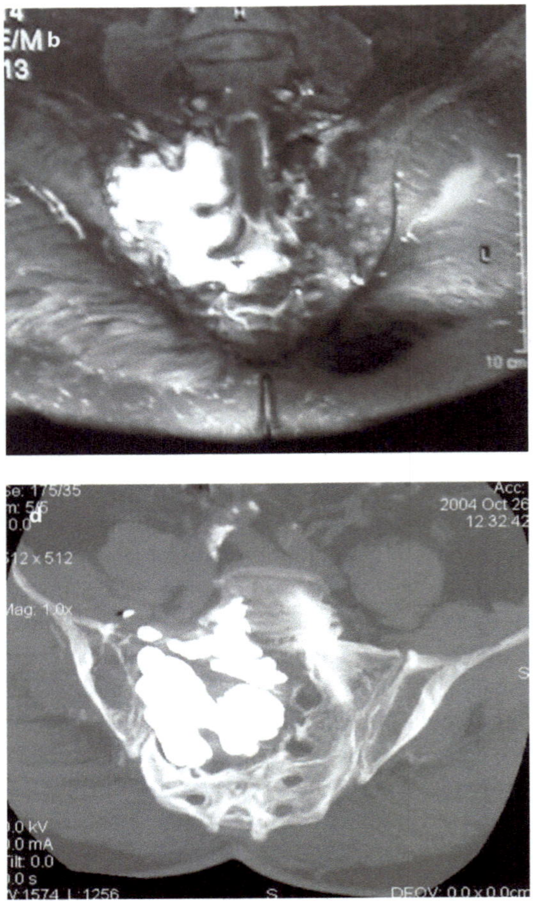

Fig. 11.19 Subtotal sacral remodeling using multiple needles in a patient with multiple myeloma and severe sacral pain. Preoperative axial CT (**a**) and T2-weighted STIR MRI (**b**) show a large osteolytic lesion with total destruction of the right sacral wing, sacral body and the right wall of the sacral canal. After treatment, remodeling of the sacral wing and posterior wall of the sacral canal can be observed, with remodeling the right first and second sacral foramina and with no leakage into the sacral canal (**c** and **d**)

take into consideration the risk of neurological and vascular lesions as well as preserving the stability (and, if possible, mobility) of the spine [65].

Surgery is the first-line treatment for these lesions, and includes resection, curettage and spinal fixation. These procedures carry the risk of significant blood loss, postoperative spinal deformity, axial deformity, and postoperative hemorrhage [68]. Some authors have proposed a simple intra-lesion excision with bone grafting. Other authors have proposed "*en-bloc*" resection of the involved vertebra as the only treatment free from the risk of local recurrence [65], but this treatment is frequently complicated by kyphoscoliosis and compression of the spinal cord and nerve roots. Deformity is frequently worsened by the surgical procedures often needed for control of these lesions, which can involve more than one level [69]. Hemorrhage and pulmonary embolism can occur during or after surgery [67, 70–72].

Other strategies include radiotherapy, sclerotherapy and endovascular treatment [73–74]. In general, radiotherapy is contraindicated because of the risk of inducing neoplasm formations (sarcomas), gonadal damage, and disruption of growth plates. Nevertheless, low-dose radiotherapy is used occasionally to treat lesions that cannot be treated by surgery [73]. Another option is selective arterial embolization, which

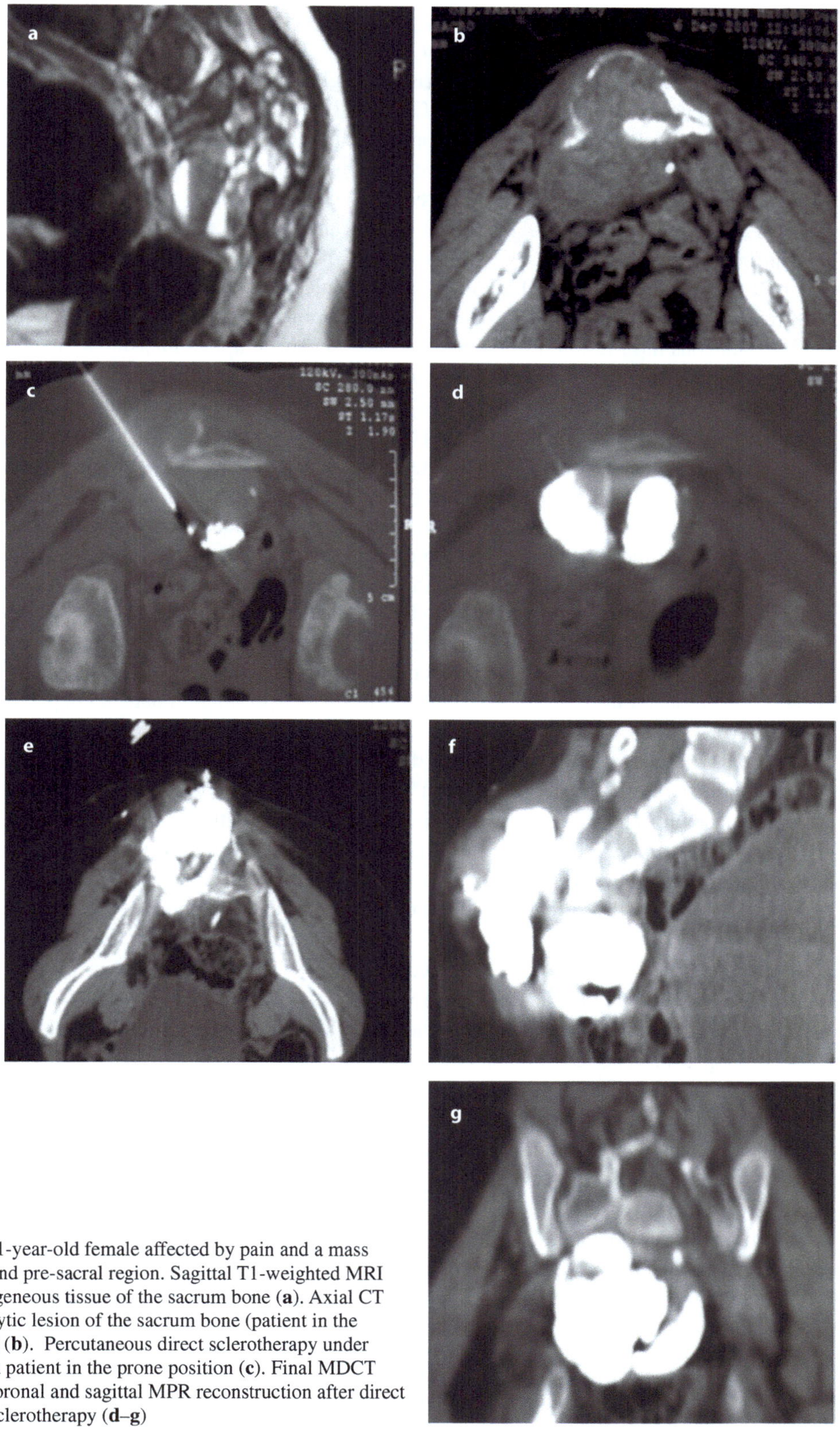

Fig. 11.20 A 11-year-old female affected by pain and a mass in the lumbar and pre-sacral region. Sagittal T1-weighted MRI shows inhomogeneous tissue of the sacrum bone (**a**). Axial CT shows a large lytic lesion of the sacrum bone (patient in the prone position) (**b**). Percutaneous direct sclerotherapy under CT guidance in patient in the prone position (**c**). Final MDCT control with coronal and sagittal MPR reconstruction after direct percutaneous sclerotherapy (**d–g**)

has a recurrence rate that is not significantly different from that observed after intra-lesion excision. However, it is associated with the risk of spinal-cord ischemia (especially if the ABC is at the thoracic level). Some authors have proposed preoperative arterial embolization followed by surgical excision with bone grafting, whereas de Kleuver et al. considered arterial embolization to be insufficient treatment [75]. de Cristofaro et al. reported a recurrence rate of 10.5% after super-selective embolization [76].

Percutaneous intra-lesion injections represent a relatively new minimally invasive therapeutic option for ABCs. They can be combined with surgical or endovascular treatments (especially for large and resistant lesions) [75–77]. The procedure comprises percutaneous injection of glue directly into the lesion to obtain obstruction at the venous side of the multiple parietal arteriolar afferents of the ABC by direct damage to the endothelial lining. This triggers a coagulation cascade and thrombotic occlusion of blood vessels [78], thereby avoiding the potential functional disabilities produced by surgery or radiotherapy (Fig. 11.20).

Several sclerotic agents have been developed. Polidocanol, Ethibloc® or Glubran® can be combined with super-selective embolization by Onyx®. The *rationale* of using these agents is to elicit arterial embolization of the feeders or venous embolization by direct injection of the cystic lesion.

Polidocanol (3% hydroxypolyaethoxydodecan) is used for the treatment of varicose veins as well as venous malformations of the head and neck. Rastogi et al. reported good outcomes with a mean clinical response of 84.5% with low recurrence rate (2%), with the avoidance of complications such as hypopigmentation, injection-site necrosis, pulmonary embolism, osteomyelitis, and allergic reactions [78].

Ethibloc is a fibrosing and sclerotic agent containing a hydroalcoholic radiopaque solution of zein, a contrast agent, oleum papaverin and propylene glycol. Falappa et al. and Adamsbaum et al. reported good outcomes in long-term follow-up in subjects treated by direct percutaneous injection of Ethibloc, demonstrating it to be a safe and efficient minimally invasive method [79–81].

Glubran is a cyanoacrylate-based synthetic glue that becomes radiopaque upon addition of Lipiodol® (which is also the diluent). Glubran polymerizes in contact with blood to elicit a sclerotic effect. The speed of polymerization is dependent upon its dilution with Lipiodol. The amount injected is dependent upon the extension of the lesion and vascular structures. However, injection requires in-depth study of the lesion, its circulation and the collateral circulation to avoid severe complications due to inappropriate use.

Onyx is a biocompatible liquid polymer that precipitates and solidifies in contact with blood, thus forming a soft and spongy embolus. The injected material is sufficiently thick to fill vessels but does not adhere to the catheter. Three concentrations are available to permit a range of precipitation rates. One drawback of Onyx is the angiotoxicity of dimethylsulfoxide. It is injected under fluoroscopic guidance if combined with direct percutaneous treatment. The procedure is employed under general anesthesia or local anesthesia (depending on patient cooperation) and under fluoroscopic guidance. In general, and especially for vertebral sites, the needle used is the same as for percutaneous injection (16 G). It can be positioned directly into the lesion followed by a slow injection of the agent for better control of flow. Very careful and considered patient selection with good understanding of vascular anatomy is recommended for correct use of this procedure [82].

11.10 Osteoid Osteoma (OO)

OO is a small, benign (but painful) reactive bone lesion that, in general, occurs in males aged 10–20 years. The tumor is characterized by a nidus of diameter <1.5 cm and comprised well-organized trabecular bone with vascular fibrous connective stroma surrounded by reactive cortical bone. Most lesions are found in the long bones of the lower extremities (particularly the metadiaphyseal regions of the femur and tibia). Intramedullary and subperiosteal lesions are less common, are usually intra- or juxta-articular, and usually demonstrate less osteosclerosis (which may appear at some distance from the nidus) [83].

Spinal OO accounts for 10–25% of all cases of OO and 1% of spinal tumors (59% in the lumbar, 27% in the cervical, 12% in the dorsal, and 2% in the sacral region). It involves the posterior elements in 70–100% of cases and the VB in 7% of cases [83]. Spinal OO typically begins with an insidious onset of pain over the affected region that may radiate distally. Scoliosis can occur at the side of the lesion due to asymmetric muscle spasm. This causes asymmetric inhibition of the growth of the vertebral epiphysis and leads to a rotaional deformity. In general, most of these lesions are asymptomatic but management can become complex if they become symptomatic. Spontaneous regression due to unknown mechanisms has been documented.

The treatment options are:

- medical therapy with aspirin;
- *en-bloc* resection;
- minimally invasive percutaneous treatment with radiofrequency ablation (RFA).

Minimally invasive percutaneous treatment with RFA was described by Rosenthal et al. in 1989 and 1992, and was undertaken with CT guidance under local anesthesia [84]. The procedure involves placement, using a bone biopsy needle, of a radiofrequency probe into the nidus. At this point, RFA is carried out by inducing thermal necrosis of the lesion. Two cycles of ablation at 90°C for 2 min are needed for lesions of diameter <1 cm whereas for lesions of diameter >1 cm, a further two 2-min cycles in a different position are required. The duration of the procedure is about 90 min, but the duration of post-procedural hospitalization for observation is 3–24 h [84–85]. All daily activities can be resumed immediately without external supportive help.

The principle of RFA is use of an alternating current of high-frequency radio waves (>10 kHz) that pass from an electrode tip in body tissue and which dissipates its energy as heat. A radiofrequency generator forms an electric current that flows from the generator, through the electrode, into the patient and out through a ground electrode back to the generator. The resistance of biological structures causes local ions to vibrate. This "ionic agitation" results in friction around the electrode tip as ions change direction due to the alternating current and create heat to the point of dessication [86].

Vanderschueren et al. [87] reported a success rate of 79% on 28 RFAs without complications. Cioni et al. [88] observed good outcome in 30/38 patients. Rosenthal et al. demonstrated a success rate of >85% [86]. The recurrence rate is 5–10% and skin burns are reported quite often [83–90].

The relative contraindications for RFA are:

- a lesion on the hand in the spine (<1 cm from vital structures such as nerves);
- pregnancy;
- cellulitis;
- sepsis;
- coagulopathy.

Lesions with a nidus >1 cm usually require multiple applications of the electrode in various positions. Percutaneous RFA ablation induces necrosis in the lesion. It is a minimally invasive alternative to surgical treatment of OOs.

11.11 Vertebral Hemangiomas (VHs)

VHs are benign tumors with a rich vasculature. They represent 2–3% of all spinal tumors, and are identified in 10–12% of all vertebral autopsies [91–93]. They are usually asymptomatic and are diagnosed as accessory findings during radiographic or MRI examinations undertaken for other purposes. They tend to remain stable over time. Only 0.9–1.2% of VHs are symptomatic [94–95]. Symptoms vary from vertebral pain (54% of cases)–sometimes resistant to conservative medical treatment–to progressive neurological deficits (45% of cases) due to a vertebral fracture or medullary compression related to extension of the lesion to the VB/vertebral arch [95–96].

The histological pattern is characterized by anomalous vascular proliferation with regular venous and capillary structures (more frequently in the vertebral soma). A cavernous and capillary pattern of VH can be distinguished. The most common type that occurs in VBs is the cavernous variety, which is characterized by large sinusoidal spaces of venous engorgement and a single stratified epithelium [93, 97, 98].

VHs become symptomatic with the onset of critical neurological deficits as: the lesion grows in the VB or vertebral arch; when they determines the compression of the dural sac or of the nerve root due to presence of epidural tissue; or due intra-lesion bleeding. Venous types of congestion impair the trabecular architecture of the vertebral bone, thereby leading to fractures [97].

The physiological changes that occur during pregnancy tend to stress the growing tendency of VHs (especially during the first trimester of gestation). In fact, venous occlusion, increased intra-abdominal pressure, and the vascular redistribution of flow in the vertebral venous plexus due to uterine enlargement predispose to VH growth and to the related onset of compression fractures [99].

The management of VHs is complex. Surgery or radiotherapy have been first-line treatments for several years, but are worsened by intraoperative and postoperative hemorrhagic complications related to the rich vascularization that characterizes this type of lesion [92–93].

Recently, vertebroplasty (with or without MRI) has been introduced as an alternative to traditional surgical and radiotherapy of symptomatic VHs . The principle of vertebroplasty is to completely fill the vertebral lesion with cement (PMMA) to achieve irreversible sclerosis of the hemangiomatous venous pool, thus obtaining an antalgic effect. Moreover, in the case of vertebral fracture due to compression from tumor growth, the cement stabilizes the movements of the trabecular microfractures of the spongious bone which is responsible for the pain, and it also makes the VB more compact and resistant [100].

The main characteristics that make vertebroplasty the first-line treatment for VHs are a minimally invasive approach, early antalgic effect, and the low prevalence of complications. The low level of invasiveness is related to the use of a 11–15 G needle (depending on the location of the VH) with a length of 10–15 cm through the vertebral pedicle. Traumatic cutaneous and muscular incisions are not required. This type of procedure reduces the duration of hospitalization and offers a faster and less painful postoperative recovery.

The procedure is the same as that used for the treatment of porotic or primary/secondary vertebral tumors. However, a bipedicular approach is recommended to guarantee complete filling of the VB with an antalgic effect. The amount of cement used is dependent upon the size of the VH. In general, filling up the VH is the most important feature to obtain complete venous embolization. During treatment of expansive cavernous VHs, the perivertebral component of the lesion can become thrombosed even if it is not directly involved in the cement injection because the thrombolization is secondary to cementification of the main vascular bed, as described by Manfrè et al. [101].

Deramond et al. [102] described the successful outcome of vertebroplasty for the treatment of symptomatic and/or VHs with neurological deficits in >80% of patients, even if the lesions showed aggressive features upon imaging. Brunot et al. [103], in the short-term and long-term follow-up of treatment with vertebroplasty of symptomatic VHs observed efficacious treatment in 90% of cases and, in the long term, 3 patients preemptively treated for aggressive VHs remained asymptomatic. None of the treated patients showed a worsening of symptoms during the follow-up. Our research team has also observed complete remission of vertebral pain within 24–72 h of treatment without major or minor complications in all patients [100].

The selection criteria for cervical VHs are very strict. Patients with persistent pain with signs of atypical VH upon MRI should undergo vertebroplasty. Treatment can be combined with laminectomy. Feydy et al. [104] described 2 cases of symptomatic and non-aggressive VHs at the C4 level treated with vertebroplasty with a good antalgic effect and good vertebral stabilization as well as prompt regression of pain. Dousset et al. [105] reported a case of non-symptomatic but collapsed VHs treated with vertebroplasty for spinal stabilization.

Some authors have described the association of PMMA injection with direct intra-lesion injection of ethanol (<15 mL). Ethanol emphasizes the sclerotizing effect of the cement, thereby producing thrombosis of vascular angiomatous lesions. Nenertheless, injection of too large much ethanol in one dose can produce vertebral collapse [106–108].

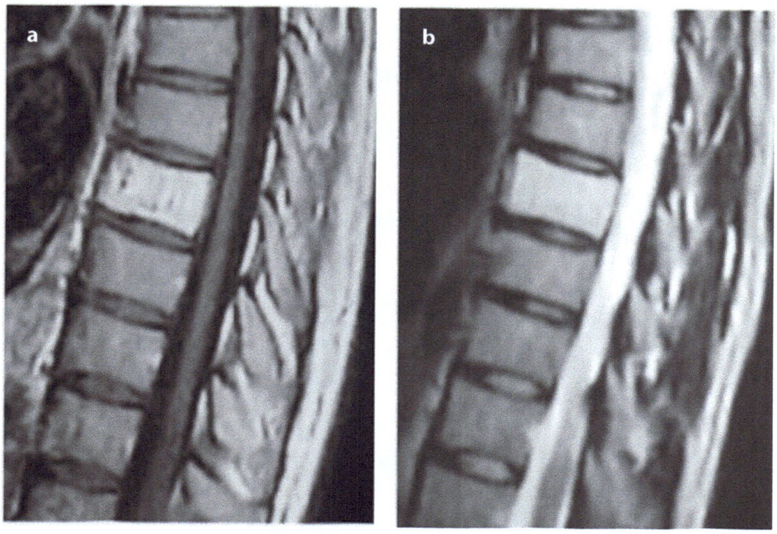

Fig. 11.21 Typical vertebral hemangioma at the dorsal level. Sagittal T1-weighted and T2-weighted MRI show the typical hyperintense signal (**a** and **b**) without epidural tissue or cortical erosion. The patient was asymptomatic

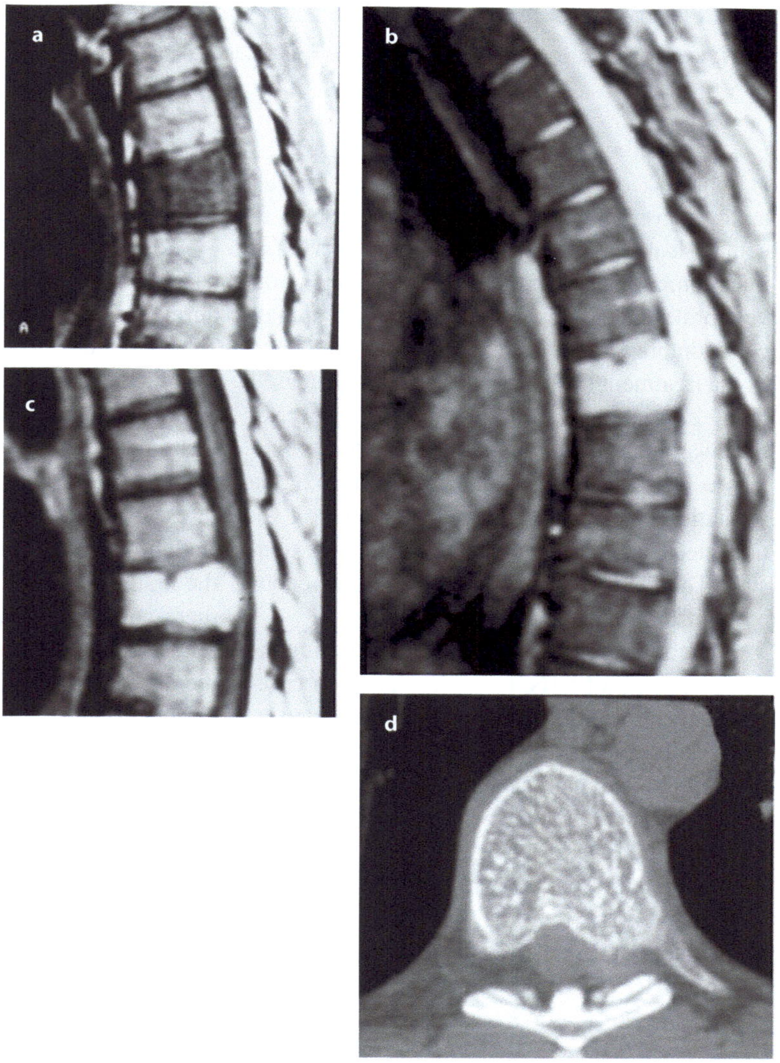

Fig. 11.22 Atypical vertebral hemangioma at the dorsal level with a hypointense signal on sagittal T1-weighted MRI (**a**) and a hyperintense signal on T2-weighted MRI (**b**) as well as homogeneous contrast enhancement on T1-weighted MRI on mild soft epidural tissue (**c**). Axial MDCT confirms the hemangioma of the vertebra at the dorsal level (**d**)

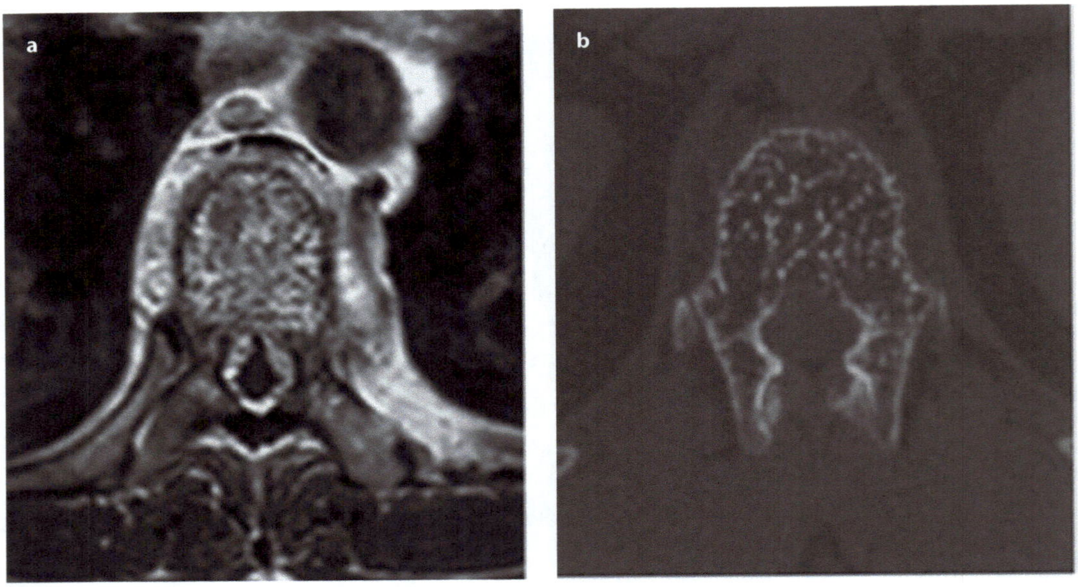

Fig. 11.23 An aggressive vertebral haemangioma with epidural tissue

The risk of complications for VHs (as well as for all vertebroplastic treatment) is related to cement leakage during extravertebral intra-canal injection, as well as in the prevertebral and paravertebral venous plexus with the risk of spinal-cord compression or pulmonary embolism [100]. In the treatment of the VHs, this risk is increased doing arterial access due to anarchic intravertebral vascularization, aggressive lesions, high-flow ectasisia (due to expansive angiomas) or the formation of intravertebral and paravertebral venous neoanastomoses related to the tumor extension. The risk is reduced by carrying out venous embolization with vertebroplasty.

To reduce the risk of complications during the vertebroplasty of VHs, restricted selection criteria are recommended. The population affected by VHs can be divided into four categories on the basis of clinical manifestations:

- asymptomatic patient with no sign of an aggressive VH (Fig. 11.21);
- symptomatic patient with no sign of an aggressive VH;
- asymptomatic patient with signs of an aggressive VH;
- symptomatic patient with signs of an aggressive VH.

The final group can be subdivided further based on the presence or absence of an epidural vascular component. Hypo-intensity on T1-weighted MRIs and hyperintensity on T2-weighted and T2 short TI inversion recovery (STIR) sequences with enhancement after contrast injection, the presence of epidural tissue, or evidence of cortical erosion are radiological features of aggressiveness (Fig. 11.22 and 11.23). Vertebroplasty is not indicated for patients in the first group. For patients in the second group, there could be an indication for vertebroplasty related to the presence of low back pain even in the absence of radiological evidence of aggressiveness. The patients in the third group must be evaluated carefully; management comprises annual MRI to check disease evolution. In fact, this treatment must be reserved only for VHs that are symptomatic and resistant to common conservative treatments, with radiological evidence of aggressiveness and/or epidural extension. All patients in the fourth group must undergo vertebroplasty [109] (Fig. 11.24).

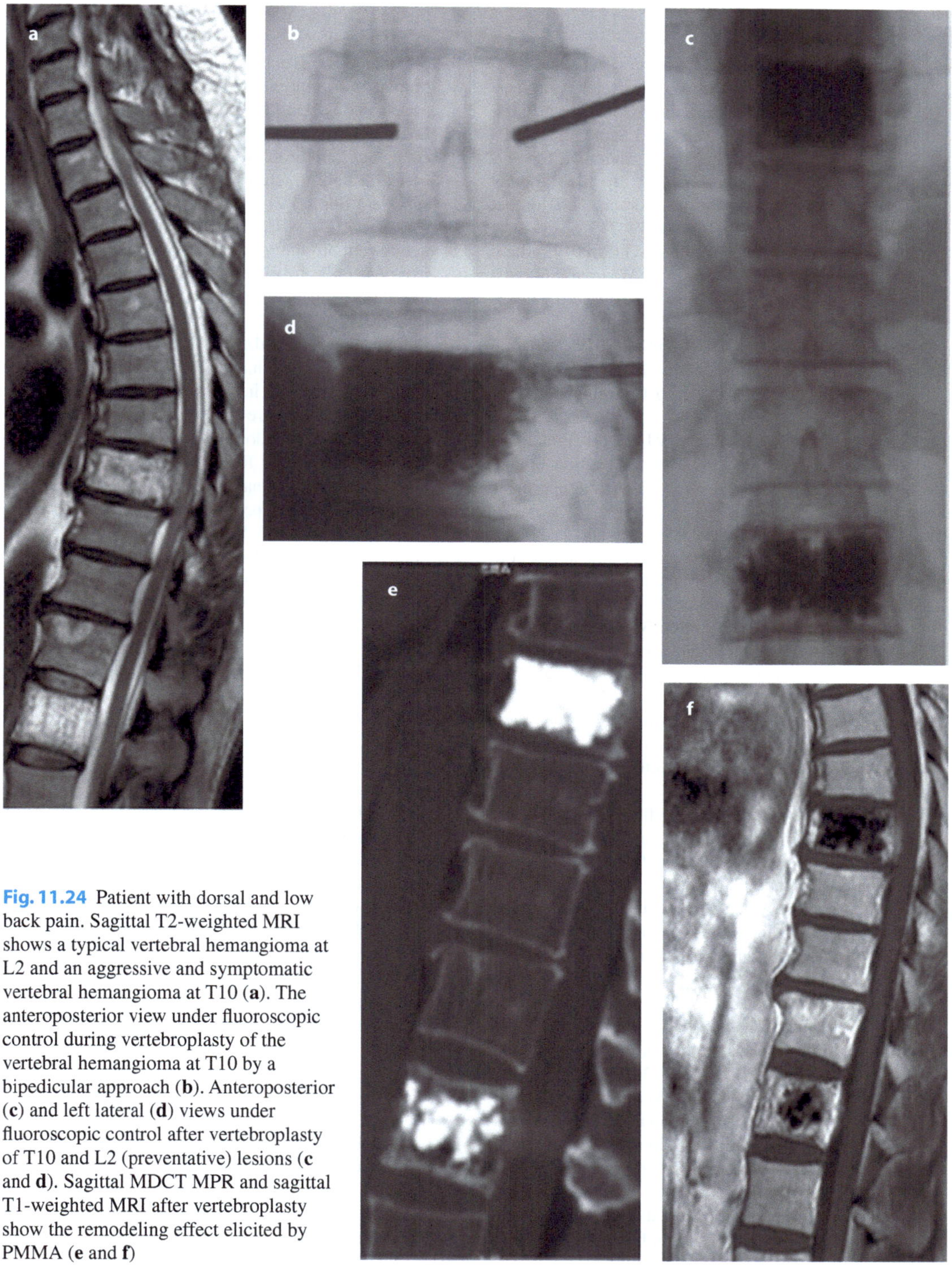

Fig. 11.24 Patient with dorsal and low back pain. Sagittal T2-weighted MRI shows a typical vertebral hemangioma at L2 and an aggressive and symptomatic vertebral hemangioma at T10 (**a**). The anteroposterior view under fluoroscopic control during vertebroplasty of the vertebral hemangioma at T10 by a bipedicular approach (**b**). Anteroposterior (**c**) and left lateral (**d**) views under fluoroscopic control after vertebroplasty of T10 and L2 (preventative) lesions (**c** and **d**). Sagittal MDCT MPR and sagittal T1-weighted MRI after vertebroplasty show the remodeling effect elicited by PMMA (**e** and **f**)

References

1. American Cancer Society: Cancer Facts and Figures 2007. Available at: http:// www.cancer.org/acs/groups/content/@nho/documents/document/caff-2007pwsecuredpdf.pdf. Accessed 3 September 2012
2. Taneichi H, Kaneda K, Takeda N, Abumi K, Satoh S (1997) Risk factors and probability of vertebral body collapse in metastases of the thoracic and lumbar spine. Spine (Phila Pa 1976) 22:239–245
3. Byrne TN, Benzel EC, Waxman SG (2000) Epidural tumors. In: Byrne TN, Benzel EC, Waxman SG (eds) Diseases of the spine and spinal cord. Oxford University Press, New York, p 166–205
4. Rastogi R, Patel T, Swarm RA et al (2010) Vertebral augmentation for compression fractures caused by malignant disease. J Nat Comp Cancer Network 8: 1095–1102
5. Schiff D, O'Neill BP, Suman VJ (1997) Spinal epidural metastasis as the initial manifestation of malignancy: Clinical features and diagnostic approach. Neurology 49:452–456
6. Maranzano E, Latini P (1995) Effectiveness of radiation therapy without surgery in metastatic spinal cord compression: final results from a prospective trial. Int J Radiat Oncol Biol Phys 32:959–967
7. Rougraff BT, Kneisl JS, Simon MA (1993) Skeletal metastases of unknown origin: a prospective study of a diagnostic strategy. J Bone Joint Surg Am 75:1276–1281
8. Lis E, Bilsky MH, Pisinski L et al (2004) Percutaneous CT-guided biopsy of osseous lesion of the spine in patients with known or suspected malignancy. Am J Neuroradiol 25:1583–1588
9. Edelstyn GA, Gillespie PJ, Grebbell FS (1967) The radiological demonstration of osseous metastases: experimental observations. Clin Radiol 18:158–162
10. Buhmann Kirchhoff S, Becker C, Duerr HR, Reiser M, Baur-Melnyk A (2009) Detection of osseous metastases of the spine: comparison of high resolution multi-detector-CT with MRI. Eur J Radiol 69:567–573
11. Taneichi H, Kaneda K, Takeda N, Abumi K, Satoh S (1997) Risk factors and probability of vertebral body collapse in metastases of the thoracic and lumbar spine. Spine (Phila PA 1976) 22:239–245
12. Katagiri H, Takahashi M, Inagaki J et al (1998) Clinical results of nonsurgical treatment for spinal metastases. Int J Radiat Oncol Biol Phys 42:1127–1132
13. Sørensen S, Helweg-Larsen S, Mouridsen H, Hansen HH (1994) Effect of high-dose dexamethasone in carcinomatous metastatic spinal cord compression treated with radiotherapy: a randomised trial. Eur J Cancer 30A:22–27
14. Patchell RA, Tibbs PA, Regine WF et al (2005) Direct decompressive surgical resection in the treatment of spinal cord compression caused by metastatic cancer: a randomised trial. Lancet 366:643–648
15. Saliou G, Kocheida M , Lehmann P et al (2010) Percutaneous vertebroplasty for pain management in malignant fractures of the spine with epidural involvement. Radiology 254:882–890
16. McDonald RJ, Trout AT, Gray LA et al (2008) Vertebroplasty in multiple myeloma: outcomes in a large patient series. Am J Neuroradiol 29:642–648
17. Fourney DR, Schomer DF, Nader R et al (2003) Percutaneous vertebroplasty and kyphoplasty for painful vertebral body fractures in cancer patients. J Neurosurg 98(1 Suppl.):21–30
18. Cheung G, Chow E, Holden L et al (2006) Percutaneous vertebroplasty in patients with intractable pain from osteoporotic or metastatic fractures: a prospective study using quality-of-life assessment. Can Assoc Radiol J 57:13–21
19. Pflugmacher R, Kandziora F, Schroeder RJ, Melcher I, Haas NP, Klostermann CK (2006) Percutaneous balloon kyphoplasty in the treatment of pathological vertebral body fracture and deformity in multiple myeloma: a one-year follow-up. Acta Radiol 47:369–376
20. Calmels V, Vallée JN, Rose M, Chiras J (2007) Osteoblastic and mixed spinal metastases: Evaluation of the analgesic efficacy of percutaneous vertebroplasty. Am J Neuroradiol 28:570–574
21. Ahn H Mousavi P, Roth S, Reidy D,. Finkelstein J, Whyne C (2006) Stability of the metastatic spine pre- and post-vertebroplasty. J Spinal Disord Tech 19:178–182
22. Leigh WB, Draffin J, Taylor P, Theis JC, Walton M (2006). Experimental studies on thermal effects of cement during vertebroplasty. J Bone Joint Surg 88B (Suppl. 2):313
23. Bai B, Yin Z, Xu Q et al (2009) Histologic changes of an injectable rhBMP-2/calcium phosphate cement in vertebroplasty of rhesus monkey. Spine (Philla Pa 1976) 34:1887–1892
24. Marcia S, Boi C, Dragani M et al (2012) Effectiveness of a bone substitute (CERAMENT™) as an alternative to PMMA in percutaneous vertebroplasty: 1-year follow-up on clinical outcome. Eur Spine J 21:S112-8
25. Fenton DS, Czervionke LF (2004) Image-guided spine interventions. Springer, New York p 69–93
26. Mathis JM. Vertebroplasty for vertebral fractures with intravertebral clefts (2002) Am J Neuroradiol 23:1619–1620
27. Schaefer O, Lohrmann C, Markmiller M, et al (2003) Combined treatment of a spinal metastasis with radiofrequency heat ablation and vertebrioplasty. Am. J Roentgenol 180:1075–1077
28. van der Linden E, Kroft LJ, Dijkstra PD, et al (2007) Treatment of vertebral tumor with posterior wall defect using image-guided radiofrequency ablation combined with vertebroplasty: preliminary results in 12 patients. J Vasc Int Radiol 18: 741–747
29. Gangi A, Buy X (2010) Percutaneous bone tumor management. Semin Intervent Radiol 27:124–136
30. Hirsch JA, Horsch AE, Jha R et al (2010) Practical management of malignant compression fractures. J NeuroIntervent Surg 2:219–220
31. Luo J, Pollintine P, Dolan P, Adams MA (2011) Creep deformity of aging human vertebrae is accelerated

following micro-damage. J Bone Joint Surg Br Proc 93B:487
32. Licht AW, Kramer W (2011) Radiofrequency kyphoplasty: a new method for the treatment of osteoporotic vertebral body compression fractures – a case report. J Miner Stoffwechs 18 (Suppl. 1):S26–S28
33. Pflugmacher R, Bornemann R, Randau T, Wirtz, DC (2011) Comparison of clinical and radiological data in treatment of patients with osteoporotic vertebral compression fractures with radiofrequency kyphoplasty or balloon kyphoplasty. GRIBOI 2011 – The 21st Interdisciplinary Research Conference On Injectable Osteoarticular Biomaterials and Bone Augmentation Procedures. Boston, 5–7 April
34. Luo J, Adams MA, Dolan P (2010) Vertebroplasty and kyphoplasty can restore normal spine mechanics following osteoporotic vertebral fracture. J Osteoporosis 1–9: article ID 729257
35. J. Gibson, et al., "Does cement distribution influence the mechanical outcome of vertebroplasty?" in Proceedings of the Society of Back Pain Research Meeting, Keele University, November 2008.
36. Baroud G, Crookshank M, Bohner M (2006) High-viscosity cement significantly enhances uniformity of cement filling in vertebroplasty: an experimental model and study on cement leakage. Spine 31:2562–2568
37. Loeffel M, Ferguson SJ, Nolte L.-P, Nolte, Kowal JH (2008) Vertebroplasty: experimental characterization of polymethyl-methacrylate bone cement spreading as a function of viscosity, bone porosity, and flow rate. Spine 33:1352–1359
38. Sun K, Mendel E, Rhines L, et al (2006) Cement filling pattern has a significant effect on biomechanics of vertebroplasty. Proceedings of the 52nd Annual Meeting of the Orthopaedic Research Society, Chicago
39. Cortet B, Cotten A, Boutry N, et al (1997) Percutaneous vertebroplasty in patients with osteolytic metastases or multiple myelomas. Rev Rhum Engl Ed 64:177–183
40. Cotten A, Dewatre F, Cortet B, et al (1996) Percutaneous vertebroplasty for osteolytic metastases and myeloma: effects of the percentage of lesion filling and the leakage of methylmethacrylate at clinical follow up. Radiology 200:525–530
41. Appel NM, Gilula LA (2004) Percutaneous vertebroplasty in patients with spinal canal compromise. Am J Roentgenol 182:947–951
42. Saliou G, Kocheida el M, Lehmann P et al (2010) Percutaneous Vertebroplasty for pain management in malignant fracture of the spine with epidural involvement. Radiology 882–889
43. Uemura et al. (2005) Case report - Reduction of tumoral volume after sacroplasty with combined injection of PMMA & n-BCA n-butilcyanacrilate) in HCC metastasis. Bone cement used as an embolic agent for active bleeding in vertebroplasty of metastatic lesions. AJNR
44. Baba Y, Hayashi S, Ueno K, Nakajo M. Bone cement used as an embolic agent for active bleeding in vertebroplasty of metastatic lesions. Acta Radiol 48:1024–1027
45. Manfrè L (2006) Ischemic changes after vertebroplasty in epidural masses. Proc Am Soc Neuroradiol 1:385
46. Deramond H, Wright NT, Belkoff SM (1999) Temperature elevation caused by bone cement polymerization during vertebroplasty. Bone 25(2 suppl):17S-21S
47. Attivazione dose-dipendente di mRNA e proteine tumore-soppressore (TNF) dopo introduzione di PMMA. Kayamura. Spine 2006
48. Taneichi H, Kaneda K, Takeda N, Abumi K, Satoh S (1997) Risk factors and probability of vertebral body collapse in metastases of the thoracic and lumbar spine. Spine (Phila Pa 1976) 22: 239–245
49. Gailloud P (2002) Pain sedation with bupivacaine infiltration after vertebroplasty failure. J Vasc Interv Rad
50. Eyheremendy EP, De Luca SE, Sanabria E (2004) Percutaneous pediculoplasty in osteoporotic compression fractures. J Vasc Interv Radiol 15:869-74
51. Gangi A, Dietemann JL, Guth S et al (1998) Percutaneous laser photocoagulation of spinal osteoid osteomas under CT guidance. AJNR Am J Neuroradiol 19:1955-8
52. Venbrux AV et al (2003) Image-guided percutaneous radiofrequency ablation for osteoid osteomas. J Vasc Interv Radiol 14: 375–380
53. Nour SG, Duerk JL, Lenin JS et al (2002) MR Imaging-guided radio-frequency thermal ablation of the lumbar vertebrae in porcine models. Radiology 224:452–462
54. Woertler K, Heindel W, Lindner N et al (2001) Osteoid osteoma: CT-guided percutaneous radiofrequency ablation and follow-up in 47 patients. J Vasc Interv Radiol 12:717–722
55. Pommershei W et al (2003) Sacroplasty: a treatment for sacral insufficiency fractures. Am J Neuroradiol 24:1003–1007
56. Garant M (2002) Sacroplasty: a new treatment for sacral insufficiency fracture. J Vasc Interv Radiol 13:1265–1267
57. Mehdizade A, Payer M, Martin JB et al (2004) Percutaneous vertebroplasty through a transdiscal access route after lumbar transpedicular instrumentation. Spine J 4:475–479
58. Gangi A et al (1994) Percutaneous vertebroplasty guided by a combination of CT and fluoroscopy. Am J Neuroradiol 15:83–86
59. Perisinakis K, Papadokostakis G, Gourtsoyannis N et al (2004) Patient exposure and associated radiation risks from fluoroscopically guided vertebroplasty or kyphoplasty. Radiology 232:701–707
60. Seibert JA (2004) Vertebroplasty and kyphoplasty: do fluoroscopy operators know about radiation dose, and should they want to know? Radiology 232:633–634
61. Jaffe HL, Lichtenstein L (1942) Solitary unicameral bone cyst with emphasis on the roentgen picture, the pathologic appearance and the pathogenesis. Arch Surg 44:1004-1025

62. Saccomanni B et al (2008) Aneurysmal bone cyst of spine: a review of literature. Arch Orthop Trauma Surg 128:1145–1147
63. Hay MC, Paterson D, Taylor TKF (1978) Aneurysmal bone cysts of the spine. J Bone Joint Surg Br 60B:406–411
64. Topouchian V, Mazda K, Pennecot GF et al (2004) Aneurysmal bone cysts in children: complications of fibrosing agent injection. Radiology 232:522–526
65. Boriani S, Bertoni F, Picci P et al (2001) Aneurysmal bone cyst of the mobile spine. Spine 26:27–35
66. Pennekamp W, Peters S, Schinkel C et al. Aneurysmal bone cyst of the cervical spine (2008) Eur Radiol 18: 2356–2360
67. Bollini G, Jouve JL, Cottalorda J, Petit P, Panuel M, Jacquemier M (1998) Aneurysmal bone cyst in children: analysis of twenty seven patients. J Pediatr Orthop B 7:274–285
68. Seller K, Jager M, Kramer R et al (2004) Occurrence of a segmental kyphosis after laminectomy of C2 for an aneurysmatic bone cysts: course and treatment strategy. Z Orthop Ihre Grenzgeb 142:83–87
69. Bush CH, Drane WE (2000) Treatment of an aneurysmal bone cyst of the spine by radionuclide ablation. Am J Neuroradiol 21:592–594
70. Ramirez AR, Stanton RP (2002) Aneurysmal bone cyst in 29 children. J Pediatr Orthop 22:533–539
71. Tokarz F, Jankowski R, Żukiel R (1993) Aneurysmal bone cyst of the skull and vertebral column treated operatively. Neurol Neurochir Pol 27: 533–540
72. Daszkiewicz P, Roszkowski M, Grajkowska W (2004) Aneurysmal bone cyst of skull and vertebrae in children. Analysis of own material and review of the literature. Folia Neuropathol 42:25–30
73. Feigenberg SJ, Marcus RB, Zlotecki R et al (2001) Megavoltage radiotherapy for aneurysmal bone cysts. Int J Radiat Oncol Biol Phys 49:1243–1247
74. Dubois J, Chigot V, Grimard G, et al (2003) Sclerotherapy in aneurismal bone cysts in children: a review of 17 cases. Pediatr Radiol 33:365–372
75. Dekeuwer P, Odent T, Cadilhac C et al (2003) Aneurysmal bone cyst of the spine in children: a 9-year follow-up of 7 cases and review of the literature. Rev Chir Orthop Reparatrice Appar Mot 89:97–106
76. De Cristoforo R, Boriani S, Roversi R et al (1992) Selective arterial embolitation in the treatment of aneurismal bone cyst and angioma of bone. Skel Radiol 21:523–527
77. de Kleuver M, van der Heul RO, Veraart BE (1998) Aneurysmal bone cyst of the spine: 31 cases and the importance of the surgical approach. J Pediatr Orthop B 7:286–292
78. Rastogi S, Varshney MK, Trikha V, Khan SA, Choudhury B, Safaya R (2006) Treatment of aneurysmal bone cysts with percutaneous sclerotherapy using polidocanol. A review of 72 cases with long-term follow-up. J Bone Joint Surg Br 88:1212–1216
79. Shisha T, Nemeth T, Szoke G et al (2007) The dangers of intraosseous fibrosing agent injection in the treatment of bone cysts. The origin of major complications shown in a rabbit model. Int Orthopaed 31:359–362
80. Falappa P, Fassari FM, Fanelli A et al (2002) Aneurysmal bone cysts: treatment with direct percutaneous ethibloc injection: long-term results. Cardiovasc Intervent Radiol 25:282–290
81. Adamsbaum C, Mascard E, Guinebretiere JM Kalifa G, Dubousset J (2003) Intralesional Ethibloc injections in primary aneurysmal bone cysts: an efficient and safe treatment. Skel Radiol 32:559–566
82. Guarnieri G, Vassallo P, Muto M. (2010) Combined percutaneous and endovascular treatment of symptomatic aneurysmal bone cyst of the spine: clinical six months. Follow-up of six cases. Neuroradiol J 23:74–84
83. Motamedi D, Learch TJ, Ishimitsu DN et al (2009) Thermal ablation of osteoid osteoma: overview and step-by-step guide. Radiographics 29:2127–2141
84. Rosenthal DI, Hornicek FJ, Wolfe MW et al (1998) Percutaneous radiofrequency coagulation of osteoid osteoma compared with operative treatment. J Bone Joint Surg Am 80:815–821
85. Rosenthal DI, Springfield DS, Gebhardt MC, Rosenberg AE, Mankin HJ (1995) Osteoid osteoma: percutaneous radio-frequency ablation. Radiology 197: 451–454
86. Rosenthal DI, Hornicek FJ, Torriani M, Gebhardt MC, Mankin HJ (2003) Osteoid osteoma: percutaneous treatment with radiofrequency energy. Radiology 229:171–175
87. Vanderschueren GM, Taminiau AHM, Obermann WR, Bloem JL (2002) Osteoid osteoma: clinical results with thermocoagulation. Radiology 224:82–86
88. Cioni R, Consoli V, Bartolozzi C (2004) CT-guided radiofrequency ablation of osteoid osteoma: long-term results. Eur Radiol 14:1203–1208
89. Lindner NJ, Ozaki T, Roedl R, Gosheger G, Winkelmann W, Wörtler K (2001) Percutaneous radiofrequency ablation in osteoid osteoma. J Bone Joint Surg Br 83:391–396
90. Laus M, Albisinni U, Alfonso C, Zappoli FA (2007) Osteoid osteoma of the cervical spine: surgical treatment or percutaneous radiofrequency coagulation? Eur Spine J 16:2078–2082
91. Dagi TF, Schmidek HH (1990) Vascular tumors of the spine. In: Sundaresan N, Schmidek HH, Schiller AL (eds) Tumors of the spine: diagnosis and clinical management. Saunders, Philadelphia, p 181–191
92. Fox M, Onofrio B (1993) The natural history and management of symptomatic and asymptomatic vertebral hemangiomas. J Neurosurg 78:36–45
93. Pastushyn A, Slinko E, Mirzoyeva G et al (1998) Vertebral hemangiomas: diagnosis, management, natural history and clinicopathological correlates in patients. Surg Neurol 50:535–547
94. Healy M, Herz DA, Pearl L (1983) Spinal hemangiomas. Neurosurgery 13:689–691
95. Nguyen JP, Djindjian M, Gaston A (1987) Vertebral hemangiomas presenting with neurologic symptoms. Surg Neurol 27:391–397

96. Krueger EG (1961) Vertebral hemangioma with com-pression spinal cord. J Neurosurg 18:331–338
97. Acosta F, Chou D, Ames CP et al (2008) Comprehensive management of symptomatic and aggressive vertebral hemangiomas. Neurosurg Clin N Am 19:17–29
98. Castel E, Lazennec JY, Chiras J et al (1993) Acute spinal cord compression due to intraspinal bleeding from a vertebral hemangioma. J Vasc Interv Radiol 8:244–248
99. Kiroglu Y, Benek B, Yagci B, Cirak B, Tahta K (2009) Surgical spinal cord compression caused by vertebral hemangioma being symptomatic during pregnancy Neurology 71:487–492
100. Guarnieri G, Muto M, Vassallo P et al (2009) Vertebroplasty as treatment of aggressive and symptomatic vertebral hemangiomas: up to 4 years of follow-up. Neuroradiology 51:471–476
101. Manfre L et al (2002) La vertebroplastica nelle neoplasie del rachide. Riv Neuroradiol 15:461–472
102. Deramond H (2003) Vertebroplasty for pain relief. Riv Neuroradiol 16:767–770
103. Brunot S, Berge J, Barreau X, Ménégon P, Dousset V (2005) Long term clinical follow up of vertebral hemangiomas treated by percutaneous vertebroplasty. J Radiol 86:41–47
104. Feydy, Cognard C, Chiras J (1996) Acrylic vertebroplasty in symptomatic cervical vertebral haemangiomas: report of 2 cases. Neuroradiology 38:389–391
105. Dousset V, Senegas U et al (1996) Asymptomatic cervical ha haemangioma treated by percutaneous vertebroplasty. Neuroradiology 38:392–394
106. Cheen L, Zhang C, Tang T (2007) Cement vertebroplasty combined with ethanol injection in the treatment of vertebral haemangioma. Chin Med J 120:1136–1139
107. Doppman J, Oldfield E, Heiss J et al (2000) Symptomatic vertebral hemangiomas: treatment by means of direct intralesional injection of Ethanol. Radiology 214:314–348
108. Gangi A, Kastler B, Dietmann JL et al (1994) Injection of alcohol into bone metastases under CT guidance. J Comput Assist Tomogr 18:932–935
109. Muto M, Muto E, Izzo R et al (2005) La vertebroplastica nel trattamento delle sindromi algiche del rachide. Radiol Med 109:208–219

Kyphoplasty and Kyphoplasty-like Devices: Indications and Results

12

Mario Muto, Gianluigi Guarnieri and Giovanni Carlo Anselmetti

12.1 Introduction

Kyphoplasty (KP) can be considered to be a development and evolution of vertebroplasty (VP). In fact, KP has been termed "balloon or mechanical-assisted VP". The first KP was carried out in the USA in 1998 [1]. The procedure involves delivering cement in the form of polymethylmethacrylate (PMMA) or other types of cement into a fractured vertebral body (VB) under fluoroscopic guidance after dedicated balloon tamps have been used to create a cavity within the compacted trabecular bone [2].

The rationale of KP is to combine the analgesic and vertebral consolidation effects of VP with restoration of the physiological height of the collapsed VB. This action reduces the kyphotic deformity of the VB, thereby eliciting normal vertebral biomechanics, improving respiratory and gastrointestinal dysfunction, and producing some of the advantageous clinical effects seen with VP.

The main indications for KP are osteoporotic and non-osteoporotic vertebral fractures. These include primary and secondary vertebral tumors, Magerl type-A1 fractures, and selected Magerl type-A2 and -A3 fractures [3–4]. As with VP, the major indication is for porotic vertebral compression fractures (VCFs) with spinal pain refractory to conservative medical and physical treatment [5–12]. Approximately 70% of eligible patients are treated with VP and 30% with KP.

M. Muto (✉)
Neuroradiology Department, A. Cardarelli Hospital, Naples, Italy
e-mail: mutomar2@gmail.com

12.2 Indications

A VCF with pain is the major indication for KP. Reduction of the kyphotic deformity is the primary goal of all KP devices because such systems can be used to recover the height of the VB. Hence, KP should be recommended in cases of loss of vertebral height of ≥50%. The diagnostic approach is similar to the one employed for VP. Patient selection is based upon examination by magnetic resonance imaging (MRI) with sagittal T2-short-term inversion recovery (STIR) with fat-suppression sequences. T2-STIR sequences are used to choose the type of treatment and the number of VBs showing bone-marrow edema that can be treated.

The absolute contraindications of KP are local or systemic infections, coagulopathy, allergy to PMMA, and a painless vertebral fracture. The relative contraindications are the same as those described for VP (see chapter 9). Multiple myeloma and spinal metastases can also be treated by KP [6, 7, 12].

Vertebral traumatic fractures can be defined as "stable" or "unstable" according to three-columns theory [13–15]. Multiple classifications of vertebral trauma are available, including those of

M. Muto (ed.), *Interventional Neuroradiology of the Spine*,
DOI 10.1007/978-88-470-2790-9_12, © Springer-Verlag Italia 2013

Table 12.1 Magerl classification of fractures

A Compression injury	A1 Impaction fracture	A1.1 Endplate impaction A1.2 Wedge impaction A1.3 With collapse
	A2 Split fracture	A2.1 Sagittal A2.2 Coronal A2.3 Pincer
	A3 Burst fracture	A3.1 Incomplete A3.2 Burst/split A3.3 Complete
B Distraction injury	B1 Post-ligament lesion	B1.1 With disk disruption B1.2 With type-A fracture
	B2 Post-bony lesion	B2.1 Transverse bi-column B2.2 With disc disruption B2.3 With type-A fracture
	B3 Anterior disk rupture	B3.1 with subluxation B3.2 with spondilolysis B3.3 with post dislocation
C Rotation injury	C1 Type A with rotation	C1.1 With wedge C1.2 With split C1.3 With burst
	C2 Type B with rotation	C2.1 B1 with rotation C2.2 B2 with rotation C2.3 B3 with rotation
	C3 Rotational shear injury	C3.1 Slice fracture C3.2 Oblique

Holdsworth, Louis, Roy-Camille, Ferguson and Allen, Magerl, Patel, and Aebi. The most utilized classification is that of Magerl. This classification divides trauma into types of injury (compression, rotation, distraction) with multiple subtypes (Table 12.1). The major indications for KP are for traumatic vertebral fractures of the Magerl A1 type; selected patients with traumatic vertebral fractures of Magerl A2 and A3 types can also be considered for KP [3–4]. Patients affected by Magerl A1-type fractures can also be treated with orthesis device, bed rest and medical/physical therapy for ≥3–6 months. One cannot exclude the possibility of development of a kyphotic deformity due to the problems related to orthesis devices such as respiratory disturbances and sleep problems. KP is a suitable treatment for Magerl A1 fractures because it can restore vertebral height and guarantee homogeneous distribution of cement with better axial resistance to loads. Patients who have suffered polytrauma, elderly subjects in whom a surgical indication is not suggested, and individuals in which the risk of surgery and anesthesia is too high can also be considered for KP. There are no absolute rules about the timing also of KP except that traumatic fractures should be treated as soon as possible [16].

12.3 Procedure

A bilateral trans-pedicular approach under fluoroscopic guidance is essential to obtain good restoration of VB height and homogeneous cement filling. High-quality fluoroscopy is also very important to have complete anatomical control of the spine (even in elderly scoliotic patients). An appropriate pedicular approach lessens the risks of complications. The dimension of the peduncles is important to direct the correct anatomical approach, and it should be checked the treatment is decided.

KP can be undertaken with local anesthetic but general anesthesia may be required if more than one level is to be treated or in trauma cases (especially if the patient is young due to their

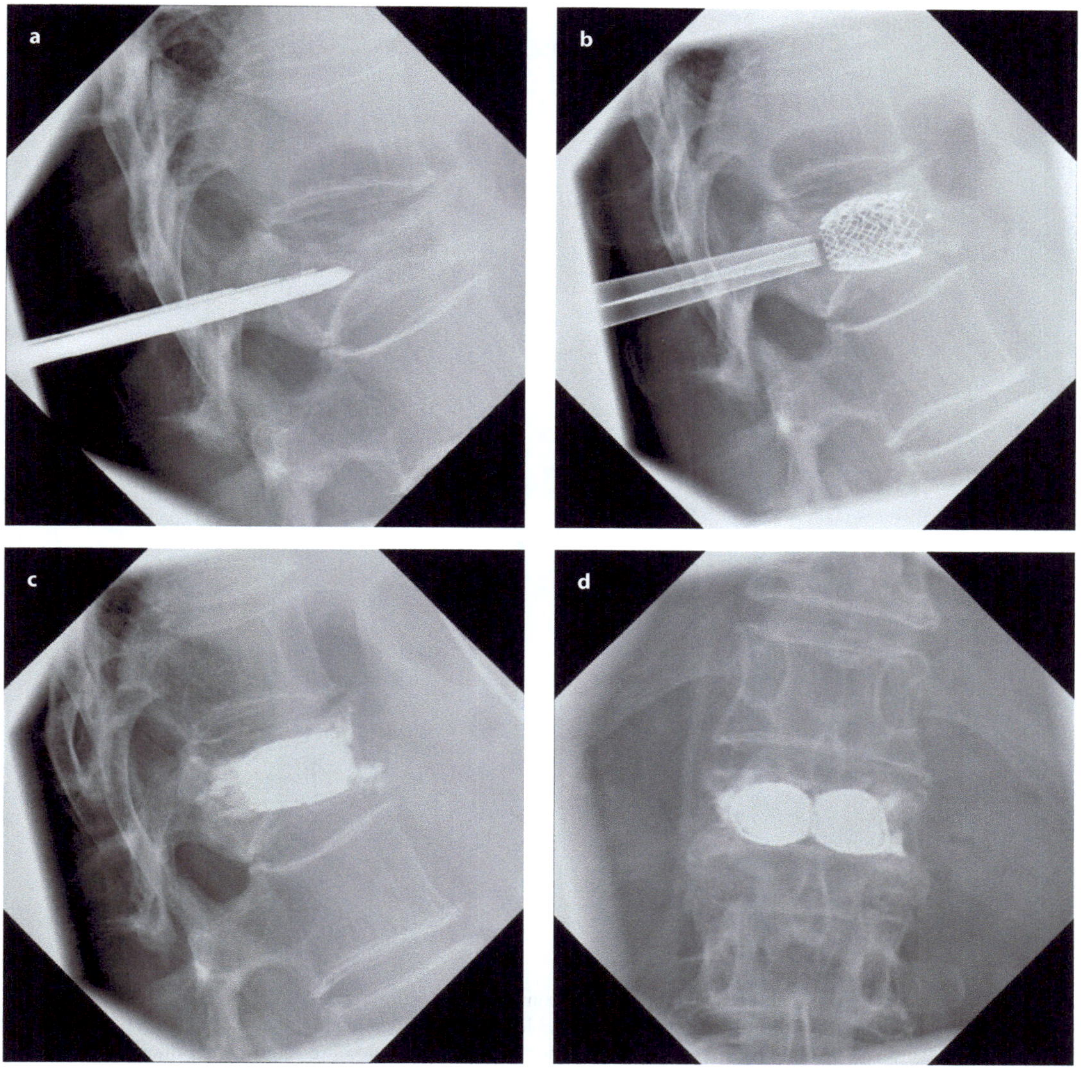

Fig 12.1 72-year-old female with severe osteoporosis and acute back pain resistant to medical therapy due to a vertebral fracture at the L1 level. Left lateral view under fluoroscopic control during KP with the vertebral body stenting system at the L1 level by a bipendicular approach shows the correct position of needles into the vertebral body (**a**). Left lateral view under fluoroscopic control after deployment of the vertebral body stent into the L1 level (**b**). Left lateral and anteroposterior views under fluoroscopic control after KP show augmentation after deployment of the vertebral body stenting system with homogeneous distribution of cement into the soma without venous or disk leakage (**c** and **d**)

different bone structure). This is because of the dimension of the cannulas are used in KP (8–12 G) compared with those utilized in VP (13–15 G). Also, KP takes longer to complete than VP. Once local anesthesia has been induced, the needle is positioned in the VB through a trans-pedicular approach until the posterior wall is reached. The medial margin of the peduncle is a crucial anatomical landmark to check in anteroposterior view before passing over the posterior wall of the VB in the left lateral view. At this point, a Kirschner wire (K-wire) can be used. The first cannula is removed, leaving the K-wire *in situ*, and the working cannula is positioned. A metallic drill can also be used to model the trabecular bone to enable insertion of the tamp. The drill is removed and the balloons inserted. The inflators are connected to the balloon and, under

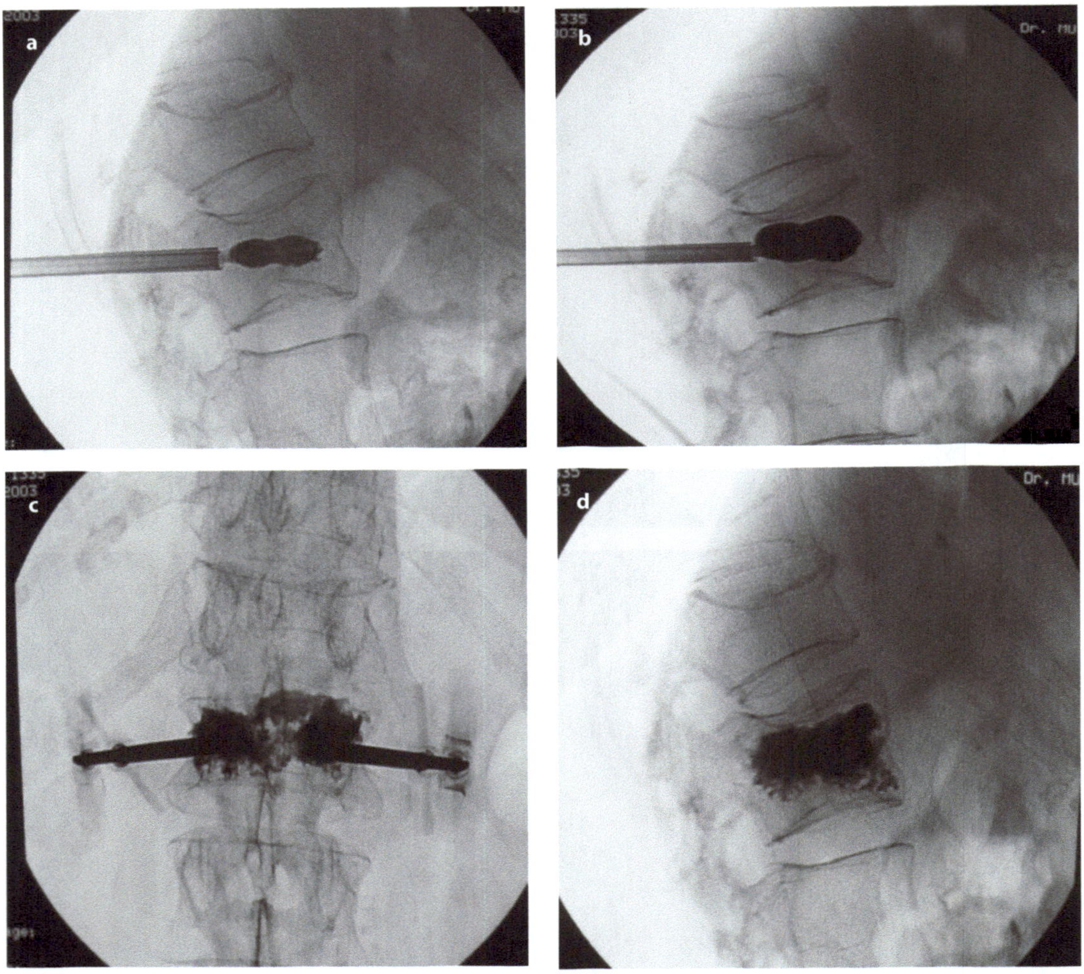

Fig 12.2 52-year-old female with a traumatic vertebral compression fracture at the L3 level. Left lateral view under fluoroscopic control during KP during balloon-KP at the L3 level by a bipendicular approach shows the correct position of needles into the vertebral body (**a** and **b**). Anteroposterior and left lateral views (**c** and **d**) under fluoroscopic control after KP show augmentation after deployment of the vertebral body stenting system with homogeneous distribution of cement into the soma without venous or disk leakage

fluoroscopic control, balloon inflation can begin with the use of diluted contrast media. In case of KP like-devices, the system is inserted through the working cannula after the use of a drill and bone compactor. A stent (or any other type of system) is inserted through the working cannula and can be released to achieve height restoration.

The amount of cement injected into the VB is extremely variable, i.e., 2–4 mL by each peduncle depending on the metamer being treated (thoracic or lumbar), and the degree of collapse in the VB. There are no absolute rules regarding the amount of cement to be injected. The cement is injected through bone filler or through a 1-mL syringe. The procedure is identical no matter which VB augmentation devices are used (Figs 12.1–12.6).

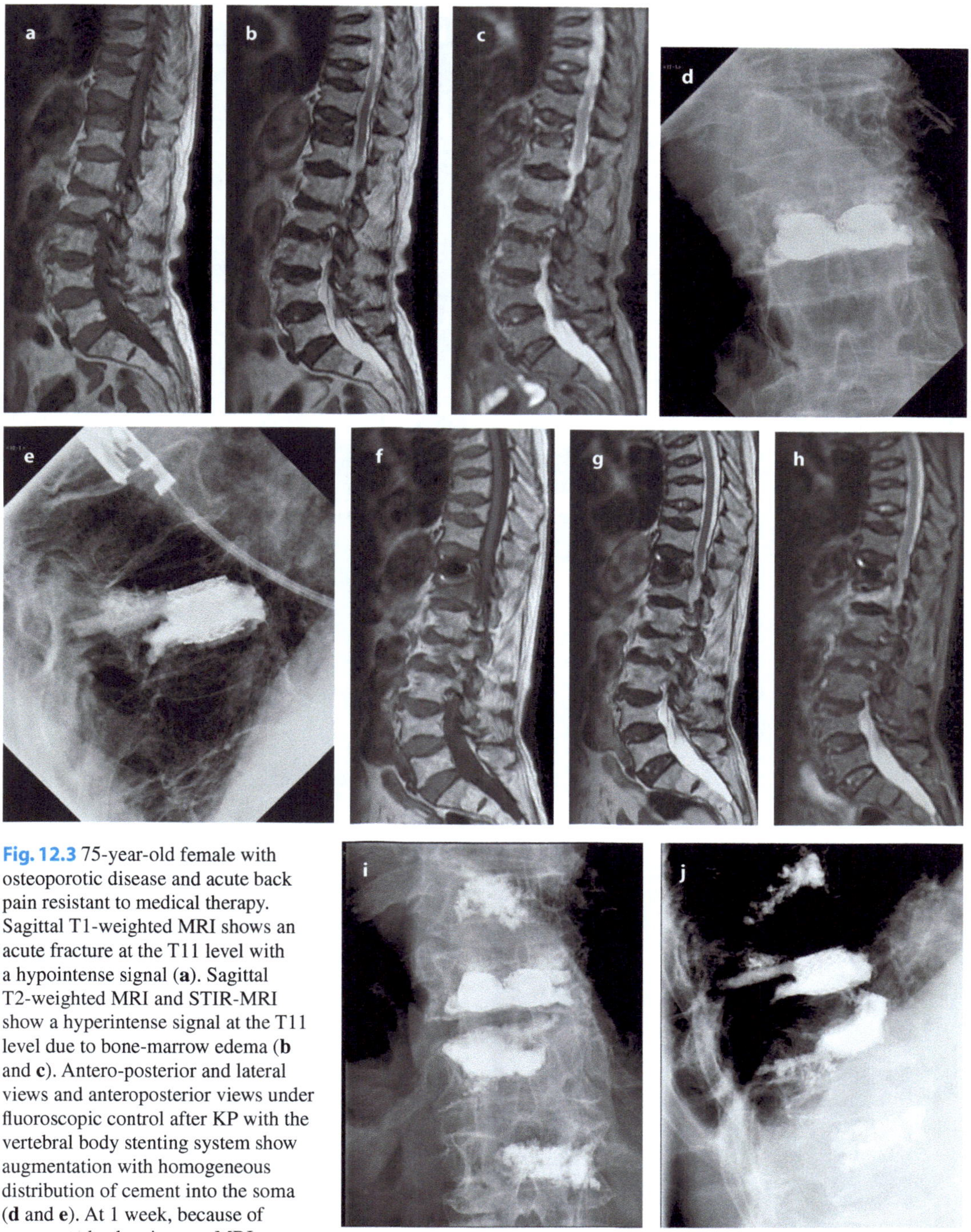

Fig. 12.3 75-year-old female with osteoporotic disease and acute back pain resistant to medical therapy. Sagittal T1-weighted MRI shows an acute fracture at the T11 level with a hypointense signal (**a**). Sagittal T2-weighted MRI and STIR-MRI show a hyperintense signal at the T11 level due to bone-marrow edema (**b** and **c**). Antero-posterior and lateral views and anteroposterior views under fluoroscopic control after KP with the vertebral body stenting system show augmentation with homogeneous distribution of cement into the soma (**d** and **e**). At 1 week, because of new acute back pain, new MRI was undertaken; sagittal T1-weighted MRI showed a new vertebral fracture at the T12 level after KP with vertebral body stenting at the T11 level (**f**). Sagittal T2-weighted MRI and STIR-MRI show a new symptomatic vertebral compression fracture after KP with vertebral body stenting at the T12 level with a hyperintense signal on STIR-MRI due to bone-marrow edema and a low signal at the T11 level due to polymethylmethacrylate (**g** and **h**). Antero-posterior (**i**) and lateral (**j**) views under fluoroscopic control after the second treatment show VP into the new vertebral compression fracture at the T12 level without venous or disk leakage as well as preventative VP at T10 and L1 levels with a good antalgic effect (**i** and **j**)

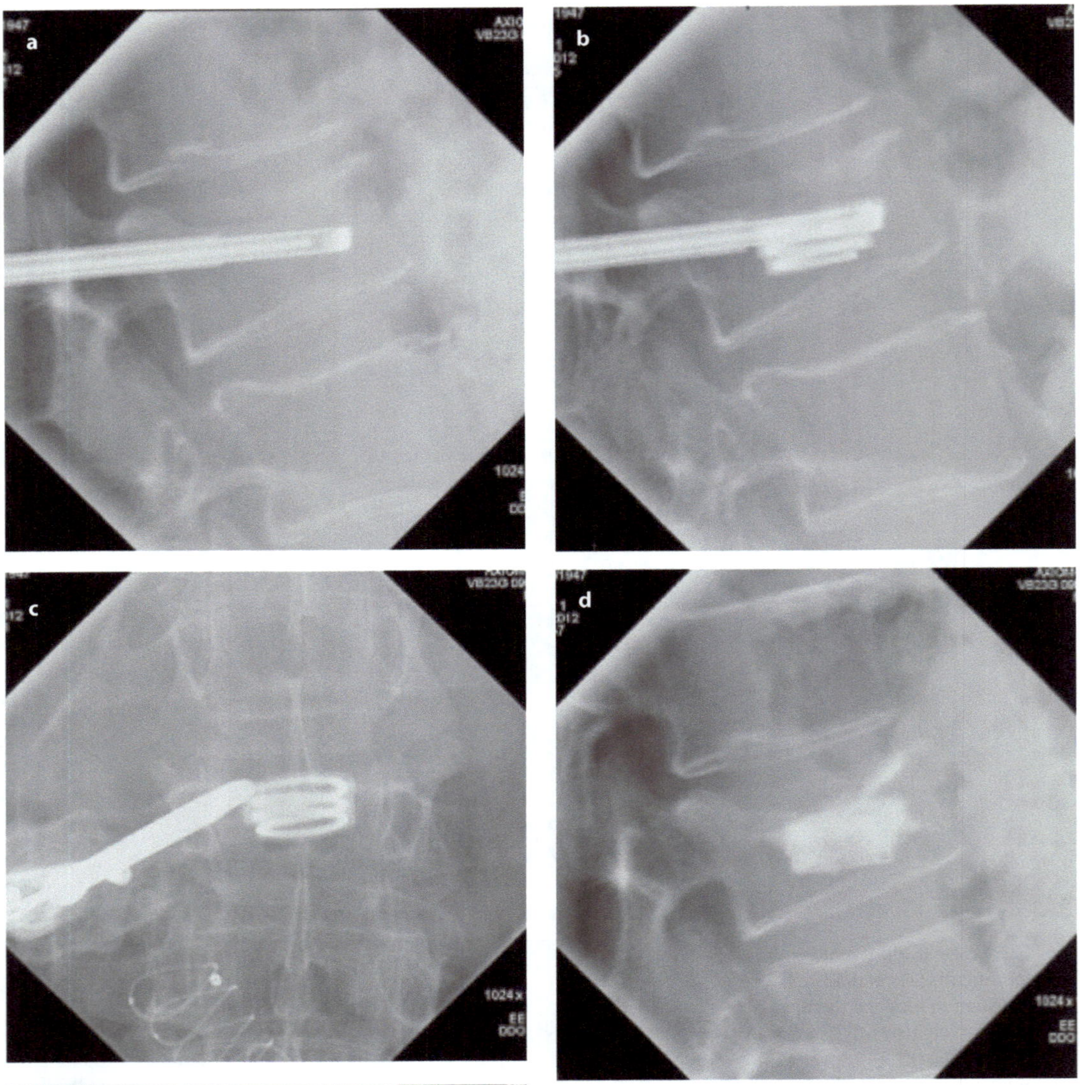

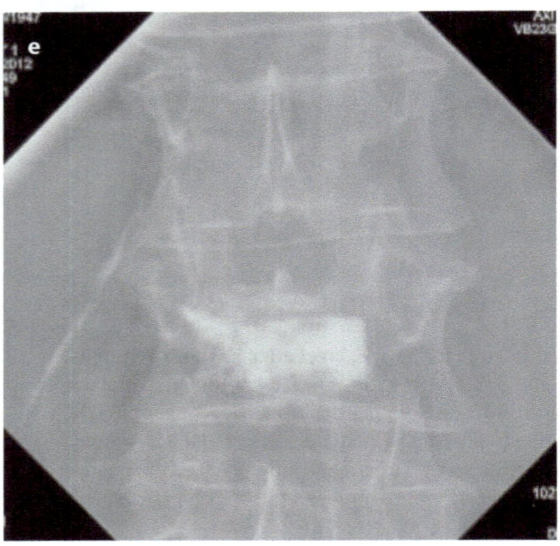

Fig. 12.4 Left lateral (**a**-**b**) and anteroposterior (**c**) views under fluoroscopic control during treatment using the Kiva® system at the L1 level using a unipedicular approach (**a**–**c**). Left lateral and anteroposterior views under fluoroscopic control during treatment using the Kiva system at the L1 level using a unipedicular approach shows good distribution of cement without venous or disk leakage (**d** and **e**)

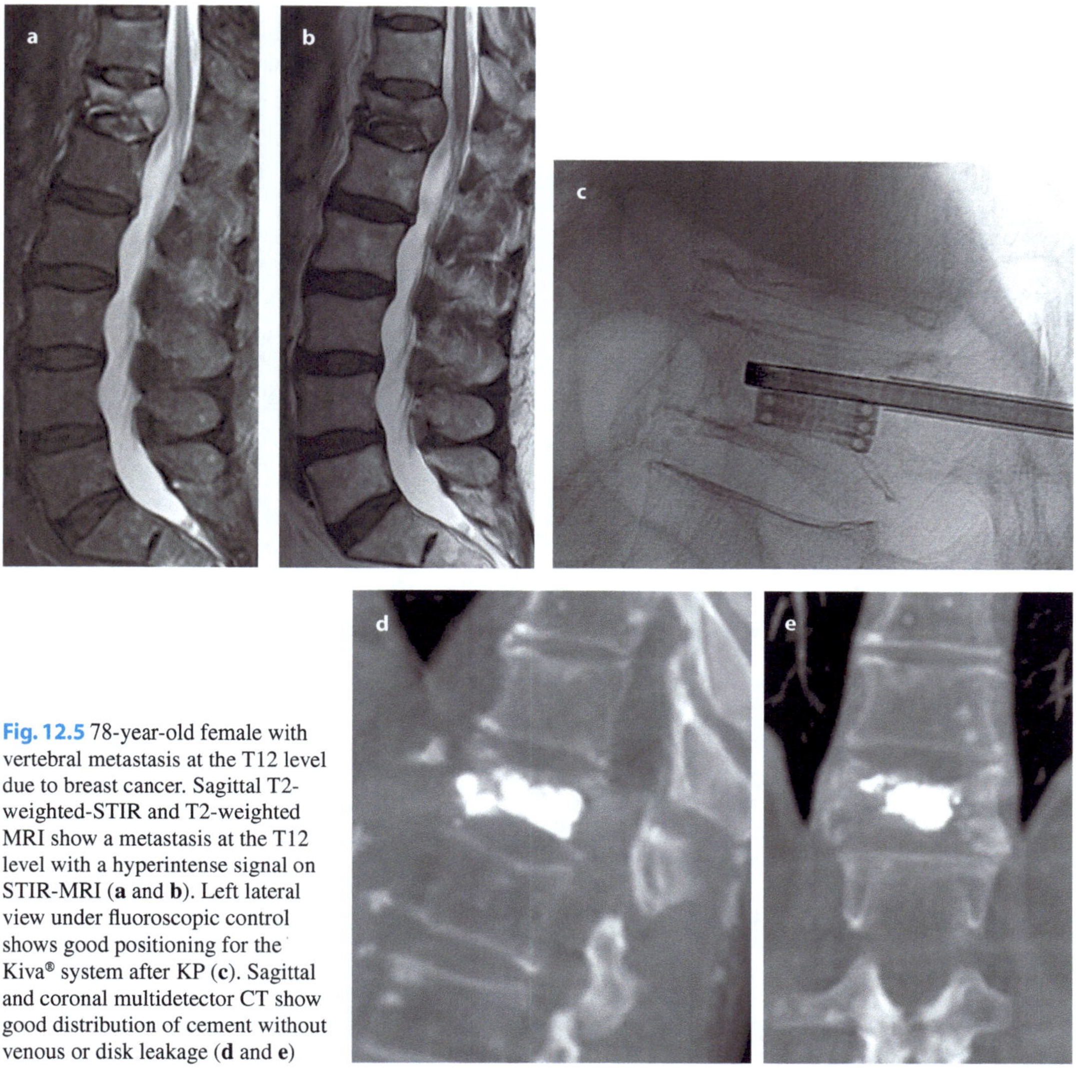

Fig. 12.5 78-year-old female with vertebral metastasis at the T12 level due to breast cancer. Sagittal T2-weighted-STIR and T2-weighted MRI show a metastasis at the T12 level with a hyperintense signal on STIR-MRI (**a** and **b**). Left lateral view under fluoroscopic control shows good positioning for the Kiva® system after KP (**c**). Sagittal and coronal multidetector CT show good distribution of cement without venous or disk leakage (**d** and **e**)

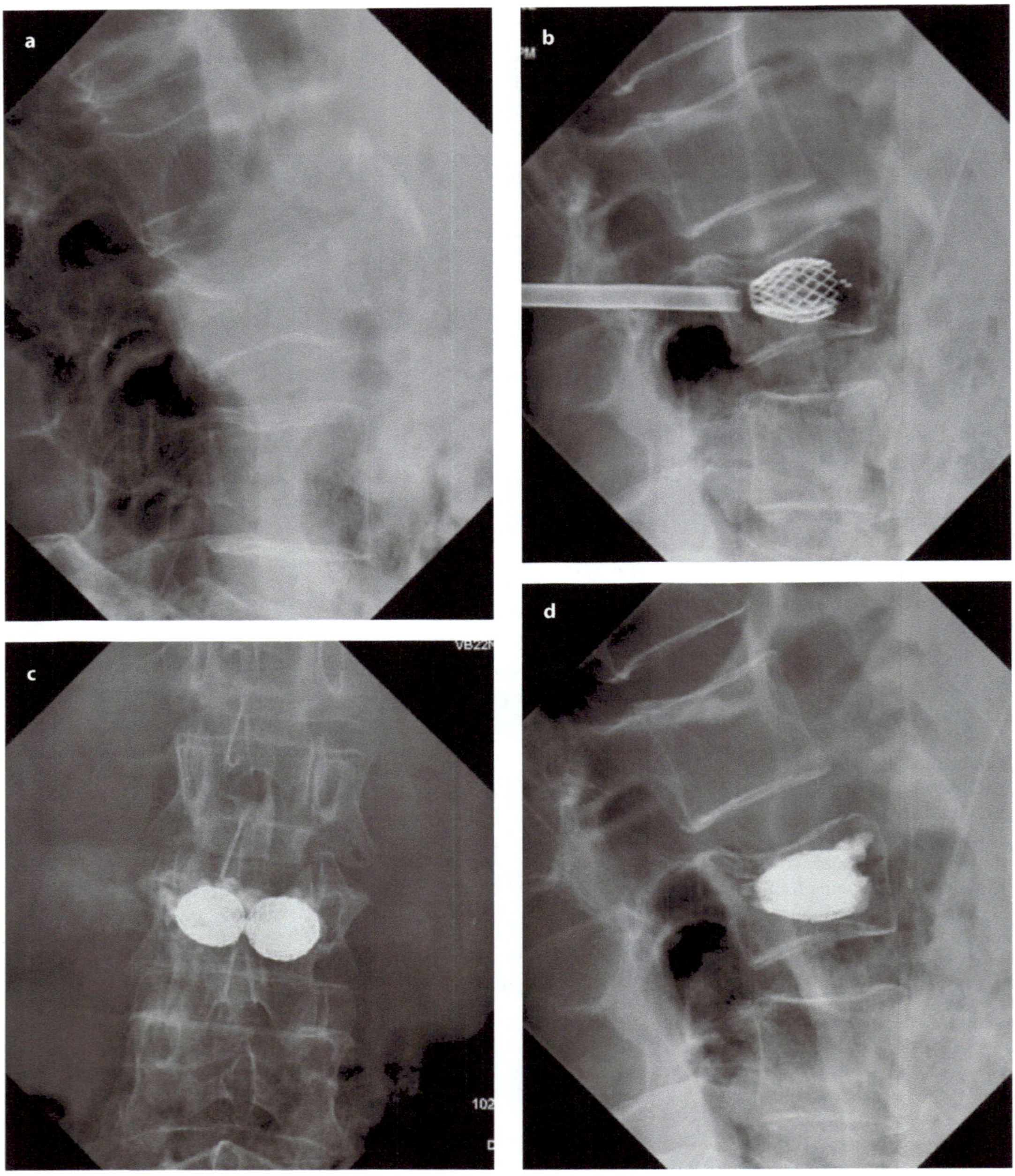

Fig. 12.6 78-year-old male with severe osteoporosis and acute back pain resistant to medical therapy due to a vertebral fracture at the L3 level. Left lateral view under fluoroscopic control during KP with the vertebral body stenting system shows a vertebral compression fracture at the L3 level (**a**). Left lateral view under fluoroscopic control during KP after stent placement into the L3 level (**b**). Anteroposterior (**c**) and left lateral views (**d**) under fluoroscopic control after KP with the vertebral body stenting shows good augmentation with homogeneous distribution of cement into the soma without venous or disk leakage (**c** and **d**)

12.4 Biomechanics of KP

KP, thanks to a balloon tamps system followed by cement injection into the newly created cavity of the fractured VB, produces an appreciable augmentation effect with rapid relief from pain [17]. As with VP, KP contributes to biomechanical alterations in the vertebral column with different axial-load distributions. However, due to re-expansion of the vertebra with balloon tamps the effect of early normal spinal alignment with normal vertebral biomechanics and reduced pathological kyphosis should be greater using KP than with using VP. Also, modification of the stiffness and failure strength of the functional spinal units (SUs) can increase the prevalence of re-fracture at adjacent or distant metamers.

The biomechanical alterations observed in the vertebral column after KP are similar to those seen with VP but with a few additional differences:

- restoration of spinal alignment;
- the cements that are used for injection have different influences on spinal stiffness due to their different properties and features;
- different distribution of axial load;
- uni- or bipedicular approaches;
- different devices used.

Strength and stiffness are important parameters for assessing the biomechanics of VBs. These parameters are influenced by the method, type of cement, and devices used. To obtain normal restoration of stiffness and the strength of functional SUs, KP must be carried out by a bipedicular approach. Chen at al. compared the different effects of unipedicular and bipedicular KP on the stiffness of compression fractured VBs and assessed how cement distribution affected the bilateral biomechanical balance of VBs. They concluded that unipedicular KP and bipedicular KP significantly increase the total stiffness of VBs. Bipedicular KP creates stiffness uniformly across both sides of the vertebrae, whereas unipedicular KP creates a biomechanical balance that is dependent upon cement distribution. If bone cement is augmented only on one side, the stiffness of non-augmented side will be significantly lower than the augmented side, which might lead to an imbalance of stress on the VB. However, if cement augmentation crosses the midline, the stiffness of both sides increases comparatively, and biomechanical balance is achieved [18].

PMMA cement produces an exceedingly high compressive strength and stiffness profile that could cause fractures to adjacent VBs. Other types of cement can produce fewer alterations in strength and stiffness compared with the effect elicited by PMMA. For example, Perry et al. [17] undertook destructive biomechanical tests using fresh cadaveric thoracolumbar VBs to evaluate the biomechanical performance of the non-toxic, osteoconductive, and bio-absorbable cement calcium sulfate (CSC) compared with that seen with PMMA. PMMA treatment restored the strength of VBs to 127% of the intact level and stiffness to 70% of the intact level, whereas CSC treatment restored the strength to 108% of the intact level and stiffness to 46% of the intact level. CSC and PMMA were not significantly different with respect to restoration of strength but the restoration of stiffness tended to be greater with PMMA than with CSC.

These biomechanical alterations could be influenced by the different devices used. Sietsma et al. compared the modification of strength and stiffness of two devices in cadaveric fractured osteoporotic vertebrae: a standard inflatable bone tamp (IBT) system and a vertebral "jack tool device" (VJT). In the VJT group, the post-restoration strength was 81% of the original strength, and it was 96% in the IBT group. The post-restoration stiffness in the VJT group was 61% of the original stiffness and it was 76% of the original stiffness in the IBT group. The vertebrae in the VJT group were restored to 101% of their original height whereas the value in the IBT group was 104% [19].

12.5 Results

By re-expanding the vertebra with balloon tamps, KP reduces pathological kyphosis in 50–60% of patients, thereby improving the restoration of normal vertebral biomechanics, early mobilization of the patient, and pain relief in 90% of cases [20–22].

As with VP, KP requires constant fluoroscopic monitoring (angiographic equipment or the portable C-arm) to ensure correct positioning of the needle. Sometimes, neuroleptoanalgesia or even general anesthesia may be required.

KP is based on creating a cavity in a VB by inflating the balloons to enable safe injection of PMMA at low pressure and with a low prevalence of cement leakage. This procedure makes KP a safe and important therapeutic option for VCFs. The risk of somatic or venous leakage of cement during KP is lower than that observed for VP because the cement is highly viscous and is pushed through the working cannula with a bone-filler device. Upon injection of PMMA into the VB, the vertebral microfractures (which are responsible for the pain) are immobilized, making the VB more compact and resistant. By inflating the balloon into the VB, the vertebral kyphosis can be corrected. However, KP has been shown to restore vertebral height in 20% of cases, with a reduction in wedge angle varying between 6° and 9° [23, 24].

Several studies have been carried out to ascertain the outcome of methods with regard to pain reduction, kyphotic correction and complications (e.g., cement leakage; disk leakage; pulmonary embolism; new vertebral fractures adjacent or distal to the VB). The risk of cement leakage is lower in KP than in VP. However, the incidence of new vertebral fractures adjacent or distal to metamers is related primarily to the porotic disease [25–26].

Recently, a new type of vertebral augmentation technique have been patented using endovertebral metallic implants. This is employed to correct the kyphotic curve not only with balloon tamps but also with a stent or a metallic cross that can restore the height of the VB.

Majd and colleagues carried out KP [26] in 360 consecutive osteoporotic patients, and they reported immediate relief of pain in 89% of patients. One patient experienced postoperative pain as a result of radiculopathy related to leakage of bone filler into the foramen. The remaining patients had persistent pain, and were diagnosed with a new fracture or underlying degenerative disk disease. Restoration of lost vertebral height (anterior) of ≥20% was observed in 63% of fractures (with an overall mean restoration of 30%) and 20% restoration of lost vertebral height (midline) was detected in 69% of fractures (with an overall mean restoration of 50%). Only 12% (30/254) of patients required additional KP procedures to treat 36 symptomatic, new adjacent and remote fractures. No device-related complications were observed.

Grafe et al. [27] compared pain reduction by evaluation using a visual analog scale (VAS) in 40 patients in the KP group compared with 20 subjects in the conservative medical treatment group. Pain scores improved from 26.2 to 44.4 in the KP group, whereas in the control group the change was from 33.6 to 34.3. After 12 months, significantly fewer patients with new vertebral fractures of the thoracic and lumbar spine were noted in the KP group than in the control group.

Several studies have suggested that KP produces greater improvement in daily activity, physical function, and pain relief when compared with optimal medical management for osteoporotic VCFs 6 months after intervention. However, there is poor-quality evidence that KP results in greater pain relief for tumor-associated VCFs [25].

In a literature review, Eck et al. observed that the mean preoperative and postoperative VAS scores for KP were 8.06 and 3.46, respectively, with a mean change of 4.60 with a risk of new fracture of 14.1% with KP and with a risk of cement leak of 7.0% with KP. This risk was lower compared with VP data [28].

Maestretti and colleagues [20] carried out a prospective study of stand-alone balloon KP with augmentation with calcium phosphate cement (Calcibon®) in traumatic fractures according to the Magerl classification. They reported preoperative, postoperative and follow-up results by applying the VAS (0–10) for pain rating and the Roland–Morris (0–24) disability score. They observed a mean initial vertebral deformity of 17° corrected to a postoperative value of 6°. All active patients returned to the same work within 3 months with the same ability to work as before. The authors concluded that, due to the intrinsic characteristics of calcium phosphate cement, application of this biological cement for standalone reduction and stabilization is recommended only in fractures of type A1 and A3.1 in young patients.

We treated, by KP, 39 consecutive patients affected by A1 and A3 Magerl vertebral fractures within 3 months of trauma, Pain relief was achieved in 90–95% of cases depending on the fracture type as well as an increase in VB height sufficient to allow early mobilization of the patient and restoration of the physiological distribution of postural forces [12].

12.6 Complications

The first step in which it is possible to observe complications is positioning of the needle and cannula. Three approaches are possible at the lumbar level (transpedicular, parapedicular, transomatic) whereas at the thoracic level a costotransverse approach is possible. These procedures must be carried out with good-quality equipment to achieve optimal anatomical control. The literature [29–32] suggests that complications are usually related to abnormal distribution of cement with leakage (disk, epidural, vascular) but that abnormal leakage is often completely asymptomatic. Some types of leakage can lead to only small amounts of radicular pain or compression of the thecal sac, whereas vascular leakage can cause asymptomatic/symptomatic pulmonary emboli, cerebral infarct or heart/vascular dissection. Disk leakage seems to be related to a higher incidence of fracture to the contiguous VB. To avoid complications, two major tricks must be considered: (i) use dense cement and (ii) inject slowly. A very important anatomical landmark is the posterior wall of the VB, which should never be passed by cement. This is a key point to avoid cement leakage within the canal with the very dramatic complications of paraplegia and tetraplegia. KP is not suggested at the cervical level so complications for this level are not so well described. There are no significant differences compared with VP in terms of new fractures to adjacent/distant metamers within 1 year after treatment.

12.7 Conclusions

KP is a safe and effective method for the treatment of vertebral compression, primary or secondary spinal tumors, and select types of traumatic fracture. Compared with VP, the advantages of KP are the increased vertebral height capacity, a low pressure of cement injection, the use of high-density cement, and a low prevalence of vascular and disk leakage. Compared with VP, the disadvantages of KP is the invasiveness of the procedure, cost (fourfold more expensive), and the requirement of general anesthesia. The literature indicates that there are no significant differences in terms of pain relief between KP and VP.

References

1. Wong X, Reiley MA, Garfin S (2000) Vertebroplasty/kyphoplasty. J Women's Imaging 2:117–124
2. Pflugmacher R, Kandziora F, Schroder R et al (2005) Vertebroplasty and kyphoplasty in osteoporotic fractures of vertebral bodies: a prospective 1-year follow-up analysis. RöFo177:1670–1676
3. Mcgirt MJ, Parker SL, Wolinsky JP, Witham TF, Bydon A, Gokaslan ZL (2009) Vertebroplasty and kyphoplasty for the treatment of vertebral compression fractures: an evidenced-based review of the literature. Spine J 9:501–508
4. Magerl F, Aebi M, Gertzbein SD et al (1994) A comprehensive classification of thoracic and lumbar injuries. Eur Spine J 3:184–201
5. Guarnieri G, Ambrosanio G, Vassallo P et al (2009) Vertebroplasty as treatment of aggressive and symptomatic vertebral hemangiomas: up to 4 years of follow-up. Neuroradiology 51:471–476
6. Peh WC, Gilula LA (2003) Percutaneous vertebroplasty: indications, contraindications, and technique. Br J Radiol 76:69–75
7. Guglielmi G, Andreula C, Muto M, Gilula L (2005) Percutaneous vertebroplasty: indications, contraindications, technique and complications. Acta Radiol May 46:256-68
8. Cotten A, Boutry N, Cortet B et al (1998) Percutaneous vertebroplasty: state of the art. Radiographics 18:311–320
9. Gangi A, Guth S, Imbert JP et al (2003) Percutaneous vertebroplasty: indications, technique, and results. Radiographics 23:10–20
10. Mathis JM, Barr JD, Belkoff SM et al (2001) Percutaneous vertebroplasty: a developing standard of care for vertebral compression fractures. Am J Neuroradiol 22:373–381
11. Ambrosanio G, Lavanga A, Vassallo P, Izzo R, Diano

AA, Muto M. (2005) Vertebroplasty in the treatment of spine disease. Interven Neuroradiol 11:309–323

12. Muto M, Guarnieri G, Lavanga A, Vassallo P et al (2008) Vertebroplasty and kyphoplasty: friends or foes? Radiol Med 113:1171–1184
13. Panjabi MM, Oxland TR, Kifune M, Arand M, Wen L, Chen A (1995) Validity of the three-column theory of thoracolumbar fractures. A biomechanic investigation. Spine 20:1122–1127
14. Leibl T, Funke M, Dresing K, Grabbe E (1999) Instability of spinal fractures – therapeutic relevance of different classifications RöFo 170:174–180
15. Denis F (1983) The three column spine and its significance in the classification of acute thoracolumbar spinal injuries. Spine (Phila Pa 1976) 8:817–831
16. De Falco R, Scarano E, Guarnieri L et al (2005) Balloon kyphoplasty in traumatic fractures of the thoracolumbar junction. Preliminary experience in 12 cases. J Neurosurg Sci 49:147–153
17. Perry A, Mahar A, Massie J, Kim C et al (2005) Biomechanical evaluation of kyphoplasty with calcium sulfate cement in a cadaveric osteoporotic vertebral compression fracture model. Spine J 5:489–493
18. Chen B, Li YQ, Xie DH, Zheng ZM et al (2011) Comparison of unipedicular and bipedicular kyphoplasty on the stiffness and biomechanical balance of compression fractured vertebrae Eur Spine J 20:1272–1280
19. Sietsma SM, Hosman AJF (2009) Biomechanical evaluation of the vertebral jack tool and the inflatable bone tamp for reduction of osteoporotic spine fractures. Spine 34: E640–E644
20. Maestretti G, Cremer C, Otten P, Jakob RP (2007) Prospective study of standalone balloon kyphoplasty with calcium phosphate cement augmentation in traumatic fractures. Eur Spine J 16:601–610
21. Fuentes S, Metellus P, Fondop J et al (2007) Percutaneous pedicle screw fixation and kyphoplasty for management of thoracolumbar burst fractures. Neurochirurgie 53:272–276
22. Theodoru DJ, Theodorou SJ, Duncan TD et al (2002) Percutaneous balloon kyphoplasty for the correction of spinal deformity in painful vertebral body compression fractures. J Clin Imaging 26:1–5
23. Deramond H, Salioub G, Aveillana M et al (2006) Respective contributions of vertebroplasty and kyphoplasty to the management of osteoporotic vertebral fractures. Joint Bone Spine 73:610–613
24. Voggenreiter G (2005) Balloon kyphoplasty is effective in deformity correction of osteoporotic vertebral compression fractures. Spine 30:2806–2812
25. Matthew J, Parker SJ, Wolinsky JP et al (2009) Vertebroplasty and kyphoplasty for the treatment of vertebral compression fractures: an evidenced-based review of the literature. Spine J 9:501–508
26. Majd ME, Farley S, Holt RT et al (2005) Preliminary outcomes and efficacy of the first 360 consecutive kyphoplasties for the treatment of painful osteoporotic vertebral compression fractures. Spine J 5: 244–255
27. Grafe IA, Da Fonseca K, Hillmeier J, et al. (2005) Reduction of pain and fracture incidence after kyphoplasty: 1-year outcomes of a prospective controlled trial of patients with primary osteoporosis. Osteoporos Int 16: 2005–2012
28. Eck JC, Nachtigall D, Humphreys SC, Hodges SD: Comparison of vertebroplasty and balloon kyphoplasty for treatment of vertebral compression fractures: a meta-analysis of the literature. Spine J 2008, 8:488–497
29. Walter J, Haciyakupoglu E, Waschke A, Kalff R, Ewald C (2012) Cement leakage as a possible complication of balloon kyphoplasty – is there a difference between osteoporotic compression fractures (AO type A1) and incomplete burst fractures (AO type A3.1)? ACTA Neurochir 154:313–319
30. Wardlaw D, Cummings SR, van Meirhaeghe J et al (2009) Efficacy and safety of balloon kyphoplasty compared with non-surgical care for vertebral compression fracture (FREE): a randomized controlled trial. Lancet 373:1016–1024
31. Prokop A, Koukal C, Dolezych R, Chmielnicki M (2012) Kyphoplasty in the treatment of osteoporotic spine fractures: experience in over 500 patients. Z Gerontol Geriatr [Epub ahead of print: in German]
32. Frankel BM, Monroe T, Wang C (2007) Percutaneous vertebral augmentation: an elevation in adjacent-level fracture risk in kyphoplasty as compared with vertebroplasty Spine J 7: 575–582

Endoscopic Treatment Approaches to Herniated Lumbar Disks

13

Jürgen Reul

13.1 Introduction

Several minimally invasive image-guided methods have been developed to treat diseases in lumbar disks (e.g., automated percutaneous lumbar diskectomy, laser diskectomy, intradiskal electrotherapy). Nearly all of these methods provide a good approach to the disk space and nucleus. However, removal of sequestered disk fragments that have into the spinal canal or neuroforamen is extremely difficult.

In orthopedic surgery, endoscopic approaches to the joints ("arthroscopy") are standard for many procedures on different joints. Such approaches are likely to transform treatments for spinal diseases. Several attempts have been made using medial transligamental approaches or lateral transforaminal access.

The outcome of each endoscopic method must be compared with those of microneurosurgical methods. These methods are well developed and have a high success rate as well as a low prevalence of complications. Several commercial companies have started to develop systems for endoscopic approaches. The main difference is if they use transforaminal lateral, transforaminal posterolateral or transligamental medial access. All methods should allow not only access to lumbar disks but also to the spinal canal and neuroforamen. Figure 13.1 details the different approaches to lumbar disks and the spinal canal as well as the types of herniation that can be treated by endoscopic methods.

J. Reul (✉)
Beta Klinik International Head and Spine Center, Bonn, Germany
e-mail: reul@betaklinik.de

13.2 Indications, Contraindications and Limitations of Endoscopic Approaches

Nearly all lumbar-disk herniations can be treated by endoscopic methods. The spectrum of indications is similar to that seen in microsurgical therapy. A foraminal stenosis can be treated. A stenosis of the spinal canal should be treated by microsurgical decompression.

The limitations are herniation in combination with osseous spinal stenosis and, especially in men, cranial sequestration at the L5-S1 level due to a high iliac crest that does not permit lateral or posterolateral access. Pure axillary herniation can also be problematic.

The contraindications are similar to those seen in microneurosurgery. These include the risk hemorrhage in patients with anticoagulation problems or anticoagulation therapy with coumadin. This method has advantages compared with open surgery because it can be carried out under local anesthesia. It can be done under analogosedation. The indications, contraindications and

M. Muto (ed.), *Interventional Neuroradiology of the Spine*,
DOI 10.1007/978-88-470-2790-9_13, © Springer-Verlag Italia 2013

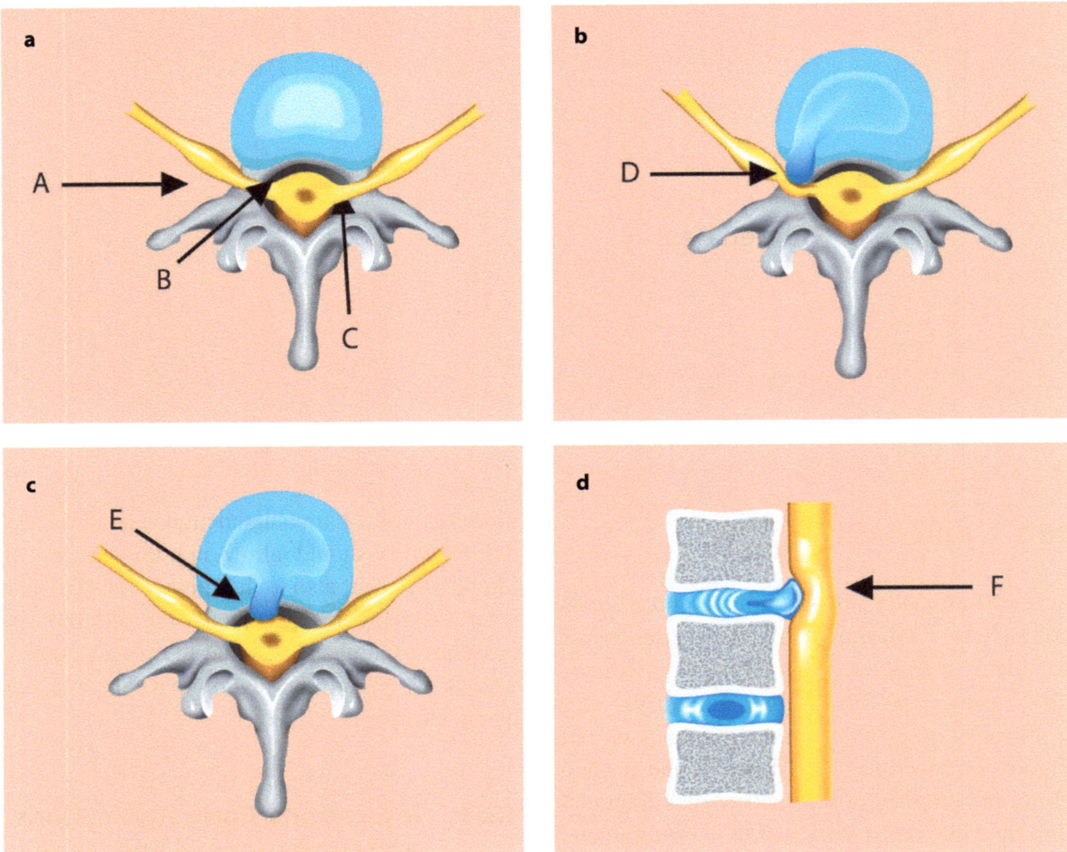

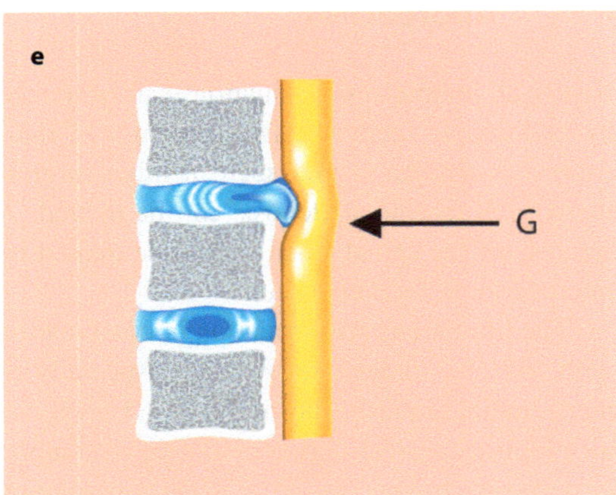

Fig. 13.1 Different approaches to the disk and spinal canal as well as the types of herniation that can be treated by endoscopic techniques. **a** *A* shows the direct transforaminal lateral approach, which is sometimes difficult because of the crossing exiting nerve root; *C* shows the dorsal transligamentary approach very similar to the microsurgical access; *B* demonstrates the dorsolateral approach used for the Max More technique. **b-e** Different types of herniations that can be treated endoscopically: *D* lateral intraforaminal; *E* medial sequestration; *F* cranial and *G* caudal sequestration

Table 13.1 Indications, contraindications and complications related to endoscopic treatment of herniated lumbar disks

Indication	Contraindications	Technical and anatomical limitations	Complications
Any lumbar-disk herniation; epidural and intraforaminal sequestered disk fragment Osteochondrosis (Modic stage I) Painful disk	Coagulation disorders High-grade stenosis of the spinal canal	High iliac crest and/or cranial sequestration at the L5-S1 level Transaxial dorsal sequestration at the L5-S1 level Severe scoliosis	Dural leak Nerve-root damage Epidural hemorrhage

Table 13.2 Technical equipment needed for endoscopic treatment of herniated lumbar disks

Fluoroscopy system (mono or biplane): if sterile conditions are guaranteed, the procedure can be done on a standard angiography table
Radiography-compatible endoscopy table
Sterile one-way set
Endoscope (3.2-mm working channel with cold light source and video connection)
Low-pressure flush pump
Suction pump
Instrument set
Lumbar puncture needle (18 G; length, 11 cm)
Dilatators (diameter, 4 mm and 6 mm)
Drills with blunt tips (diameter, 4, 6, 7, 8 and 9 mm)
Working tube (diameter, 8 mm)
Different types of forceps

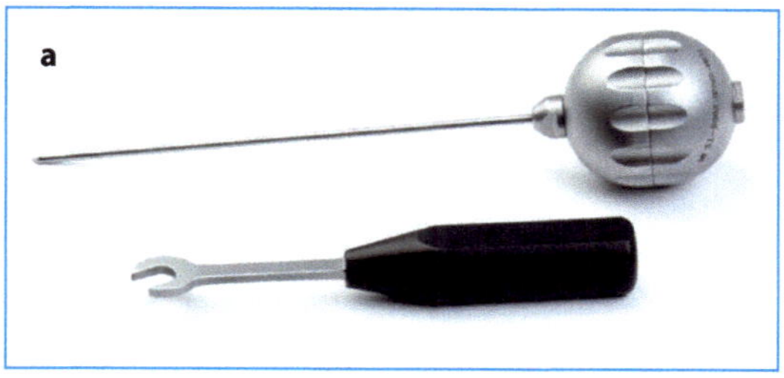

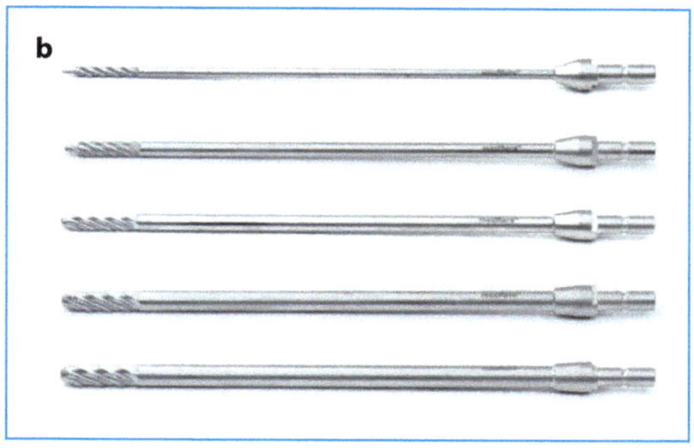

Fig. 13.2 Tom Shidi® needle (**a**) and drills of different diameters (**b**). Note the blunt tip, avoiding dural sack damage

limitations of endoscopic approaches to disk herniation are shown in Table 13.1.

13.3 Diagnosis

Overall, the success of the intervention is determined mainly by a fluoroscopy-guided approach to the target (sequestered disk fragments). Therefore, this must be considered at all steps of the procedure. There is a very limited field of view and, if the working tube is not placed close to the sequestered disk fragment, it will be missed.

The most important diagnostic tool is MRI. MRI of the lumbar spine should comprise good-quality T1- and T2-weighted images (with T2-weighted images in at least sagittal and axial planes). Sometimes, T1-weighted images with fat suppression and administration of contrast media can be helpful.

In some cases, CT may also be required. If too much calcification of the sequestered disk fragment is observed, a switch to a microsurgical procedure may be indicated.

Rarely, conventional myelography (e.g., in patients with heart pacemakers) can be undertaken. Sometimes, diskography can be useful. This can be done with access to the disk during the endoscopic procedure. In cases with a "black disk" and "pure" back pain, a pressure test with saline is helpful to confirm the relationship between pain and MRI findings. In such cases, an endoscopic nucleotomy and/or endoscopic abrasion ("shaving") can be done (see section 13.5.5).

If MRI suggests scoliosis or severe osseous degenerative changes, radiography of the lumbar spine in two planes can be used to obtain clearer information about the width of the foramen.

13.4 Preparation

Blood cell count, kidney function, liver function, electrolytes, and coagulation status are neces-

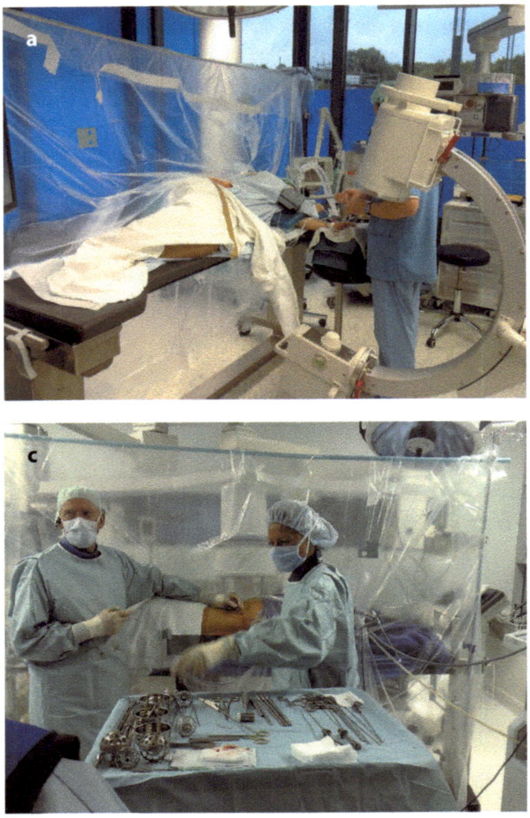

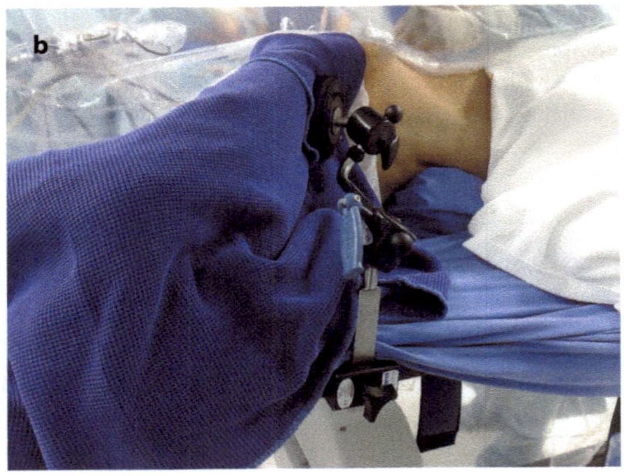

Fig. 13.3 Patient position (**a**), access for anesthesia (**b**) and interventionists looking at the monitor (**c**)

sary. Anticoagulants and antiaggregants (acetylsalicylic acid, clopidogrel) should be stopped 3–5 days before the intervention. The patient is then prepared for anesthesia (see section 13.5.1). The technical equipment needed is listed in Table 13.2, some of which is shown in Figure 13.2.

13.5 Procedure

13.5.1 Anesthesia

The intervention is a challenge for the anesthesiologist because the patient must be able to respond during the entire procedure. While obtaining access to the epidural space through the foramen, the patient must respond when the drills touch the excited nerve root. We use a combination of remifentanil and propofol by continuous controlled injection with an injection pump and monitoring by the anesthesiologist.

13.5.2 Patient Positioning

There are two possibilities: lateral or prone. The latter is useful if bilateral access is required (rare). Usually, the lateral position is more comfortable for the induction of anesthesia and for the patient (Fig. 13.3) To avoid movement, the patient is fixed with special holders. The table is specially designed for endoscopic surgery: a carbon table allowing 360° fluoroscopy and reduced doses of radiation.

13.5.3 Access to the Disk

Access to the disk and/or epidural space through the neural foramen is achieved from a dorsolateral approach. Lateral access is more difficult, more dangerous and sometimes anatomically impossible.

The distance from the midline (processus spinosus) to the lateral position is dependent upon

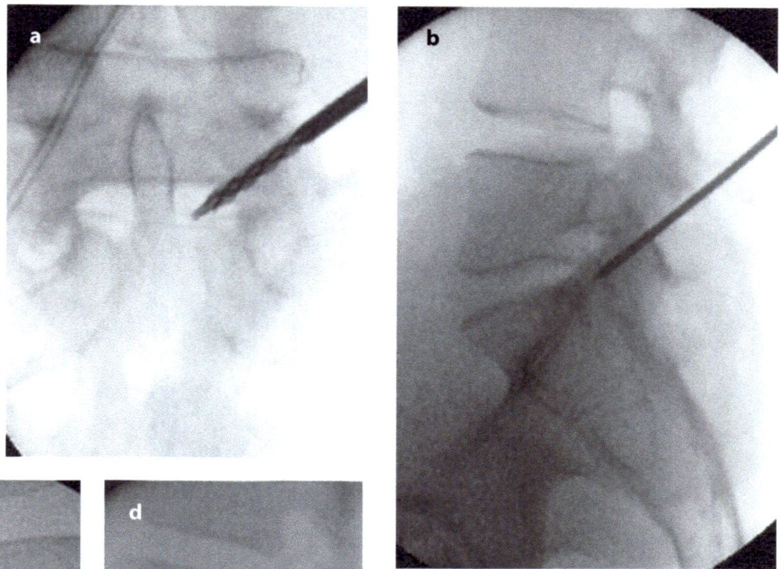
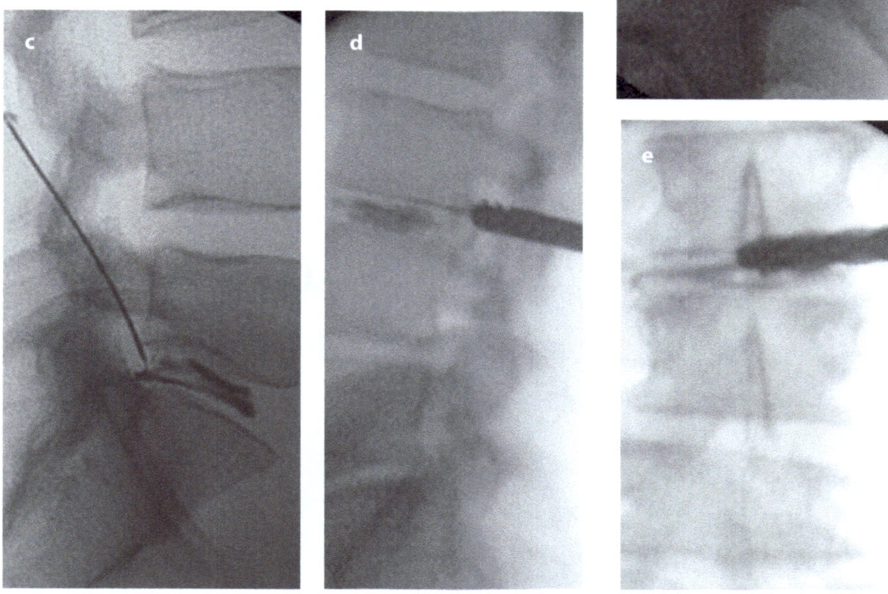

Fig. 13.4 Access point and passage to the disk and epidural space. The instrument tip is always behind the bone and disk in both projections. Additionally, discography can be done *via* the lumbar puncture needle. A horizontal or caudocranial direction is selected if a cranial sequestered disk fragment is targeted. In **a** and **b** the access to a caudally sequestered piece is shown; in **c** the additional discography is visible; in **d** and **e** the approach to a cranially sequestered disc is illustrated

the level of disk herniation. In L5-S1 it is 12–14 cm; in L4-L5 it is 10–12 cm; in L3-L4 it is 7–9 cm; and in L2-L3 it is about 5–6 cm. The angle in the craniocaudal direction is dependent upon the type of sequestration. If a caudal sequester is present, a caudal direction is used; if the sequestered disk fragment has moved in a cranial direction, horizontal access is employed. This has limitations at the L5-S1 level because of anatomical reasons (especially a high iliac crest).

To navigate through the foramen, one must be aware that the nerve root is excited in the cranial part of the foramen (at a 12 o' clock position) and that access with the instruments is at the 5–6 o' clock position). Careful analyses of the pre-procedure MRI is important to exclude anatomical variants and anomalies (e.g., conjoined root).

13.5.4 Steps of the Procedure

Local anesthesia and placement of the puncture needle: After skin marking, scandicain is administered to skin and muscle. A standard lumbar-puncture needle is guided under fluoroscopy to the facet joint. Local anesthesia is induced at the facet joints. If discography is required, the needle can be advanced to the disk and contrast

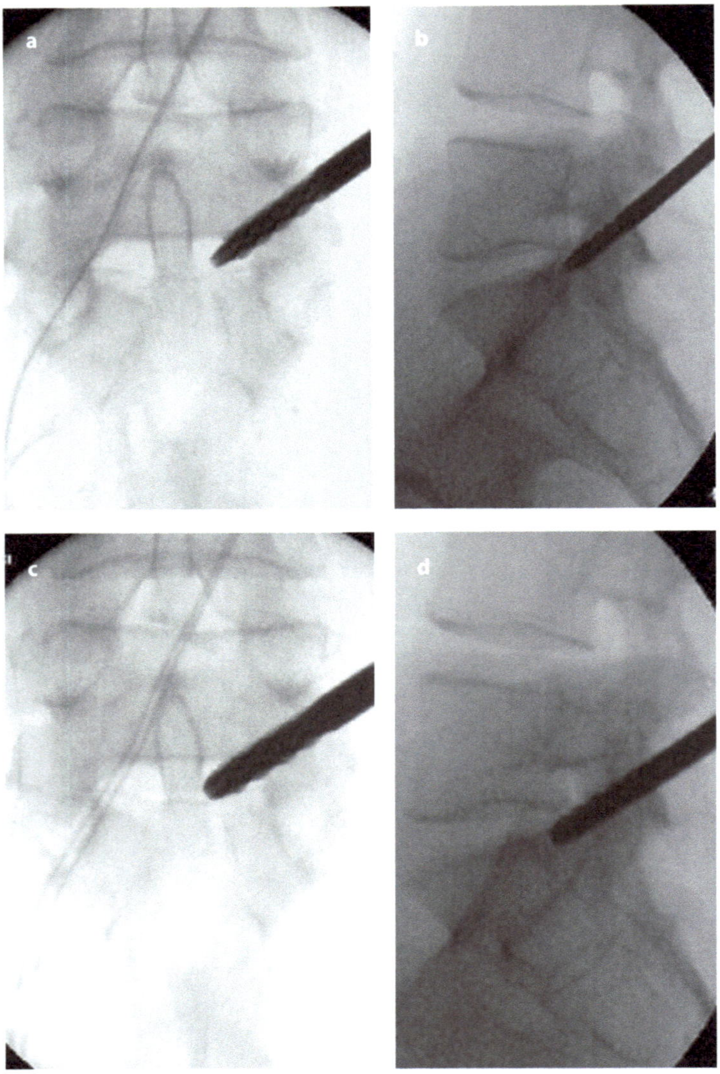

Fig. 13.5 The different steps of drilling during fluoroscopy. Note the blunt tip of the drills

media applied. After that, the needle is pulled back with the tip close to the facet joint.

Guidance of the K-wire and pre-dilation: A K-wire is positioned through the needle at the facet joint. Pre-dilation with a 4 mm^2 and 6 mm^2 tube is undertaken. During all maneuvers, the K-wire is left *in situ*. If possible, it should be advanced through the foramen into the epidural space. This can be done if the foramen is large and if significant drilling is not necessary.

Placement of a Tom Shidi® needle: In most cases, the wire is in contact with the facet joint. A diamond-tipped Tom Shidi needle is advanced. After control of its position, it is hammered carefully into the bone of the superior process of the facet joint and advanced until the tip reaches the inner peduncular line (anteroposterior projection during fluoroscopy). With its blunt tip, the needle can be advanced carefully into the epidural space (Fig. 13.4).

Stepwise drilling with drills of diameter 4–9 mm: Special atraumatic drills with blunt tips are used (Fig. 13.5). The advantage of blunt tips is that they lessen the risk of dural leaks and damage to the nerve root due to cutting effects. The

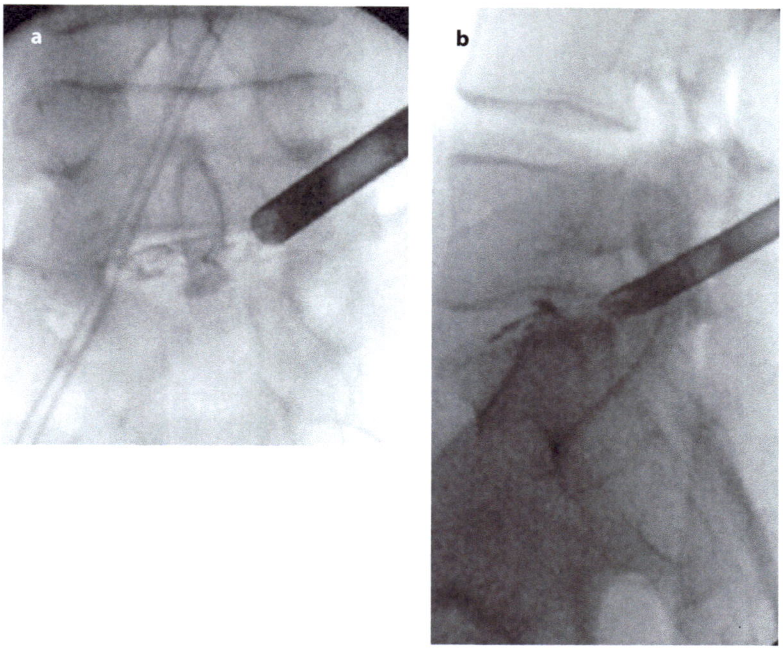

Fig. 13.6 Fluoroscopy of the working tub

K-wire is left *in situ* and used as a guide. One must not enter the disk but instead reach the epidural space and be directed to the sequestered disk fragment. During these steps the patient must be observed closely. He/she must be sedated but able to respond. If the excited nerve in the foramen is touched, leg pain and/or radicular sensations will be experienced. At this point, the position of the instrument must be controlled and changed (usually it is to the cranial position in the foramen). If, during drilling, local pain in the back is reported, it is normal and due to bone drilling. Ideally, the patient is without pain and able to respond/speak adequately.

Placement of the working tube with guidance by a 6-mm dilator: After the final drilling, a 6-mm dilator is advanced. Using the dilator, a working tube is placed with the tip inside the spinal canal. It is placed in the lateral projection with the opening towards the sequestered disk fragment (dorsal and cranial or caudal) and behind the dorsal margin of the disk and vertebrae and in anteroposterior projection medial from the inner peduncular line (Fig. 13.6).

Removal of the sequestered disk fragment under video guidance: The endoscope is advanced through the working tube by continuous flushing. If the tube is placed correctly, the view is now on the sequestered disk fragment. It can be grasped with small forceps and removed. Large fragments are pulled through the working tube by pulling back the endoscope and forceps simultaneously (Fig. 13.7).

Ideally, anatomical structures can be identified: dorsal margin of the disk (annulus); dorsal longitudinal ligament; capsule of the facet joint, excited nerve root; descending nerve root; dural sack. If there is an axillary herniation, the forceps can be advanced carefully between the nerve root and dural sack. In normal caudal or cranial sequestration with anterior compression of the nerve root, access is between the annulus and nerve root.

Sometimes the disk fragment is one large piece and can be removed in one step. However, often there are four or five pieces which must be identified and removed. For inspection of the annulus and to advance into the disk, the working tube is turned with the opening in an anterior direction

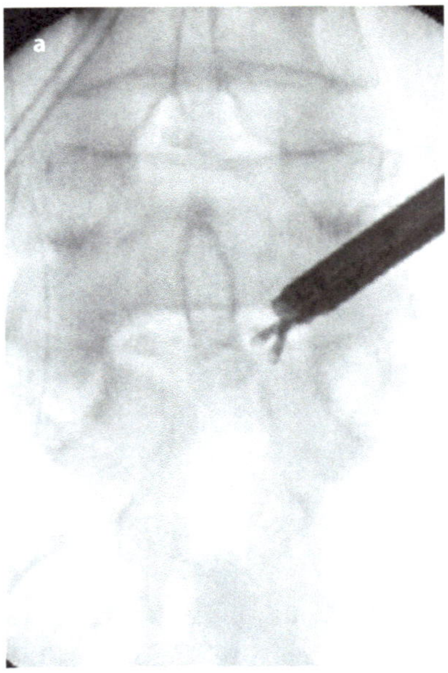

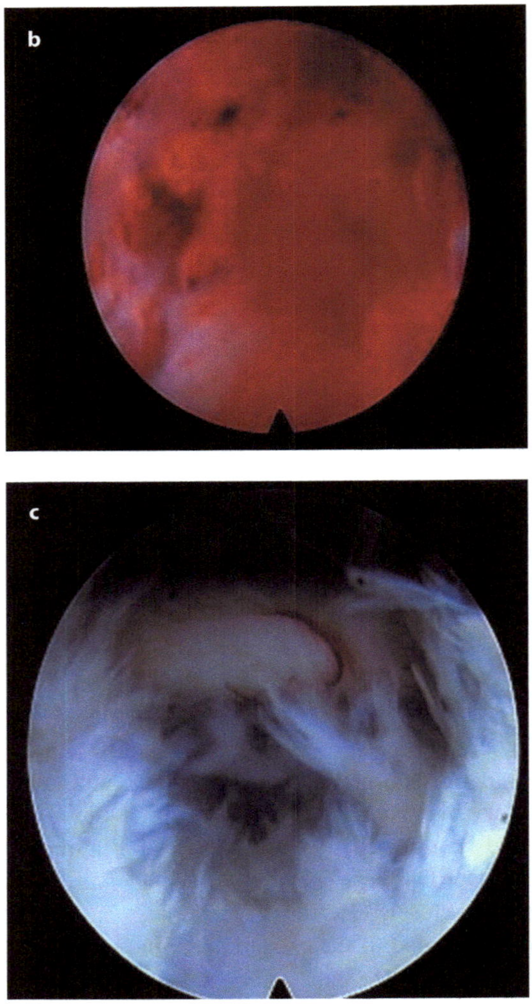

Fig. 13.7 Endoscopic views. Panel **a** shows the open forceps in the spinal canal; panel **b** shows the sequester covering the nerve and **c** shows the free nerve after removal of the piece of cartilage

towards the disk space. Usually, the hole in the annulus can be identified and the forceps can enter the disk space through the hole. Additional loose fragments can be removed, thereby reducing the risk of early recurrence of disk herniation.

13.5.5 Endoscopic Nucleotomy and Abrasion Therapy

Indications: The indications for endoscopic nucleotomy and abrasion therapy are treatment-resistant back pain or findings of a black disk on MRI or Modic changes (stage I). To confirm the indication in such cases, discography with pressure testing must be done (at the diseased level and ≥1–2 normal segments). During pressure increases, the patient should not know which level is being tested. If the correct level can be identified, access to the disk is similar to removal of the disk fragment. However, the positioning is easier because it is at the disk level and can be a done more laterally and directly by targeting the center of the disk.

After removal of the avitalized parts of the nucleus with forceps, the endplates of the vertebrae are refreshed and revitalized using small instruments for shaving. The efficacy of this procedure has been demonstrated in one study in >80 patients with success rates of approximately 70%.

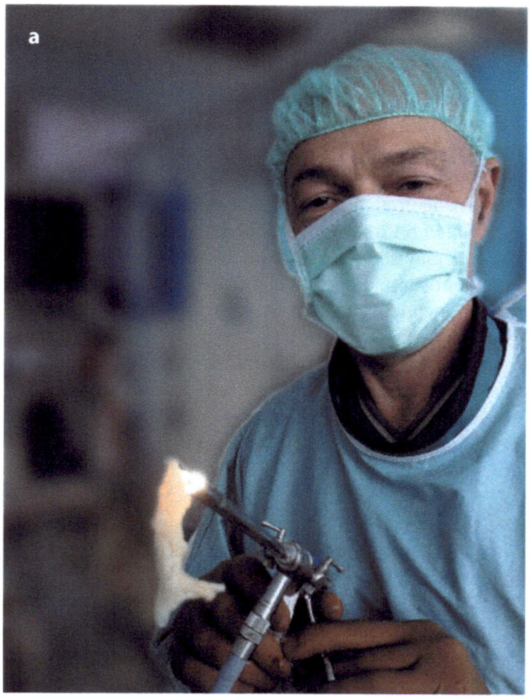

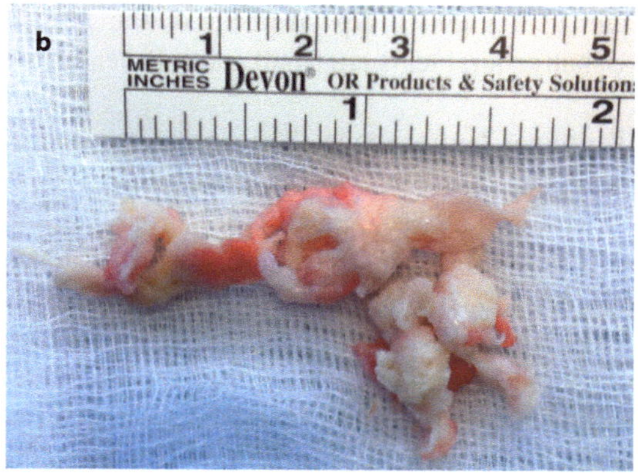

Fig. 13.8 In **a** the captured sequester is shown. **b** The size of the pieces

13.6 Post-intervention Care

The patient is monitored for 2 h after the procedure, and can be mobilized after 4 h. Usually, discharge from hospital is on the following day. If an abrasion has been carried out, a brace is provided to stabilize and protect the spine for about 4–6 weeks. The patient also receives a special rehabilitation program.

13.7 Causes of Failure, Pitfalls and Complications

Suboptimal or incorrect positioning: Correct positioning is the most important step for the success of the intervention. It starts with positioning of the Tom Shidi needle. If this is not placed correctly and the bone is punctured and drilled, it is very difficult to achieve another direction.

High iliac crest and cranial sequester/transaxial sequestration at the L5-S1 level is a clear indication to switch from endoscopic intervention to microsurgery.

Severe scoliosis is an indication to switch to microsurgery.

Anesthesiological management: The procedure must be stopped if the patient is not awake and unable to respond. There is no control of damage to the nerve root in the fully anesthetized patient. Using analog-sedation with remifentanil and propofol, one can be wait until the patient wakes up and the intervention can be continued. The lateral position is much better for anesthetic control. The prone position is tolerated by fewer patients and higher doses of anesthetics are required, thereby leading to complete loss of consciousness.

Calcified sequestered disks and facet joint ganglions should be identified before the intervention using the relevant diagnostic tools (e.g., additional CT) and should lead to a switch to microsurgery.

Damage to nerve roots and leakage from the dural sack are, in most cases, related to suboptimal analog-sedation (lack of patient response)

and to aggressive advancement of the needle. Usually, dural tears are small and self-healing.

Epidural hemorrhage: The epidural space in segments L3-L4 to L5-S1 contains fewer venous structures than the epidural space from L2-L3 to Th12/L1. The venous epidural plexus is much more expansive in the upper levels. Therefore, bleeding in the lower levels is seen very rarely. Small bleeds can be controlled by transient increases in the pressure of the flush pump. At upper levels, damage to venous structures with the K-wire and/or with the first 4-mm drill may be possible. In the worst-case scenario, a change to microsurgery may be necessary.

Suggested Reading

Hoogland T (2003) Transforaminal endoscopic discectomy with foraminoplasty for lumbar disc herniation. Surg Techn Orthoped Traumatol C40:55–120

Iprenburg M (2006) Percutaneous transforaminal endoscopic discectomy. Twentieth meeting of the International Intradiscal Therapy Society, Phoenix

John M (2007) Die perkutane transforaminale endoskopische Diskus-Abrasion zur Behandlung der schmerzhaften Osteochondrose. Dissertationsschrift der Medizinischen Fakultät der RWTH Aachen

John M, Hoogland T, Reul J (2006) Transforaminal disc abrasion: a new minimal surgical method for the regeneration of painful degenerative lumbar discs. Twentieth meeting of the International Intradiscal Therapy Society, Phoenix

Lühmann D, Burkhardt-Hammer T, Borowski C, Raspe H (2005) Minimally invasive surgical procedures for the treatment of lumbar disk herniation. HTA Report/Executive Summary, Deutsche Institut für Medizinische Dokumentation und Information, Köln

Rütten S (2006) Interlaminar and lateral transforaminal full endoscopic operation of recurrent lumbar disc herniations in patients with conventional previous operations. Twentieth meeting of the International Intradiscal Therapy Society, Phoenix

Schubert M (2005) Endoscopic transforaminal nucleotomy in combination with low-dose chemonucleolysis: results of a prospective study with 2-year follow-up. Eighteenth Meeting of the International Intradiscal Society, San Diego

Schubert M, Hoogland T (2005) Die transforaminale endoskopische Nukleotomie mit Foraminoplastik bei lumbalen Bandscheibenvorfällen. Operative Orthopädie und Traumatologie 17:641–661

Tsou PM, Alan Yeung C, Yeung AT (2004) Posterolateral transforaminal selective endoscopic discectomy and thermal annuloplasty for chronic lumbar discogenic pain: a minimal access visualized intradiscal surgical procedure. Spine J 4:564–573

Yeung AT, Yeung CA (2003) Advances in endoscopic disc and spine surgery: foraminal approach. Surg Technol Int 11:255–263

Yeung AT, Tsou PM (2002) Posterolateral endoscopic excision for lumbar disc herniation: surgical technique, outcome and complications in 307 consecutive cases. Spine 27:722–731

Percutaneous Lumbar Posterior Stabilization for Low Back Pain

14

Giuseppe Bonaldi and Alessandro Cianfoni

14.1 Introduction

Low back pain (LBP) is a leading cause of chronic disability and psychological distress. In Europe, estimates of the lifetime prevalence of back pain range from about 60% to 90% [1–3]. Back pain can be a sign of degenerative segmental instability, defined as "an abnormal response to applied loads, characterized by motion in motion segments beyond normal constraints" by the American Academy of Orthopedic Surgeons [4–6]. Motion in degenerated joints (i.e., beyond the normal limits of the joint itself) generates pain; eliminating abnormal motion seems to eliminate pain. Therefore, surgical spinal fusion (locking of two or more vertebrae as a single unit) with or without instrumentation has been the mainstay of surgical approaches for these forms of LBP. However, despite improvement in the rate of radiographically demonstrated fusion, conventional fusion methods entail several potential complications (e.g., infection, cerebrospinal fluid (CSF) leaks, harvest-site pain, instrumentation failure) and biomechanical disadvantages (e.g., loss of mobility and curvature, altered sagittal balance, transitional disease). In fact, fusion may increase the biomechanical stresses imposed on the adjacent segments, resulting in overload and early degenerative changes in adjacent facet joints and disks [7–11]. Ghiselli and colleagues [12] estimated a prevalence of symptomatic adjacent-level disease of 36% at 10 years after lumbar fusion. An improvement in fusion rates does not necessarily correspond to an improvement in outcomes [13, 14], and fusion surgery is not readily reversible. These issues have led to attempts to develop new motion-preservation technologies for the surgical treatment of spinal instability, commonly referred to as "dynamic stabilization".

Dynamic stabilization has been defined as "a system that would alter favorably the movement and load transmission of a spinal motion segment, without the intention of fusion of the segment" [15]. Dynamic stabilization (or "soft stabilization") is intended to restrict motion in the direction or plane that produces pain ("painful motion"), otherwise allowing a full range of motion. Dynamic stabilization techniques introduce a more gradual, intermediate therapeutic step between abnormal movement of the spinal unit (SU) (instability) and total absence of movement (fusion). The most significant advances in dynamic stabilization techniques were made in the past 10–15 years. During the same period a gradual shift toward a minimally invasive approach of spinal surgery was developed and accepted. The attention of biomechanics experts and spine surgeons has been focused mainly on the posterior structures of the spine, facets, and spinous processes, for two main reasons: (i) these

G. Bonaldi (✉)
Interventional and Diagnostic Neuroradiology, Ospedali Riuniti, Bergamo, Italy
e-mail: bbonaldi@yahoo.com

M. Muto (ed.), *Interventional Neuroradiology of the Spine*,
DOI 10.1007/978-88-470-2790-9_14, © Springer-Verlag Italia 2013

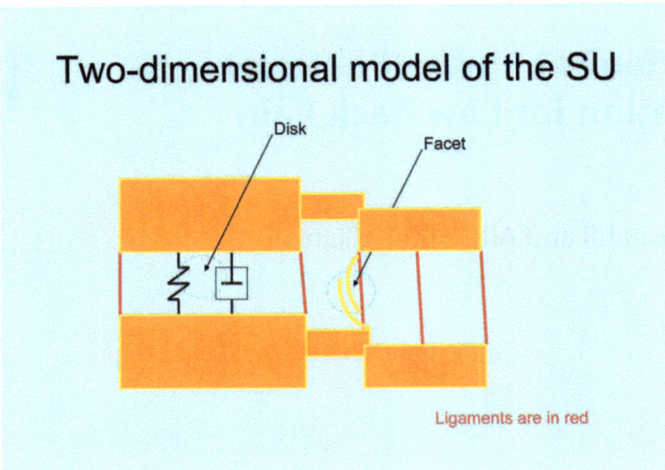

Fig. 14.1 The lumbar spinal unit is simplified in a two-dimensional model in which torque and lateral bending movements are eliminated. Such movements are not (or only partially) affected by the dynamic stabilization devices

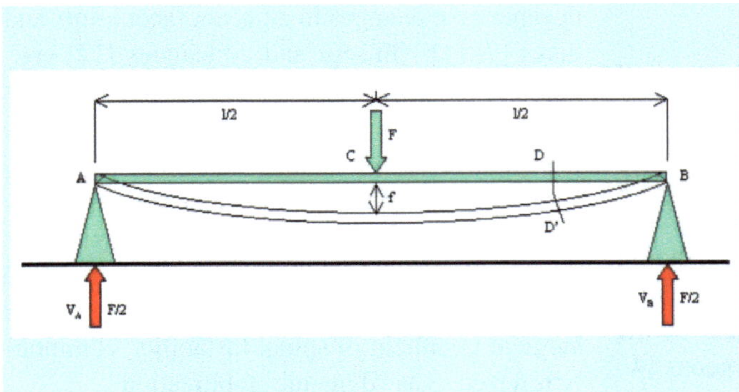

Fig. 14.2 A bending moment is present in a structural element if a moment is applied to the element so that the element bends. Moments and torques are measured as a force multiplied by a distance: M = Fd

structures are readily accessible by a minimally invasive approach and (ii) actions upon them determined by different devices can modify the functional behavior of the SU. The combination of preservation of motion and minimal surgical invasiveness seems to be opening a new era in the surgery of symptomatic degenerative spine instability.

14.2 Basic Biomechanics

The basic functional SU is the smallest physiological unit of motion of the spine. It is therefore termed a "motion segment". It consists of two adjacent vertebrae, the disk, and all the connecting ligaments. Individual motion segments contribute to the total motion of the spine. The components and movements of the SU are extremely complex. Thus, there may be many different sources of pain in pathologic situations. Unfortunately, the biomechanics of SUs are neither fully understood nor simple to explain. We will try to summarize the main concepts on which the designs of the different devices are based. This involves simplifying the three-dimensional (3D) anatomy and physiology of the SU to a two-dimensional (2D) model (Fig. 14.1) and moving only in the sagittal plane (essentially eliminating the torque and lateral bending movements, which are not influenced significantly by dynamic stabilization devices).

In flexion and extension, muscles apply a bending moment to the SU. A bending moment (M) corresponds to two vector forces applied in opposite directions with a distance between them different from 0, and is measured as a force (F) multiplied by a distance (d): M = Fd (Fig. 14.2). During flexion of the lumbar spine, muscles ap-

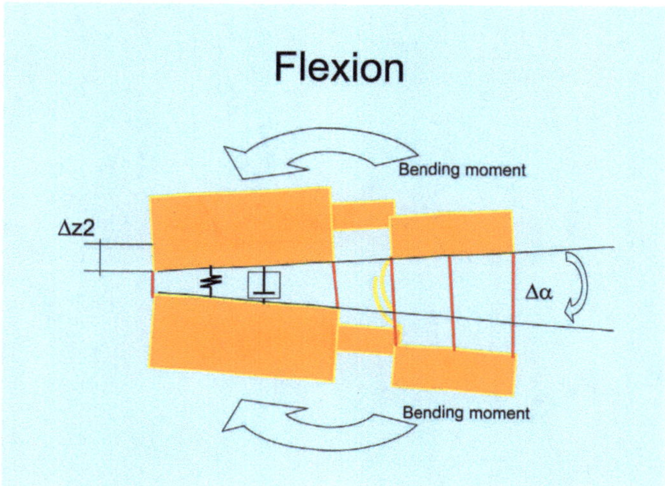

Fig. 14.3 The bending moment applied by muscles in flexion to the spinal unit determines an asymmetric decrease in the height of the disk and an opening of the posterior bony elements

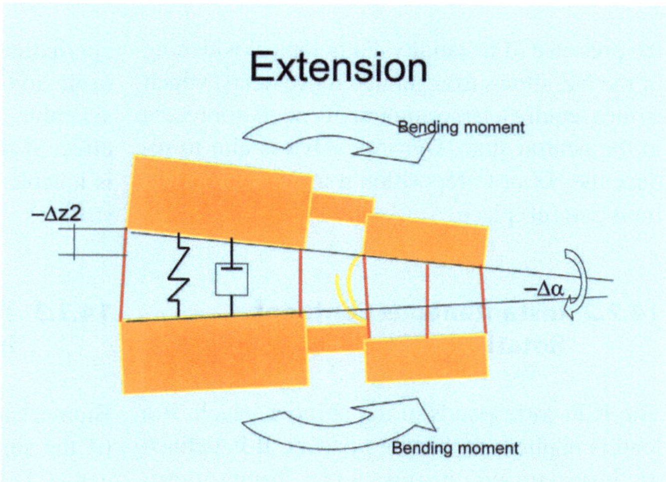

Fig. 14.4 In extension, the bending moment determines an asymmetric increase in the height of the disk, whereas the posterior bony elements get closer, with the angle determined by the two spinous processes becoming negative

ply a bending moment to the SUs (Fig. 14.3). The total motion obtained (modification of posture from neutral to flexion) is the sum of the modifications obtained at the level of each single SU (i.e., a decrease of the anterior disk height [Δz2] and a widening [defined by the angle between the spinous processes: Δa] of the posterior structures, which are stretched and moved apart). The supraspinous ligament is the structure limiting flexion more effectively. The opposite happens in extension, with an increase in the anterior disk height and closing of the interspinous space, with the angle becoming negative (Fig. 14.4).

14.2.1 Neutral Zone (NZ)

The NZ (Fig. 14.5) is the position of the SU in which a small bending moment can result in a large movement (i.e., a large change in the angles between the two vertebrae). In a normal SU, the center of the NZ corresponds to the middle position between flexion and extension. A small moment is required to start flexion (or extension). However, with a progressive increase in the movement it becomes increasingly harder to obtain new flexion (or extension). The NZ is a measure of the laxity of the SU, and it widens in

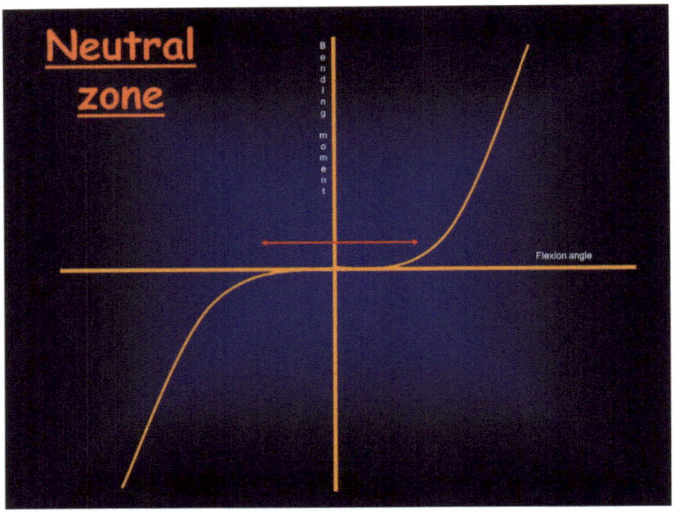

Fig. 14.5 Bending moment *versus* flexion angle of a spinal unit. In the neutral zone, small differences in bending moment result in large changes the flexion angle

the presence of instability. Pathological widening of the NZ allows exaggerated movements, which in turn require a large amount of energy for return to the neutral state. Dynamic devices aim to reduce the NZ or to reposition it in the appropriate (non-painful) place.

14.2.2 Instantaneous Center of Rotation (ICR)

The ICR corresponds to the point at which, if a load is applied, no bending occurs. It is defined as "instantaneous" because it can change at every instant during different types of movements. As an example, think of a bicycle wheel. When the wheel does not touch the ground and turns around the central pivot, the latter represents the center of rotation and does not change with time; on the contrary, in a moving bicycle, the only non-moving part is the one touching the ground, and it changes at each instant (imagine the wheel turning as a whole around the fixed point in contact with the ground). Predicting the ICR in structures as complex as the SU is difficult. The ICR changes with different movements and these changes become more unpredictable in the presence of instability. More often, in a healthy SU, in the standing, inactive position, the ICR is located posterior to the center of the disk, just above the inferior end plate [16] (corresponding approximately to the center of gravity). It moves in flexion–extension, and the variability is considerable. There are no simple rules to predict the effect of stabilization devices on the ICR, but one is notable: the ICR moves toward an increase of stiffness.

14.2.3 The Changes that Occur When an Interspinous Spacer is Deployed

Biomechanics are not modified during flexion (if the supraspinous process is preserved surgically). During extension, the biomechanics are not modified until the spacer is under compression. When the spacer undergoes compression (Fig. 14.6), provided the spacer is rigid and the osseous structure does not fail (see Fig. 14.6 for the weakest points of the posterior arch, which are possible sites of failure), the anterior annulus is stretched, and an additional increase in the anterior height of the disk is obtained ($-\Delta z3$). To allow and compensate for this, the facets move opposite to the normal direction, opening instead of closing. That is, the movement, which is no longer obtainable at the expense of the interspinous space (decrease of the angle in extension, see Fig. 14.4), is now obtained at the level of different, elastic structures. An immediate consequence is that back pain induced in extension by pressure originating in the facets or posterior annulus of

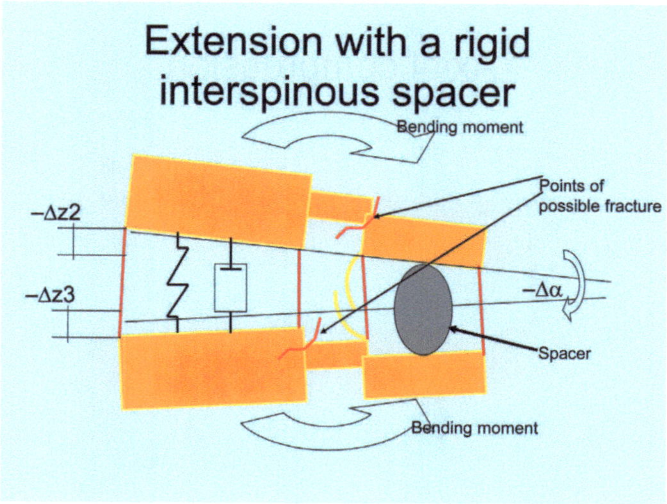

Fig. 14.6 Extension with a rigid interspinous spacer. An additional increase in disk height is obtained, whereas the facets move opposite to the normal situation (opening instead of closing). The weakest bony structures are indicated by the red lines (arrows).

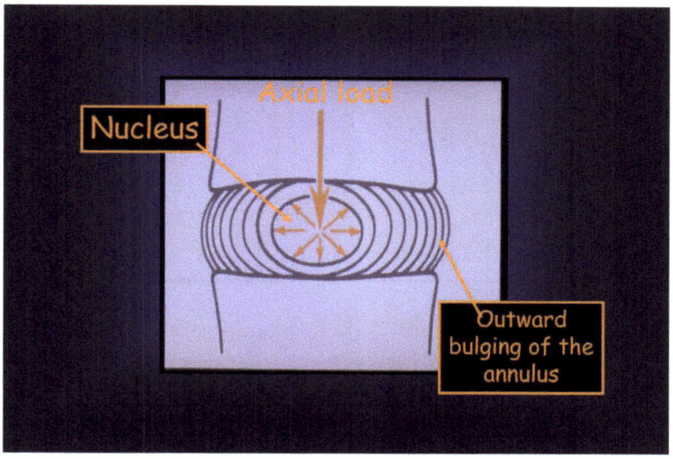

Fig. 14.7 Normal disk. The pressure exerted by the compressive loads on the hydrated nucleus is transmitted in a radial direction. This results in outward bulging of the fibers of the annulus in the horizontal plane

the lumbar spine may be relieved by unloading of the facets or posterior annulus generated by interspinous decompression [17].

In a similar way, can the whole disk be unloaded if it is surmised to be the pain source? Intervertebral disks consist of three main components: annulus fibrosus, nucleus pulposus and cartilaginous endplates. They act as a "shock absorbers" to transmit loads through the spinal column. In the healthy disk, the annulus resists the hydrostatic pressure transmitted by the radial expansion of the nucleus, which is compressed during physiological loads, with outward bulging of its fibers in the horizontal plane, thereby acting in tension rather than compression (Fig. 14.7). The disk is extremely stiff, and only minimal changes in disk height can be obtained under axial compression–distraction ($\Delta z1$ in Fig. 14.8). The disk can be unloaded only if the load is transferred to a device/instrument, but implants are not sufficiently stiff to accomplish this task. Hence, stand-alone instrumented fusions fail in the long-term if bony fusion does not occur. This is a general rule of fusion surgery: solid, effective and lasting elimination of motion in one or more SUs cannot be expected to be obtained simply by hardware (screws and rods) because the action of the hardware is temporary. Its action is to allow bone fusion to occur. Otherwise, instrumentation (even metallic ones) and contact surfaces with bone will fail in the mid- or long-term.

The disk, however, is compliant in flexion–

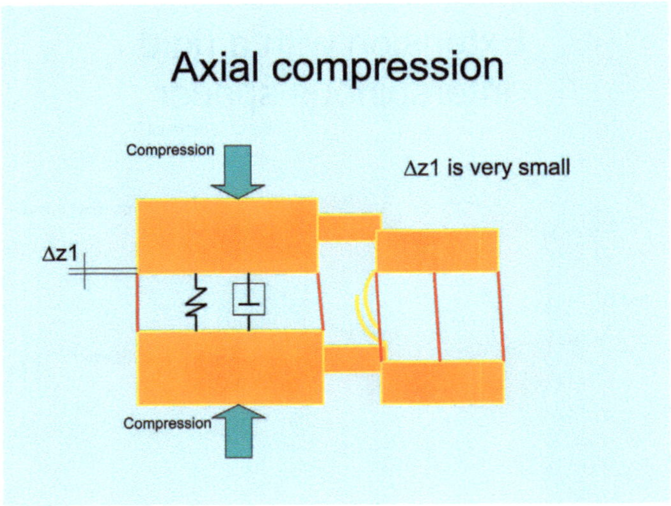

Fig. 14.8 Axial compression of a spinal unit. Only a small decrease in disk height is obtained

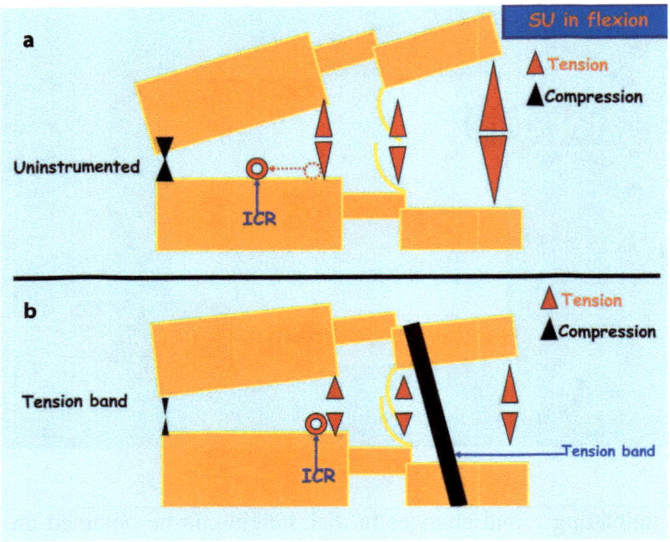

Fig. 14.9 A tension band will give an additional moment that resists bending, thus reducing compression on the anterior annulus and tension on the posterior annulus and facets

extension because of posterior and anterior shifting of the nucleus pulposus in flexion–extension. Thus, if posterior stabilization devices cannot have a primary role in unloading the disk, they can have a profound effect on the loads of specific regions of the disk. Figure 14.9 depicts the effects of a tension band (tying the upper and lower spinous processes to the interspinous device), which give an additional moment to resist bending.

In the normal/uninstrumented condition, the ICR in flexion moves anteriorly, whereas the action of the tension band keeps the ICR more posterior, thereby limiting its shifting. This action results in a reduction of compression forces on the anterior annulus and a reduction of tension on the posterior annulus and facets. Conversely, (Fig. 14.10), the rigid interspinous spacer in extension moves the ICR posteriorly behind the facets (i.e., toward the increase in stiffness determined by the device), thereby modifying the loads on the different parts of the SU: the load on the facets and posterior annulus is reduced instead of increased (tension instead of compression). In a cadaveric study on the effects of an interspinous implant on disk pressures, Swanson and colleagues reported that the pressures of the posterior annulus and nu-

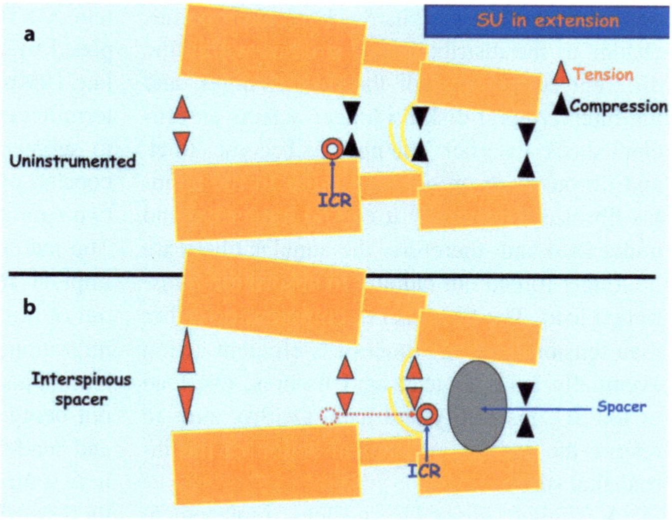

Fig. 14.10 The rigid interspinous spacer moves the instantaneous center of rotation in a posterior direction, thereby modifying the loads on the different parts of the spinal unit

cleus pulposus were reduced by 63% and 41%, respectively, during extension, and by 38% and 20%, respectively, in the neutral, standing position [18].

14.3 Design Rationale of Different Devices and General Surgical Principles

With respect to dynamic stabilization devices, because of anatomical reasons, the only surgical approaches that can be considered to be minimally invasive (and widely available in clinical practice) are the posterior ones. Anterior approaches for non-fusion procedures, such as the ones for total disk replacements (prostheses), require open procedures.

14.3.1 Nucleus Pulposus Replacement Devices

Nucleus pulposus replacement devices are based on replacement of the nucleus only. They have the advantage of cartilage and annulus preservation. Such devices are under ongoing development and evaluation. Disk nucleus replacement devices date back to the 1980s, when Charles D. Ray conceptualized a two-pillow hydrogel device. The original Raymedica prosthetic disk nucleus (PDN) was first used in humans in 1996. It was subsequently replaced by single-pillow designs: the PDN-SOLO and HydraFlex devices. These implants require open intervention. Several devices are in the conceptual or developmental stage and different materials have been proposed, the most promising among them being injectable polymers. Recently, a minimally invasive, injectable nucleus-augmentation system became available: GelStix™ (Replication Medical). It is a prosthetic device designed for implantation inside a degenerated intervertebral disk for the treatment of early-stage disk degeneration (degenerative disk disease [DDD]). GelStix is made of a water-insoluble, hydrophilic polymer (hydrogel) which, after implantation, absorbs water, with consequent swelling and expansion. Hydrogels are used in a wide range of medical products thanks to their physical properties combined with low toxicity and high biocompatibility. The hydrogel can be implanted in the low-volume, dehydrated state with a minimally invasive approach using a spinal needle. In young disks, the nucleus pulposus is composed of 90% water. Aging leads to biochemical changes affecting the water-binding capabilities of the nucleus pulposus. This results in dehydration, volume reduction, changes in cellular activity and, ultimately, a loss in function. As the nucleus pulposus dehydrates and degenerates, its mechanical properties change as the distribution of stresses within the different components of the disk changes, and the intervertebral disk no longer acts as an efficient shock absorber. The nucleus becomes thick and fibrous with properties similar to the annulus fibrosus. Eventually it can no longer expand under load and, therefore, the annular fibers are no longer forced out radially to absorb the transmitted load. The fibers act in compression rather than tension, and this much-less-efficient action eventually leads to tears and fissures, overload of the SU, instability and pain. GelStix aims to restore the normal mechanical action of the intradiskal space.

A similar injectable nucleus replacement based on polymer/synthetic technologies is NuCore® (Spine Wave). NuCore is a synthetic recombinant protein hydrogel designed to mimic the natural nucleus. The hydrogel is adherent to the annulus and nucleus pulposus and thus resistant to extrusion. NuCore is injected into the disk during open microdiskectomy, after removal of the disk herniation, with the aim to restore the natural biomechanics of the spine. Patient enrollment in clinical trials for NuCore includes subjects from Switzerland, Germany, Australia and the USA.

14.3.2 Posterior Stabilization Devices

Posterior stabilization devices fall into two main categories of design: interspinous spacers (with or without tension bands) and pedicle screw-based systems. The tension bands are passed around the upper and lower spinous processes and then tied to the interspinous component, with the double purpose of securing the device and (in some devices) limiting flexion/rotation. Rigid, non-deformable interspinous spacers have a constant effect on the distraction of the spinous processes. Alternatively low-rigidity, deformable spacers act more as shock absorbers, with a consequently more physiological action on range of motion of the SU together with an increase in bone compliance.

The interspinous process decompression system X-STOP (Fig. 14.11) (Medtronic) was proposed by Zucherman and colleagues [19] in the late 1990s for treatment of the symptoms of intermittent neurogenic claudication (INC) due to segmental spinal stenosis [20–22]. X-STOP consists of an oval spacer positioned between the two spinous processes at the symptomatic level. The lateral wing is then attached to prevent the implant from migrating anteriorly or laterally out of position. Anterior migration and posterior migration are also limited, respectively, by the lamina and the supraspinous ligament (the latter not being violated). The central pivot was rigid and made of titanium in the first version. Now it is semi-rigid thanks to a layer of polyetheretherketone (PEEK) (see below) external to the metal. It is deployed through a small posterior surgical approach. It is intended to prevent extension of the stenotic levels, yet allowing flexion, axial rotation, and lateral bending [23]. The intervention can be undertaken under local anesthesia and mild sedation without removing bone or soft tissues with preservation of the supraspinous ligament. Leaving the supraspinous ligament in place and intact has the double effect of not only preventing posterior migration of the device but also of not modifying the behavior of the SU in flexion. The procedure is typically done with hospitalization for 24 h.

Biomechanical studies have shown that the implant significantly reduces intradiskal pressure and facet load, as well as preventing narrowing of the spinal canal and neural foramens [17, 18, 24]. It is an alternative therapy to conservative treatment and decompressive surgery for patients suffering from INC. Its safety and effectiveness have been confirmed in a randomized, controlled trial [19, 25, 26].

Similar devices on the European market which have not yet been approved in the USA are available:

- Superion™ (VertiFlex);
- Aperius™ (Medtronic);
- In-Space™ (Synthes);
- Flexus™ (Globus Medical);
- BacJac™ (Pioneer Surgical Technology);
- Falena™ (Mikai, Italy);
- Prow™ (Non-Linear Technology Spine).

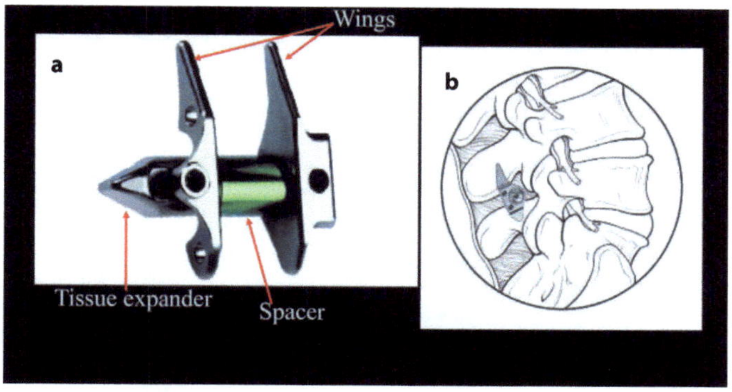

Fig. 14.11 X-Stop depicting the lateral wings, central spacer and tissue expander (**a**). The device is deployed in the interspinous ligament, with the wings limiting lateral migration (**b**)

Superion and Aperius are rigid, being made of titanium, and both are deployed through a percutaneous approach. In-Space, Flexus, BacJac and Falena, similar to the X-STOP, are made of PEEK in the part of the device in contact with bone. PEEK is a semi-crystalline thermoplastic that exhibits strength, stiffness, resilience, and biocompatibility, which is ideal for use in orthopedic surgery. It allows stress to be distributed more evenly on the surrounding bony structures, limiting an overload that could lead to acute fracture or chronic bone porosity and resorption. They are deployed percutaneously or through mini-open surgical access (like X-STOP).

Prow is made of ultra-high-molecular-weight polyethylene (UHMWPE), a material used extensively for >40 years in total joint replacements. Similar to PEEK, it has an elasticity modulus close to that of bone, granting support to adjacent bone with a lessened chance of subsidence.

Coflex™ (Paradigm Spine) is a U-shaped titanium device based on different concepts. It is inserted surgically between the spinous processes. This entails removal of all interspinous and supraspinous ligaments. It is more rigid (less dynamic in its action) and, because of its shape, has more contact surface with bone. This could be an advantage over other interspinous/interlaminar decompression devices, thereby reducing the risk of delayed bone subsidence (see below in the "Complications" paragraph).

Wallis™ (Abbot Spine) [27–29] and the DIAM™ (Medtronic) [30, 31] are double-action devices in which the interspinous spacer is secured with two tension bands wrapped around the upper and lower adjacent spinous processes. The bands also give support to the supraspinous ligament in limiting flexion of the SU (hence the double-action of the devices; more intense for Wallis and less for DIAM, whose surgical insertion does not entail sectioning of the supraspinous ligament).

The spacer of Wallis is made of PEEK. The core of DIAM is made of silicone, whereas the outer mesh and tether are made of polyethylene terephthalate (polyester). Silicone is more resilient and compressible, and is preloaded by compression before insertion. This permits posterior tensioning of the ligaments and disk, allowing a type of ligamentotaxis (particularly of the posterior annulus fibrosus).

Similar to DIAM is IntraSpine (Cousin Biotech), which is made of the same silicone covered with a polyester textile. The silicone core has a shape based on a different concept compared with other interspinous devices. The central core fitting the interspinous space has an anterior part, designed to suit the interlaminar space. This kind of "nose", covered with a layer of silicone to avoid fibrosis in the yellow ligament area, gives the device a more anterior (ventral) point of action directly between the laminae, with a consequently more efficient action on the ICR (similar to that of the PercuDyn system, see below).

Screw-based posterior stabilization devices fall in a different category of design. Most of them, like Dynesys™ (Zimmer Spine) or Stabilimax NZ™ (Applied Spine Technologies),

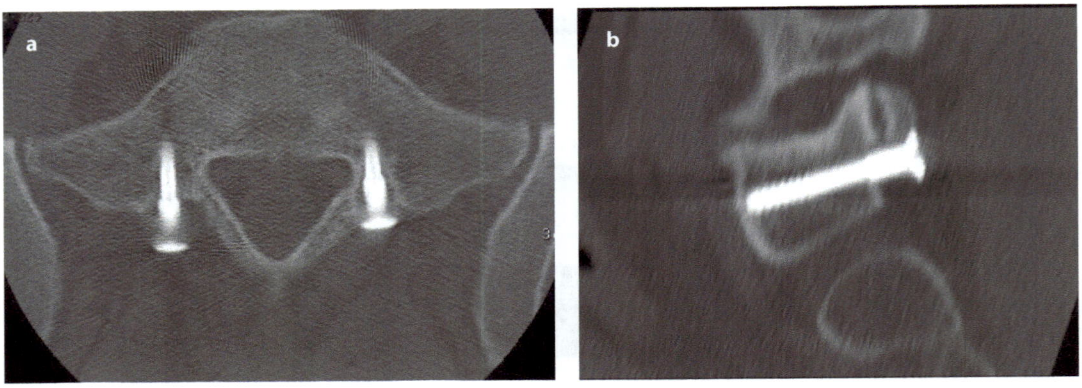

Fig. 14.12 MRI images showing the screw-based PercuDyn system: titanium screws are anchored in the S1 pedicles (**a**), whereas the polycarbonate-urethane heads of the screws support and cushion the inferior facet complex of the upper metamer (**b**), thereby limiting its extension and unloading the disk

are not minimally invasive. They require an open surgical approach similar to the one used for instrumented fusions.

Dynesys is built in analogy with the posterior screws and rod instrumentation systems. However, the spacers are made of flexible plastic tubes (polyurethane) surrounding a thin nylon-like cord (polyethylene). After implantation the system creates a dynamic push–pull relationship that stabilizes the affected joints without fusion. The device was developed and has been used in Europe since 1994, with mixed results [32, 33]. Clearance for the Dynesys system by the Food and Drug Administration (FDA) in the USA is limited to use as an adjunct to spinal fusion of the thoracic, lumbar and sacral spine for degenerative spondylolisthesis with neurological impairment, and for a prior failed spinal fusion (pseudoarthrosis). Clinical trials are ongoing for use of Dynesys as a stand-alone device in the absence of spinal fusion.

Stabilimax NZ features dual concentric springs combined with a ball-and-socket joint to enhance spinal stability and to increase the resistance of the passive spinal system around the neural zone while permitting controlled motion in flexion and extension. Stabilimax NZ is inserted by pedicle screws in exactly the same way as fusion devices. However, a bone graft is not placed to promote bone growth for fusion.

PercuDyn™ (Interventional Spine) (Fig. 14.12) is a screw-based posterior stabilization device. Two screws are inserted with a totally percutaneous, fluoroscopy-guided approach through the pedicles into the vertebral body. The polycarbonate-urethane-resilient heads provide support to the inferior articular facets of the upper vertebra, thereby limiting their range of motion in extension. This device can be used if a spinous process is not present (L5–S1 or post-laminectomy). Moreover, the device might be better at treating diskogenic pain. The device is mounted more anteriorly with respect to a true interspinous device. Consequently, it exerts a more efficient action in moving the ICR outside the disk, forcing the segment into flexion into a neutral position and keeping the posterior annulus as distracted as possible. Thus, on a theoretical, biomechanical basis, it should decrease intradiskal pressure, reduce annular compression, and preserve posterior disk height in a more efficient way than more posteriorly applied devices [34].

Several trials are being conducted to evaluate the safety and efficacy of many of the devices described above (Flexus, Prow, In-Space, Superion, Wallis, DIAM, Aperius, Coflex, Stabilimax NZ). In addition to the above-described technologies, a lot of other dynamic stabilization devices are in various stages of development. In addition, some companies are developing technologies that would allow a combination of posterior dynamic stabilization devices and total disk replacement as an alternative to spinal fusion.

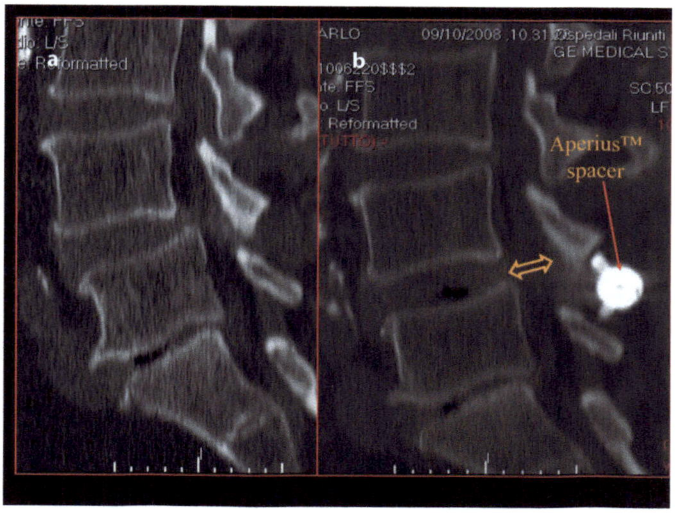

Fig. 14.13 The rigid, percutaneous Aperius™ interspinous spacer reduces degenerative spondilolisthesis and widens the sagittal diameter of the spinal canal (preoperative MRI in **a**, postoperative MRI in **b**)

14.4 Patient Selection

Rigid or semi-rigid interspinous devices such as the X-STOP, Aperius or In-Space were developed originally for the treatment of INC symptoms due to segmental spinal stenosis [20–22]. INC symptoms are pain and discomfort radiating to the buttocks, thigh, and lower limbs during standing and walking. This is exacerbated by lumbar extension and relieved by flexion. Standing narrows the neural foramina and canal area, resulting in the impingement of nerve roots, whereas flexing (such as when sitting or riding a bicycle) increases the cross-sectional area of the spinal canal, thereby relieving this impingement.

In extension, the implant significantly increases the canal area, subarticular diameter, canal diameter and area/width of the foramen [18, 35, 36]. The final effect is that the implant prevents narrowing of the spinal canal and foramina in extension, thereby reducing or eliminating compression of the nerve root. Figure 14.13 illustrates reduction of the anterolisthesis and widening of the spinal canal after insertion of an interspinous device (Aperius).

This indication for implantation of an interspinous device has been validated by a randomized, controlled, prospective, multicenter trial comparing patients treated with X-STOP with patients treated by non-surgical means [19, 25, 26].

The indications for control of axial pain are poorly defined and left to the surgeon's personal opinions and experience. Reliable data are lacking but hopefully ongoing trials will provide the necessary evidence for appropriate choices. Most studies are focused on moderate degenerative lumbar stenosis at one or two levels or treatment of mild-to-moderate degenerative disk disease (DDD) of the lumbar spine.

The most frequent indications are early disk degeneration ("black disk", which is an incorrect, non-radiological definition that is widely used in surgical communities), contained disk herniations, mild segmental instability (postoperative or not), and facet syndrome (with hypertrophy, osteophytosis, cysts, incongruity). The indications proposed by Sénégas for the Wallis system are significant loss of disk material after surgery, a degenerative disk adjacent to a fused segment, and an isolated Modic 1 lesion [37] thought to be the cause of chronic LBP. Another indication is providing a cushioning mechanism to SU adjacent to fused levels.

The principles of biomechanics (see paragraph 14.2) should direct surgical strategy. Rigid or semi-rigid interspinous components limit extension, moving the ICR and loads away from the facets and posterior annulus. The tension bands limit flexion and rotation, adding stability and helping to restore the alignment of the metamers.

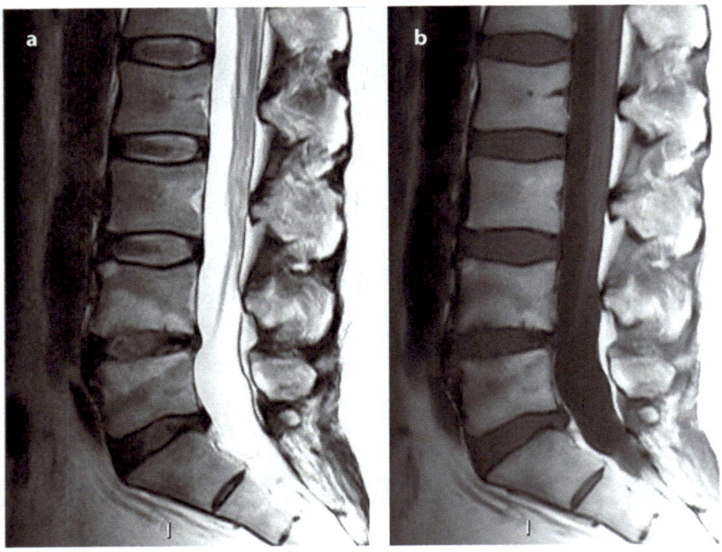

Fig. 14.14 Anterior osteocondrosis of the L4–L5 disk space as shown on MRI. **a** T2-weighted image shows intense hypersignal of the endplates and adjacent bone marrow, compared to the T1-weighted image (**b**), that shows prevalence of hyposignal; this indicates a prevalence of Modic 1 modifications (inflammatory) with a less intense Modic 2 component

Changes in the location of the ICR change the deformation of local areas of tissue, moving the distribution of the loads. In the case illustrated in Figure 14.14, the pain source is presumably the anterior inflammatory osteochondrosis. The surgical strategy should rely more on limitation of flexion (i.e., on the posterior tension band to reduce the anterior disk load). The interspinous spacer partially limits the load on the anterior disk, however, forcing the facets to open instead of closing in extension (as discussed above). For this reason, almost all devices with a tension band are double-action devices, coupling bands and an interspinous spacer. Such systems tend to add stability to the vertebral segment, while simultaneously limiting the extremes of flexion and extension (i.e., reducing the NZ that was widened by the pathologic conditions) and restoring a range of motion that is as physiological as possible. Such systems increase resistance to compression and stretch, not (or only partially) affecting rotation and lateral bending.

Nucleus augmentation materials and/or devices such as GelStix could play a part in reversing diskogenic pain in the early phases of disk degeneration (Pfirrmann grades 2–4 [38] without evidence of Modic modification of the endplates and/or evidence of intradiskal granulation tissue). Section 14.2 showed that as the nucleus pulposus dehydrates and degenerates, it no longer acts as an efficient shock absorber because it cannot expand under loads. Therefore, the annular fibers are no longer forced out radially to absorb the transmitted loads. Annulus fibers are compressed under physiological loads and this condition leads to tears, fissures and painful granulation tissue (Fig. 14.15). GelStix aims to reverse the degenerative process by restoring pressure, hydration and normal mechanical action to the intradiskal space. The indications for its use should therefore be limited to the early stages of disk degeneration.

As disk degeneration progresses, there is sprouting of vessels accompanied by nociceptive fibers from the outer toward the inner disk. This sprouting becomes painful owing to the presence of nodules of granulation tissue (sometimes evident on MRI as nodular zones of high signal) usually in the posterior annulus [39]. In some cases, as in Fig. 14.16, the origin of pain could be presumed to be from the hyperintensity zone (HIZ) in the posterior annulus. In such situations, the aim is to move the load away from the posterior annulus by means of the action on the ICR of a rigid posterior interspinous device. The action of the device could, in theory, reverse the wrong load condition on the annulus, favoring its regeneration and rehydration of the nucleus.

Among the advantages of motion preserva-

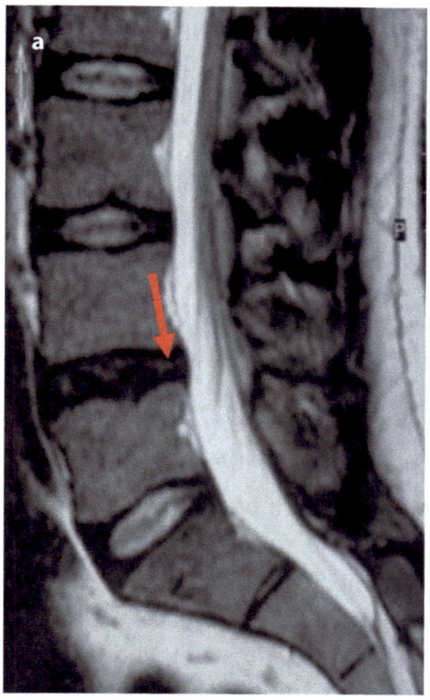

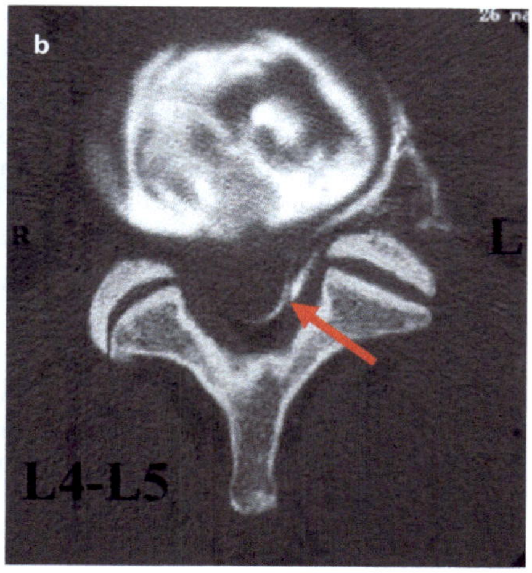

Fig. 14.15 MRI showing early disk degeneration (Pfirrmann grade 3) with dehydration of the nucleus pulposus but minimal reduction of disk height. The distinction between the nucleus and annulus fibrosus is unclear because the nucleus is fragmented and "creeps" through tears in the inner annulus (*arrow*) (**a**). This condition is confirmed in **b** by the corresponding CT diskography: the contrast medium does not remain (as it should in normal anatomy) centrally confined to the nucleus but diffuses in a circumferential annulography. Tiny tears in the external annulus are also present, justifying the epidural leak (*arrow*)

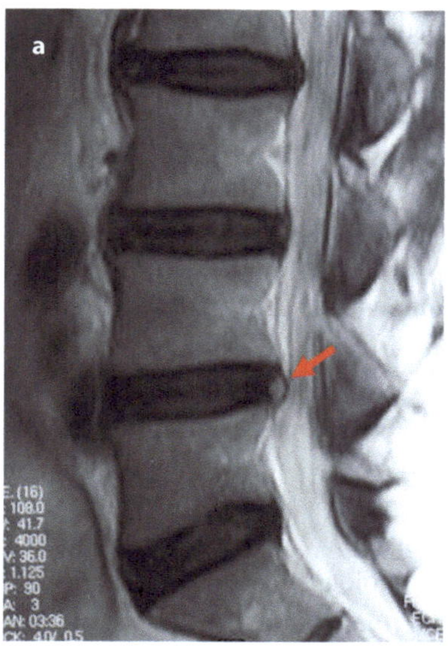

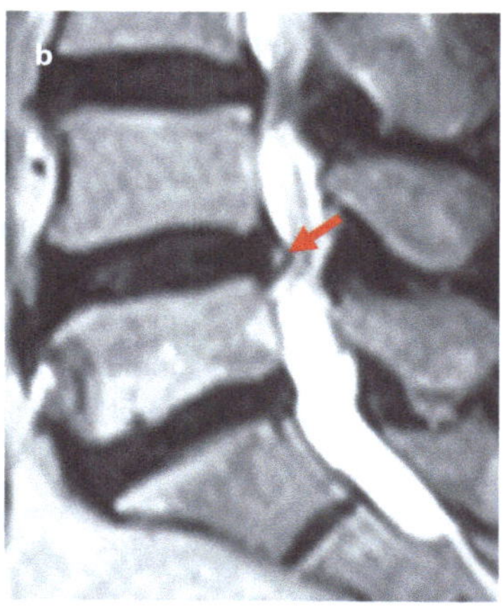

Fig. 14.16 MRI showing hyperintensity zones in the posterior annulus representing tears and granulation tissue (*arrows*). In **b**, note the asymmetric outward bulging of the external, innervated fibers of the annulus, being loaded in compression rather than radially, owing to nuclear degeneration

tion that must be considered is the positive effect that normal load and motion have in maintaining all joints in good health, thereby providing ideal nutrition for the articular components. This is true for intervertebral disks, which are not vascularized and consequently rely for nutrition and oxygenation on osmotic diffusion from the surrounding tissues (particularly through the permeability of the cartilage endplates). Nutrients are pumped into the disk, and movement plays a major part in this process. When treating diskogenic pain, disk degeneration must be limited

Table 14.1 Contraindications to the use of interspinous implants

1. Allergy to titanium or titanium alloys (or any component of the implant).
2. Spinal anatomy or disease that would prevent implantation of the device or cause the device to be unstable in situ (such as a fracture, significant scoliosis (Cobb angle >25°), degenerative spondylolisthesis greater than grade 1.0 (on a scale of 1 to 4) or true spondilolisthesis due to isthmic lysis) because the action of the device would widen and aggravate the lysis and not modify the degree of the olysthesis.
3. Ankylosed segment at the affected level(s).
4. Cauda equina syndrome (defined as neural compression causing neurogenic dysfunction of the bowel or bladder).
5. Active systemic infection or infection localized to implantation site.
6. A diagnosis of severe osteoporosis (defined as bone mineral density (from dual-energy X-ray absorptiometry or a comparable study) in the spine or hip that is >2.5 standard deviations below the mean of normal adult values.

to Pfirrmann grades 1–4, and diffused Modic changes should be excluded (though small spots of limited Modic degeneration of the endplates are acceptable).

Rigid or semi-rigid interspinous spacers may help reduce minimal degrees (grade 1.0 on a scale of 1 to 4) of degenerative spondilolisthesis (see Fig. 14.12) due to spondylotic facet deformation (but not a true olysthesis due to lysis, see below).

Degenerative retrolisthesis with diskopathy, reduction in the height of the posterior annulus, and possible associated Baastrup syndrome ("kissing" spinous processes with progressive, painful interspinous degenerative alterations) are good indications for an interspinous spacer.

14.5 Contraindications and Complications

There are several contraindications to the use of interspinous implants (Table 14.1) [40]. An osteoporotic condition must be considered to be a contraindication because of the risk of fractures consequent to the pressures generated against bony surfaces.

Barbagallo et al. [41] analyzed complications in a series of 69 patients. At a mean follow-up of 23 months, 8 complications (11.5%) were recorded: 4 device dislocations and 4 fractures of spinous processes. A prospective observational study found a high prevalence of fractures of spinous processes in 38 patients (50 implants) after implantation of interspinous stand-alone devices [42]. A fracture was not identifiable on plain radiographs, but postoperative computed tomography identified non-displaced spinous-process factures in 11 patients (28.9% of patients, 22% of levels). Direct interview of patients as well as review of medical records indicated that 5 fractures were associated with mild-to-moderate lumbar back pain, and 6 fractures were asymptomatic. Three of the 11 patients underwent device removal and laminectomy for persistent pain. Fractures in the other 3 patients had healed by 1 year.

In a recent study [43], we assessed the feasibility and efficacy of cement augmentation of the posterior vertebral arch (spinoplasty) before Aperius implantation in preventing perioperative and post-implant fractures of spinous processes. Spinoplasty seemed effective in preventing delayed fractures of the posterior arch after placement of interspinous spacers in patients at risk for fragility fractures.

14.6 Conclusion

Dynamic stabilization (non-fusion or motion-preservation technologies) aims to provide stabilization while maintaining the mobility and function of the SUs by favoring realignment, preventing extremes of flexion and extension, and unloading painful areas within the SU (especially discs or facets), through modification of distribution of loads.

Dynamic unloading of the overall SU is not possible (it is equivalent to a rigid fusion). Often, pain occurs not from an increase in the quantity of motion but from abnormal distribution of loads across sensitive areas of the SU. Changes in the location of the ICR change the deformation of local areas of tissue, moving the distribution of loading away from painful areas.

Dynamic stabilization could relieve stress peaks in facets and the anterior and posterior annulus provided adequate designs and sizes of spacers are chosen. Thus, dynamic stabilization may provide pain relief by altering the transmission of abnormal loads across the degenerated structures.

The indications for surgery remain poorly defined and reflect largely the opinions of individual surgeons. The main issue is that diagnostic techniques cannot be used to identify exactly the pain source, and our understanding of pain etiology is poor. The same issue underlies fusion surgery, which is considered to be the "gold standard" for the treatment of instability. The dynamic stabilization techniques discussed in this chapter are limited to the lower grades of instability, thereby representing the first, low-invasiveness tool in the armamentarium of the spine surgeon. Dynamic, minimally invasive implants should be used to avoid or delay more aggressive procedures, and their use as "intermediate" solutions is justified as long as iatrogenic trauma during implantation is minimal. From a speculative and prospective viewpoint, early correction of low grades of instability by minimally invasive, dynamic devices, could not only stop or delay, but even reverse degeneration of the components of the SU.

As clinicians dealing with spinal diseases, we see patients suffering from instability while simultaneously understanding the lack of diagnostic certainty. In this situation, the main advantage of dynamic stabilization systems is that they are they are minimally invasive, can be customized, and are readily reversible. They maintain motion and spinal alignment, and are cheaper and safer than instrumented fusion procedures. Furthermore, dynamic stabilization systems do not preclude further therapeutic options.

Nevertheless, many questions are yet to be answered. Further studies are required to determine the optimal design of implants. This is the beginning of a new era of surgery for the degenerative spine. Radiologists are the best trained for the correct use and application of percutaneous or minimally invasive (often radiograph-guided) surgical methods and devices. Several of these surgical methods and devices have been proposed and developed by radiologists. Orthopedic surgeons and neurosurgeons share a long tradition of invasive treatments of the degenerative spine. These "two worlds" are getting closer, and an open and unbiased cooperation of these communities should represent good news for our patients.

References

1. Airaksinen O, Brox JI, Cedraschi C et al (2006) European guidelines for the management of chronic nonspecific low back pain. Eur Spine J 15:S192–S300
2. Burton AK, Balague F, Cardon G et al (2006) European guidelines for prevention in low back pain. Eur Spine J 15:S136–S168
3. Palmer KT, Walsh K, Bendall H, Cooper C, Coggon D (2000) Back pain in Britain: comparison of two prevalence surveys at an interval of 10 years. Brit Med J 320:1577–1578
4. Paris SV (1985) Physical signs of instability. Spine 10: 277–279
5. Pope MH, Panjabi MM (1985) Biomechanical definition of spine instability. Spine 10:255–256
6. American Academy of Orthopaedic Surgeons (1981) A glossary of spinal terminology. American Academy of Orthopedic Surgeons, Chicago
7. Park P, Garton HJ, Gala VC, Hoff JT, McGillicuddy JE (2004) Adjacent segment disease after lumbar or lumbosacral fusion: review of the literature. Spine 29:1938–1944
8. Schlegel JD, Smith JA, Schleusener RL (1996) Lumbar motion segment pathology adjacent to thoracolumbar, lumbar and lumbosacral fusions. Spine 21:970–981
9. Aota Y, Kumano K, Hirabayashi S (1995) Postfusion instability at the adjacent segments after rigid pedicle screw fixation for degenerative lumbar spinal disorders. J Spinal Disord 8:464–473.
10. Etebar S, Cahill DW (1999). Risk factors for adjacent segment failure following lumbar fixation with rigid instrumentation for degenerativeinstability. J Neurosurg 90:163–169
11. Kumar MN, Jacquot F, Hall H (2001) Long-term follow-up of functional outcomes and radiographic changes at adjacent levels following lumbar spine fusion for degenerative disc disease. Eur Spine J 10: 309–313
12. Ghiselli G, Wang JC, Bhatia NN, Hsu WK, Dawson EG (2004) Adjacent segment degeneration in the lumbar spine. J Bone Joint Surg Am 86:1497–1503
13. Boos N, Webb JK (1997) Pedicle screw fixation in spinal disorders: a European view. Eur Spine J 6:2–18

14. Gibson JN, Grant IC, Waddell G (1999) The Cochrane review of surgery for lumbar disc prolapse and degenerative lumbar spondylosis. Spine 24:1820–1832
15. Sengupta DK. Dynamic stabilization devices in the treatment of low back pain (2004) Orthop Clin North Am 35:43–56
16. McNally DS (2006) Rationale for dynamic stabilization. In: Kim D, Cammisa FP, Fessler RG (eds) Dynamic reconstruction of the spine. Thieme, New York, p 237–243
17. Wiseman C, Lindsey DP, Fredrick AD, Yerby SA (2005) The effect of an interspinous process implant on facet loading during extension. Spine 30:903–907
18. Swanson KE, Lindsey DP, Hsu KY, Zucherman JF Yerby SA (2003) The effects of an interspinous implant on intervertebral disc pressures. Spine 28:26–32
19. Zucherman JF, Hsu KY, Hartjen CA et al (2004) A prospective randomized multi-center study for the treatment of lumbar spinal stenosis with the X-Stop interspinous implant: 1-year results. Eur Spine J 13:22–31
20. Katz JN, Harris MB. Lumbar spinal stenosis (2008) N Engl J Med 358:818–825
21. Arbit E, Pannullo S (2001) Lumbar stenosis: a clinical review. Clin Orthop 384:137–143
22. Blau JN, Logue V (1978). The natural history of intermittent claudication of the cauda equina. A long term follow-up study. Brain 101:211222
23. Lindsey DP, Swanson KE, Fuchs P, Hsu KY, Zucherman JF, Yerby SA (2003) The effects of an interspinous implant on the kinematics of the instrumented and adjacent levels in the lumbar spine. Spine 28:2192–2197
24. Richards JC, Majumdar S, Lindsey DP, Beaupre GS, Yerby SA (2005) The treatment mechanism of an interspinous process implant for lumbar neurogenic intermittent claudication. Spine 30:744–749
25. Zucherman JF, Hsu KY, Hartjen CA et al (2005) A multicenter, prospective, randomized trial evaluating the X STOP interspinous process decompression system for the treatment of neurogenic intermittent claudication. Two-year follow-up results. Spine 30:1351–1358
26. Kondrashov DG, Hannibal M, Hsu KY, Zucherman JF (2006) Interspinous process decompression with the X-STOP device for lumbar spinal stenosis. A 4-Year follow-up study. J Spinal Disord Tech 19:323–327
27. Sénégas J, Etchevers JP, Baulny D, Grenier F (1988) Widening of the lumbar vertebral canal as an alternative to laminectomy, in the treatment of lumbar stenosis. Fr J Orthop Surg 2:93–99
28. Sénégas J (1991) Surgery of the intervertebral ligaments, alternative to arthrodesis in the treatment of degenerative instabilities. Acta Orthop Belg 57 (Suppl. 1):221–226 [In French]
29. Sénégas J (2002). Mechanical supplementation by non rigid fixation in degenerative intervertebral lumbar segments: the Wallis system. Eur Spine J 11(Suppl. 2):164–169
30. Taylor J (2001) Nonfusion technologies of the posterior column: a new posterior shock absorber. Presented at the International Symposium on Intervertebral Disc Replacement and Non-Fusion Technology. Munich, May 3–5
31. Taylor J, Ritland S (2006). Technical and anatomical considerations for the placement of a posterior interspinous stabilizer. In: Mayer HM (ed) Minimally invasive spine surgery. Springer, Berlin, p 466–475
32. Stoll TM, Gilles Dubois G, Schwarzenbach O (2002) The dynamic neutralization system for the spine: A multi-center study of a novel non-fusion system. Eur Spine J 11(Suppl. 2):S170-S178
33. Grob D, Benini A, Junge A, Anne F, Mannion AF (2005) Clinical experience with the Dynesys semirigid fixation system for the lumbar spine: surgical and patient-oriented outcome in 50 cases after an average of 2 years. Spine 30:324–331
34. Palmer S, Mahar A, Oka R (2007) Biomechanical and radiographic analysis of a novel, minimally invasive, extension-limiting device for the lumbar spine. Neurosurg Focus 22:1–6
35. Siddiqui M, Nicol M, Karadimas E, Smith F, Wardlaw D (2005) The positional magnetic resonance imaging changes in the lumbar spine following insertion of a novel interspinous process distraction device. Spine 30:2677–2682
36. Siddiqui M, Karadimas E, Nicol M (2006) Influence of X-Stop on neural foramina and spinal canal area in spinal stenosis. Spine 31:2958–2962
37. Modic MT, Steinberg PM, Ross JS, Masaryk TJ carter JR (1988) Degenerative disk disease: assessment of changes in vertebral body marrow with MR imaging. Radiology 166 (1 pt. 1):193–199
38. Pfirrmann CW, Metzdorf A, Zanetti M, Hodler J, Boos N (2001) Magnetic resonance classification of lumbar intervertebral disc degeneration. Spine 26:1873–1878
39. Aprill C, Bogduk N (1992) High intensity zone: a diagnostic sign of painful lumbar disc on magnetic resonance imaging. Brit J Radiol 65:361–369
40. Rolfe KW, Zucherman JF, Kondrashov DG, Hsu KY, Nosova E (2010) Scoliosis and interspinous decompression with the X-STOP: prospective minimum 1-year outcomes in lumbar spinal stenosis. Spine J 10:972–978
41. Barbagallo GM, Olindo G, Corbino L, Albanese V (2009) Analysis of complications in patients treated with the X-Stop Interspinous Process Decompression System: proposal for a novel anatomic scoring system for patient selection and review of the literature. Neurosurgery 65:111-119 (discussion 119-120)
42. Kim DH, Tantorski M, Shaw J et al (2011) Occult spinous process fractures associated with interspinous process spacers. Spine 36:E1080–E1085
43. Bonaldi G, Bertolini G, Marrocu A, Cianfoni A (2012) Posterior vertebral arch cement augmentation (spinoplasty) to prevent fracture of spinous processes after interspinous spacer implant. Am J Neuroradiol 33:522–528

New Treatments for Spinal Tumors

15

Salvatore Masala, Giovanni Nano,
Tommaso Volpi and Giovanni Simonetti

15.1 Introduction

About 70% of cancer patients develop spinal metastases, and the peak age is 40–70 years (with 10–20% of these cases involving compression of the spinal cord). Given the steady ageing of the population in western countries, treatment is burdensome with appreciable economic costs [1, 2]. Common malignances with metastatic involvement of the spine are those of the breast, lung, prostate gland and bone marrow (lymphoma and multiple myeloma). These account for about 60% of the overall metastases seen in the spine, with tumors of the gastrointestinal tract and kidney accounting for 5% [3]. Primary neoplasms of the spine are relatively rare (<10% of the entire spectrum of spinal neoplasms) and are classified usually according to their origin (i.e., osseous, cartilaginous, vascular). Further classification into "benign" or "malignant" is based usually on overall evaluation of their clinical progression, histopathological evidence of invasiveness, and response to therapy. Some primary tumors that may be considered benign under strict histological evaluation show certain "aggressive" behaviors related to their usual site of origin close to neural structures and due to their tendency to recur (e.g., osteoblastomas, aneurysmal bone cysts, giant cell tumors) [4].

Tumor spread may be vascular (arterial or *via* the Batson venous plexus), through direct contiguous extension from paraspinal soft tissues, or by seeding through cerebrospinal fluid. The intense vascularization of the vertebral bodies (VBs), particularly at their posterior third, accounts for their targeting by metastases. Pedicles, articular apophyses and laminae are usually involved later due to direct tumor extension through the VB. Whatever the site of metastasis nesting (anterior or posterior vertebral elements), they are extradural in 94–99% of cases, with epidural involvement secondary to direct contiguous growth. All spinal segments may be involved, with higher frequencies observed for dorsal and lumbar segments compared with cervical and sacral segments. In ≤30% of cases, the involvement is multisegmental, but usually only one segment is symptomatic, with localized, non-radicular, dull pain being the most common complaint. The pathophysiological mechanism of such pain is based on the release of chemical agents by overturned bone and tumor cells. This action results in: the stimulation of endosteal nerves and inhibition of osteoblastic activity; periosteal stretching; and the infiltration and compression of nerves and surrounding tissues. The net effect is pathological fractures. In a cancer patient, new-onset pain in the neck and back with relentless progression are pathognomonic of spinal metastasis. Radicular pain or neurologic deficits (motor-

G. Nano (✉)
Department of Diagnostic and Molecular Imaging, Interventional Radiology and Radiotherapy, University Tor Vergata, Rome, Italy
e-mail: gionano@gmail.com

M. Muto (ed.), *Interventional Neuroradiology of the Spine*,
DOI 10.1007/978-88-470-2790-9_15, © Springer-Verlag Italia 2013

sensory or visceral) arise depending on the extent and location of neural impingement. Mechanical spinal instability, defined by the Spine Oncology Study Group as "loss of spinal integrity as a result of neoplastic process that is associated with movement related pain, symptomatic or progressive deformity and neural compromise under physiologic loads" (i.e., secondary to intersegment altered load transfer) is another common sign that usually directs the treatment toward less conservative interventions (i.e., conventional or minimally invasive) [5, 6].

In general, conservative treatment (drug- or radiation-based) has led to prolonged life expectancy with positive effects on quality of life (QoL). However, in many cases, spinal tumors manifest mechanical issues that cannot be solved conservatively, thereby leading to surgical or, for our part, interventional treatment.

Evaluation of the most suitable treatment is based on diagnostic imaging (radiography, computed tomography (CT), magnetic resonance imaging (MRI), radionuclide imaging), tumor histology, and thorough clinical evaluation. Many classification systems are available to aid evaluation. A useful mnemonic has been proposed by Paton et al. called the LMNOP system, where: "L" stands for the location-levels-extent of lesion involvement (L); "M" represents evaluation of mechanical stability according to the Spine Instability Neoplastic Score (SINS); "N" is neural structure compromise; "O" is tumor radiosensitivity; and "P" is patient clinical status and previous treatments [5, 7].

The aim of treatment of spinal metastasis is inherently palliative. Hence, it is usually indicated in the case of single lesions or, if multiple lesions are present, towards those lesions which are clinically expressive. However, one must consider if the patient is fit enough to undergo treatment (particularly in the case of conventional surgery). For example, a patient with a single, painful lesion embedded in a VB without neural impingement and good clinical status will be able to undergo each treatment up to the corpectomy with spinal instrumentation. Conversely, a patient with poor clinical status with multiple spinal lesions, one of which has clinically relevant and progressive neural impingement, will benefit from less invasive options in which the primary goal is to reduce the mass effect of the lesion.

15.2 Basic Principles of Available Treatments

The aim of the treatment is to relieve pain and to preserve or restore (even partially) neurological function. The fulfillment of this mission is of enormous value for the patient. When dealing with spinal metastasis, the first non-surgical treatment radiotherapy. For thorough coverage of these issues, cross-refer to specific chapters because here we discuss the basic principles. Radiotherapy is indicated as first-line treatment in cases of symptomatic radiosensitive lesions without neurological compromise or signs of instability. Tumors whose spinal metastases are radiosensitive are lymphoma, multiple myeloma, small-cell lung carcinoma, seminoma, neuroblastoma amd Ewing's sarcoma [8]. In general, conventional radiotherapy loads a 25–40-Gy dose fractionated over 10–14 days, beaming an area the width of about 2 VBs (a margin of about 5 cm around the target lesion). The low radiation tolerance of the spinal cord (including cauda equina rootlets at the lumbar level) is the main limiting factor in most cases, and yields suboptimal radiation of lesions [9,10].

Radiotherapy may also be delivered through the stereotactic method, the goal of which is to obliterate a relatively small lesion in a single, high-dose fraction. Conventional radiotherapy is based on the intrinsic radiosensitivity of the tumor and therefore involves multiple, small-dose fractions. Stereotactic radiotherapy is not based on such sensitivity. The *rationale* of the stereotactic method is to focus many radiation fields simultaneously onto the volume of interest (VOI) to achieve a steep decreasing dose gradient around its margins. To simplify the difference between conventional and stereotactic radiotherapy, we can assume that, whereas in conventional radiotherapy the dose is fractionated over time (i.e. multiple small doses over several days), in stereotactic radiotherapy the dose is fractioned over

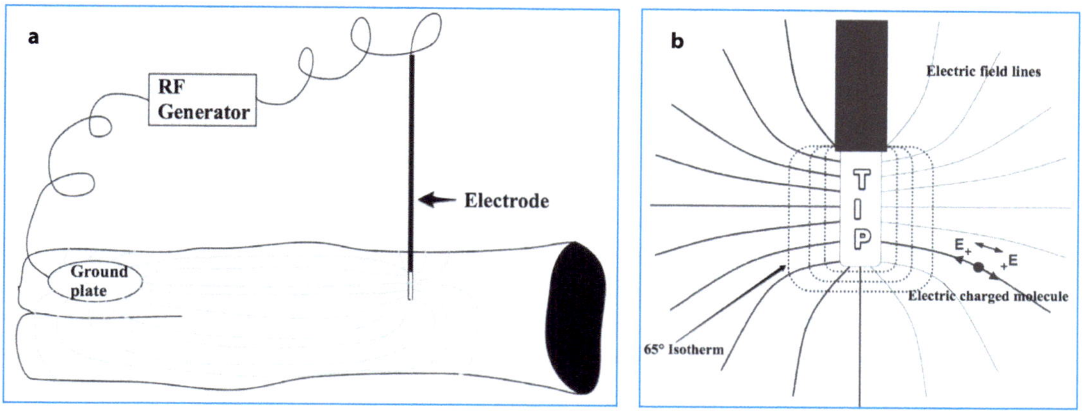

Fig. 15.1 Main components of a radiofrequency ablation system (schematic): electrode, and ground plate with the patient's body close to the circuit of the field lines (light gray) (**a**). Active tip on which surface field lines converge tightly, letting the surrounding charged molecules to vibrate to-and-fro with consequent temperature rise by the Joule effect (**b**)

space (i.e. multiple doses focusing at the same time on the VOI). Focusing almost all the dose inside the target volume allows the surrounding tissue to be spared and able to tolerate the low-intensity convergent beams. The typical dose is approximately 8–20 Gy in 1–2 sessions in the outpatient setting. The advantages of this method are that patients who were irradiated unsuccessfully and those who cannot tolerate surgery due to poor clinical status can be treated. The disadvantage is that lesion shrinkage may be delayed over several weeks, so several re-treatments may be required [11, 12].

Surgery is strongly recommended if radiotherapy is unsuccessful and if the primary tumor is not known. In such cases, surgery can be diagnostic and therapeutic. The essence of surgery in these cases is decompression of the spinal cord and spinal roots and stabilization of the spinal column. The specific types of surgical intervention are dependent upon several factors, including the location inside the vertebral element, the level and extent of involvement, bone integrity, and patient debility. The approaches may be anterior (indicated for cervical and upper thoracic segments) or posterior (indicated for the cranial–cervical junction, mid-thoracic and lumbar segments). Decompression may be the only treatment but more frequently it is associated with spinal instrumentation.

The surgical options mentioned above are "aggressive" interventions. However, some less invasive methods are available, each with their specific indications, advantages and disadvantages. Some of these (e.g., vertebroplasty, kyphoplasty) have been tackled in other chapters, to which the reader is directed. Others, such as spinal alcoholization (which was the first method to be employed successfully) have been almost completely abandoned because of poor outcomes and higher prevalence of complications.

15.3 Radiofrequency Ablation (RFA)

Each RFA apparatus comprises a ground plate, generator, and electrode, each with its own connection cable. The patient lies between the ground plate and the electrode (Fig. 15.1a). When this circuit is closed, an alternating electric current with a frequency around 5MHz is running. The prototypical monopolar electrode is completely insulated except its tip. Many types of electrodes are available, each with its own unique characteristics. However, they differ appreciably in terms of the length and thickness of the tip, which are the main determinants for lesion size. In the case of a single electrode system, the active tips usually range between 2 mm and 30 mm in length and 0.7 mm and 2 mm in radius. The lesion size is in linear proportion with the length, but not for the radius: there are reasons for this. When the circuit is closed and the generator activated, a RF electric field runs through the patient's body: it alternates in and out of the ground plate and electrode tip. The entire surface area of the electrode tip, however, is many orders of magnitude narrower than the ground plate. Hence, the density of the field lines that are forced through the electrode tip is huge. Now, because the alternating electric field acts on the charged molecules of the body, letting them vibrate to-and-fro in proportion to the density of the field lines, such vibrations will be very high at the tip and point of the ground plate (Fig. 1b). At the molecular level, to vibrate under alternating RF electric current means to "heat" ("Joule effect"), i.e. to denaturate, which is the intended purpose: coagulative necrosis of the lesion.

The "ideal" temperature for coagulative necrosis of the lesion is approximately 60–65°C. A lower temperature leads to sublethal lesions. A temperature >100°C leads to tissue dehydration and vaporization with increased impedance and hence electric current insulation, which prevents further deposition of energy. However, the tissue around the electrode absorbs such heat. Hence, the tissues around the electrode tip must be heated at higher-than-ideal temperatures (around 85–90°C) to obtain a lesion wide enough to be effective. Generator algorithms fed by detectors for temperature, voltage or impedance control the power output, pulse duration and saline flush for specific electrodes to maximize energy deposition inside the target tissue. Such variables may also be pre-set by the operator, who can determine the duration of the pulses or the minimum temperature that has to be reached to achieve complete coagulation of a specific tissue. As a general rule, in a single-electrode system, the span of coagulated tissue around the tip must be the width of about two electrodes to produce a spheroid lesion whose long axis is about the same length of the uninsulated electrode tip (Fig. 15.2a).

A single lesion produced by an electrode is usually very small compared with the diameter of the tumor. Hence, several lesions must be produced to achieve complete coagulation of the tumor. This can be accomplished by two methods: (i) multiple consecutive lesions produced by a single electrode at different positions or (ii) multiple electrodes are placed simultaneously. If a single electrode is placed, the width of each single lesion will be dependent upon the tip length and radius of the electrode, and the final width of the lesion will be the sum of all the single lesions formed. For multiple electrodes placed simultaneously, the overall lesion width will be slightly wider than would be expected by the sum of all lesions. That is because if two electrodes are placed approximately 6–10 mm from each other and if the 65°C isotherm of each electrode does not overlap, they lie close enough to create a single lesion. Hence, for very large tumors, placement of multiple electrodes is desirable (unless technically unfeasible) because of their faster and wider tumor coagulation compared with treatment using multiple consecutive single lesions.

RFA systems are available with single or multitined electrodes. Single electrode systems produce spheroid lesions whose size is dependent upon the surface area of the active tip. Some companies produce hollow electrodes through which the cavity is flushed with saline to outside the tip with the aim of control of temperature and impedance (Fig. 15.2b and d); saline flow is regulated by generator algorithms. In other models, the saline flush is in a closed circuit without external flushing (i.e., internally cooled electrodes). As stated above, the lesion size is dependent upon the surface area of the electrode. Hence, in some single electrode systems, to achieve such increases in surface area, the electrode is very long and spring-shaped (Fig. 15.2e). Some companies produce bipolar electrodes in which the distal end has two non-insulated surfaces located serially that act as double poles ("bipolar electrodes"). Alternatively, two different electrodes act as opposite poles. In both cases, a ground plate is not necessary because the circuit is closed by the two electrodes (Fig. 15.2c).

In the case of multitined electrodes, a "bundle" of narrow electrodes is deployed inside the lesion, thereby increasing the overall surface area of the electrode. The size and shape of the lesion is dependent not only on the tip size of a single tine, but also on the number and geometry of the expanded cluster of electrodes. Multitined expanding electrode systems range from 3 to 12

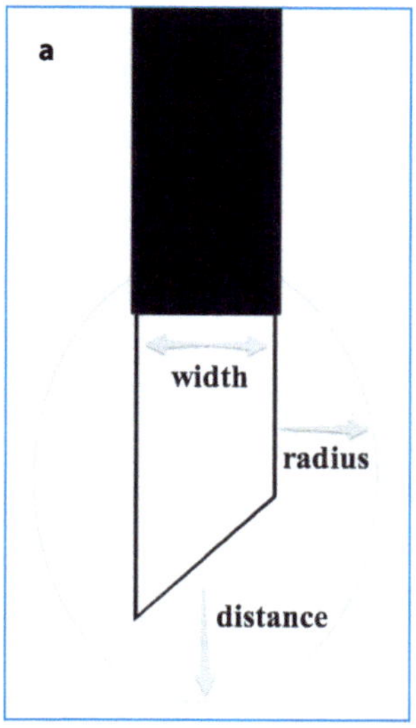

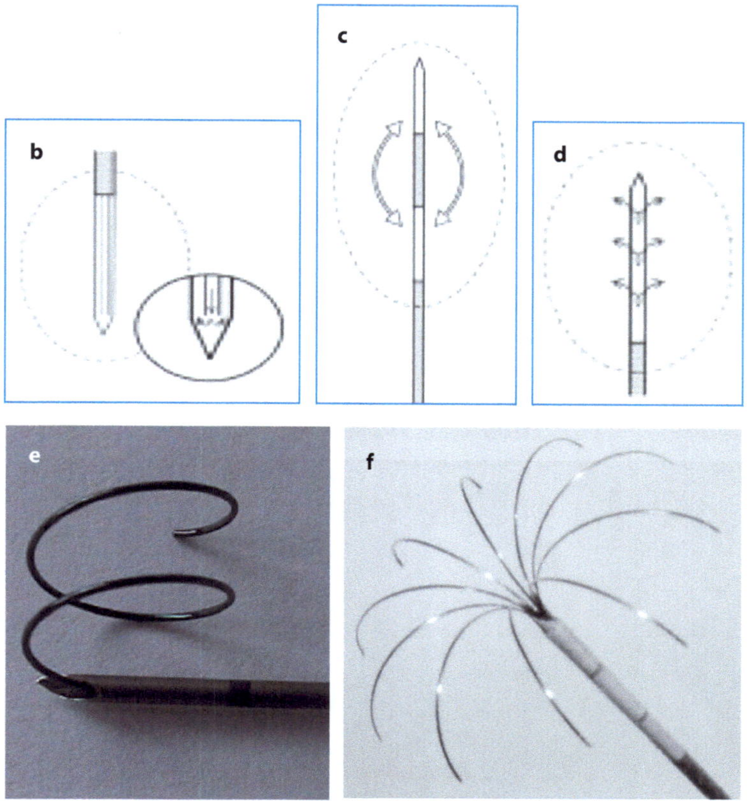

Fig. 15.2 Plain electrode highlighting the determinants of lesion size, diameter and length of the active uninsulated tip (schematic) (**a**). Plain closed circuit cooled electrode (**b**). Serial bipolar electrode (**c**). Hollow straight open circuit saline cooled electrode (**d**). Spring-shaped electrode deployed through a straight introduction cannula (**e**). Multitined electrode fully deployed through straight injection cannula (**f**)

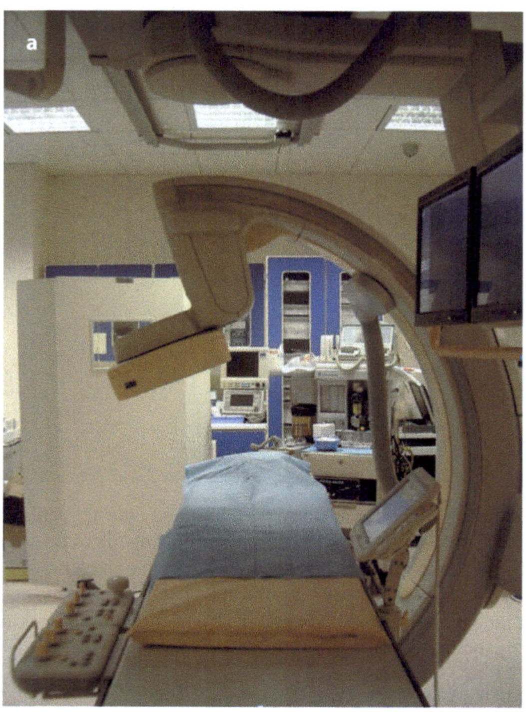

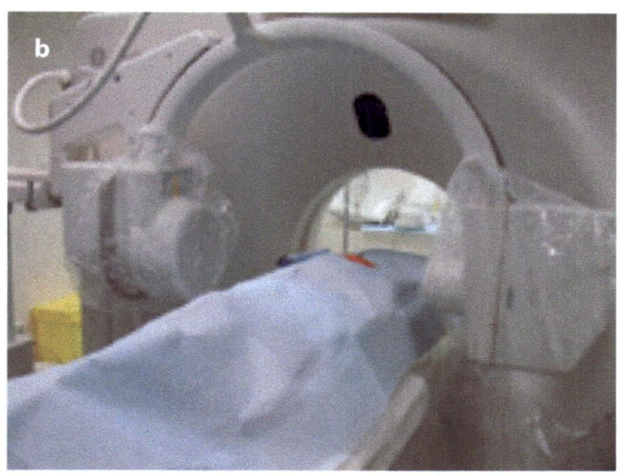

Fig. 15.3 Angiographic fluoro-CT suite (**a**) and 64-row CT with a portable X-ray system (**b**) for combined fluoroscopic-CT procedures

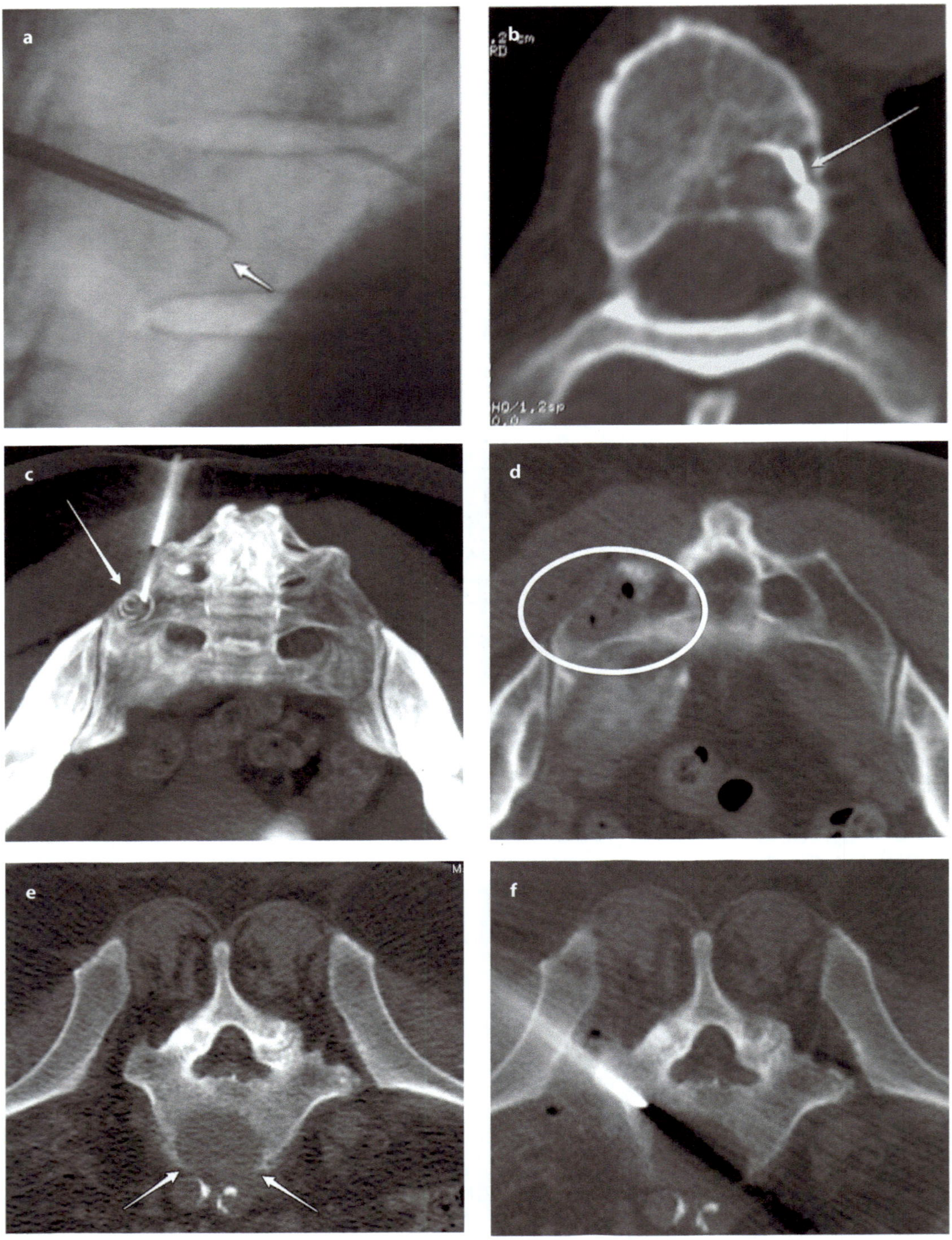

Fig. 15.4 Lateral fluoroscopic view of a spring-shaped radiofrequency electrode inside a vertebral body during deployment (*arrow*) by the transpedicular route in a case of breast-cancer metastasis (**a**). Axial CT slice showing the same case with one wire of the electrode highlighted (*arrow*) (**b**). Axial CT slices showing radiofrequency ablation of a colorectal-cancer metastasis of the right sacral wing with a spring-shaped electrode (*arrow*) *in situ* through a posterior paravertebral approach with gas inside the hollowed lesion at the end of the procedure (*circle*) (**c** and **d**). Radiofrequency ablation of a L5 somatic metastasis of myeloma (*arrows*) approached by the trans-iliac route (**e** and **f**)

active tips spanning outward, thereby leading to lesions up to 40-mm wide (Fig. 15.2f). Also, the electrodes can be "simple" or "cooled". In general, multitined electrodes are not indicated for the ablation of lesions in close contact with neural structures because of the less controllable and more invasive nature of the lesion they produce. If a small lesion with highly predictable geometry has to be created (e.g., neoplastic tissue close to a nerve root that must be spared), the electrodes of choice should be single monopolar or bipolar, whereas the bulk of the tumor can be ablated safely with multitined electrodes.

Electrode placement can be accomplished under fluoroscopy or fluoroscopy/CT guidance (Fig. 15.3a and b) with patients under local anaesthesia and sometimes mild sedation (general anaesthesia is needed very rarely). Electrodes are deployed through an introduction stiff cannula whose diameter usually ranges from 18 G to 13 G depending on the type of electrode employed (Fig 15.4 a–f).

The complications associated with RFA can be the general complications related to all percutaneous procedures (e.g., infections, hematoma at the entry site) or specific complications related to heat damage of healthy tissues. For the latter, some authors claim that posterior wall "wracking" lesions with soft-tissue involvement are not amenable for percutaneous RF treatment. In some cases, difficulties related to electrode retraction (particularly with multitined electrodes) associated with the adherence of coagulated tissue have been reported. Care must be taken in placing the ground plate because of the potential risk of skin burns in cases of uneven adhesion to the skin surface. Moreover, in the case of an already instrumented spine, electrodes should not be placed in close proximity to metallic devices because of the risk of short circuits [13].

15.4 Cryoablation

Over the past few years, image-guided minimally invasive percutaneous tumor ablation using thermal-based methods has received growing attention for the treatment of primary and secondary many malignancies.

Cryosurgery was introduced in the mid-1960s for the treatment of tumors that were readily accessible by endoscopy or direct visualization (skin, oral cavity, prostate gland). However, the first use of extreme cold in the treatment of musculoskeletal tumors dates back to 1970 [14]. Initially, this method was employed as an adjuvant in the management of various bone tumors. It comprised curettage and burr-drilling of the tumor cavity, direct injection of liquid nitrogen into the cavity, and reconstruction of the cavity using implants and polymethylmethacrylate (PMMA). However, application of liquid nitrogen directly into the cavity had several drawbacks: (i) there was no control of the overall freezing time or of the temperature at different sites within the cavity; and (ii) the liquid could not reach the areas of the tumor cavity which were situated above the fluid level because it was a gravity-dependent procedure. For these reasons, several attempts to improve this method were undertaken. In the late 1990s, a new technique was introduced to achieve accurate determination of the temperature and freezing time within a cavity of any geometrical shape. That is, after tumor removal by curettage, the cavity was filled with a gel followed by insertion of metal probes through which argon gas was delivered. Further development led to argon-based "third-generation" systems featuring unique 17-G needles which, together with advances in imaging methods, have enabled minimally invasive percutaneous procedures to be carried out under image guidance.

The aim of thermal-based tumor ablation is to destroy tumor tissue by increasing temperatures ("hyperthermic ablation") or decreasing temperatures ("cryoablation") to induce irreversible cellular damage. Cryoablation takes advantage of the Joule–Thomson effect, which describes the change in temperature of gasses if they are subject to expansion or compression. The tip of a cryoprobe contains a small chamber in which gas expansion occurs, thereby providing the necessary "heat sink" during freeze cycles and the heat source during thaw cycles. In this way, using argon (which provides a heat sink of approximately

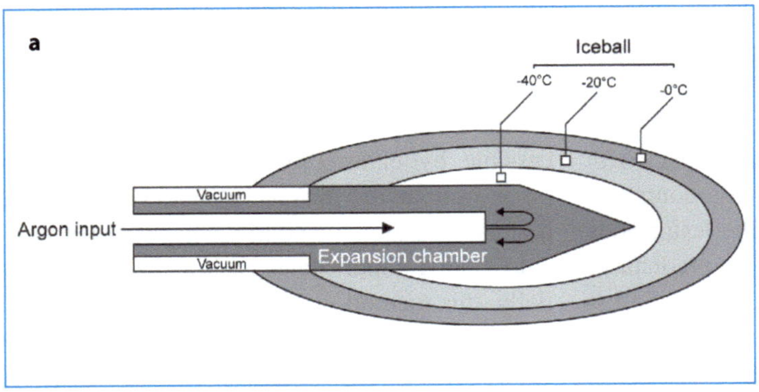

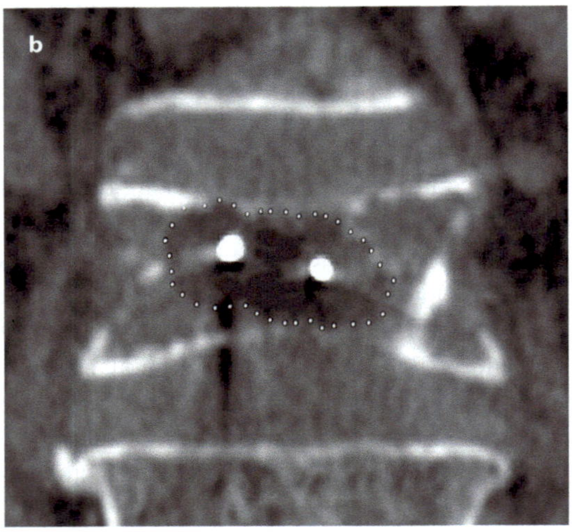

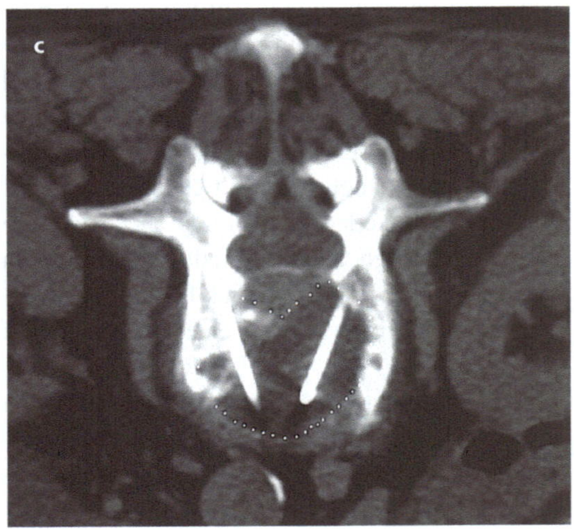

Fig. 15.5 Tip of a cryoprobe with an expansion chamber through which argon and helium produce a heat sink and thawing cycles (schematic) (**a**). Coronal (**b**) and axial (**c**) multi-planar reformatting-computed tomography images of a case of vertebral metastasis from cholangiocarcinoma showing cryoprobes inside the vertebral body, each with its own ice ball (*dotted line*) merging to produce a single lesion. Cryoprobes have been placed by the transpedicular route

9 kJ to generate a temperature as low as –140°C), an "ice ball" is generated.

In cryoablation, the freeze cycle is followed by a passive thaw cycle, a second freeze cycle and, finally, an active thaw cycle carried out by replacing argon with helium (which heats during expansion). The destructive effects of freezing tissue can be grouped into two major mechanisms: immediate and delayed. The immediate cause of damage is the effect of cooling and warming cycles on cells. That is, as temperature falls into the moderate freezing range (–20°C), formation of ice crystals occurs in the extracellular spaces, causing water withdrawal from the system, thereby creating a hyperosmotic extracellular environment. As this process continues, ice crystals grow and water is drawn from cells, which shrink, causing damage to the membranes and constituents of the cells. However, the onset of dehydration and higher concentrations of intracellular solutes are not always lethal to cells but, at lower temperatures (–40°C), ice crystals form within cells (especially with rapid decreases in temperature). Subsequently, if the temperature increases (–20°C/–25°C), ice crystals fuse to form large crystals ("recrystallization") which, in tissues characterized by closely packed cells, causes membrane disruption. All of these processes are enhanced by rapid cooling (which increases intracellular ice formation) followed by slow thawing (which maximizes the growth of crystals and is a prime destructive factor: a second freezing cycle). After the tissue thaws, the delayed cause of injury is the progressive failure of the microcirculation with subsequent vascular stasis, apoptosis and coagulative necrosis.

To achieve complete and adequate destruction of the target tumor by thermal ablation, the entire tumor and ablative margins must be exposed to cytotoxic temperatures. Hence, be-

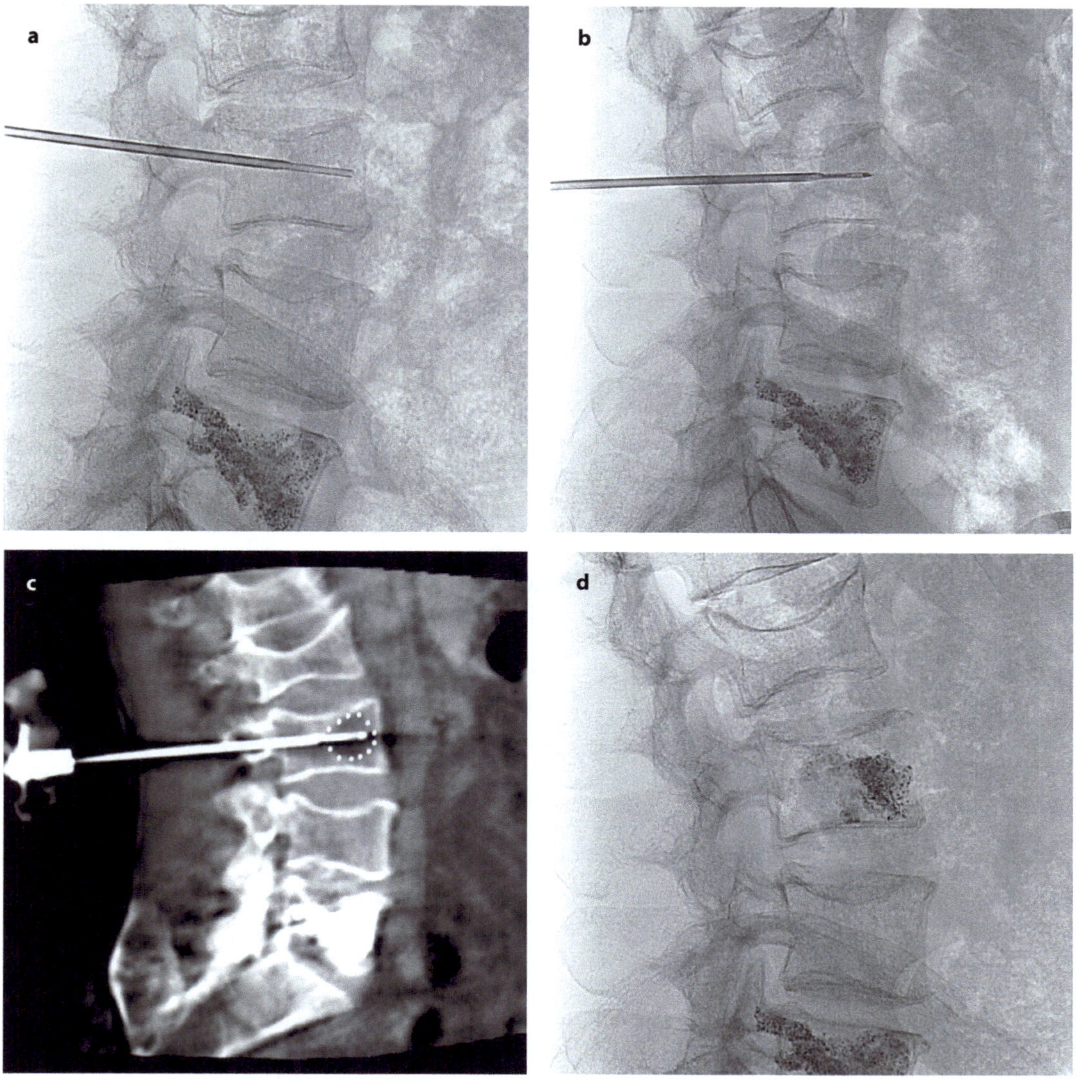

Fig. 15.6 L3 treatment of a metastatic lesion in a 50-year-old male with colorectal cancer. After biopsy (**a**), a 17-G cryoprobe was inserted coaxially through the same 13-G needle (**b**) and fluoro-CT-guided cryoablation undertaken (ice ball is shown as a *dotted oval shape*) (**c**). This was followed by cement injection to ensure vertebral stability; lateral fluoroscopic view shows good cement impregnation of the cryoablated vertebral body (**d**)

cause necrosis of malignant tissue is achieved at –40°C and cytotoxic effects are achieved at the core of the ice ball (and because the temperature increases rapidly by moving towards the ice-ball surface), imaging guidance is necessary to guarantee complete coverage of the lesion. For curative cryoablation, the margins of the ice ball should extend 3–5 mm beyond the tumor margins. Hence, multiple cycles and/or more cryoprobes placed in the geometric configuration that provides the best coverage of the tumor may be necessary (Fig. 15.5a–c). It has been demonstrated that longer thawing phases cause greater cell damage, and that repetition of the treatment cycle is associated with more extensive and more certain tissue destruction. Furthermore, different types of cryoprobes are available, resulting in different volumes and shapes of ice balls.

One of the advantages of cryoablation over RFA is the chance of precise visual monitoring of the ice ball with CT or MRI during the procedure. This reduces the risk of thermal damage

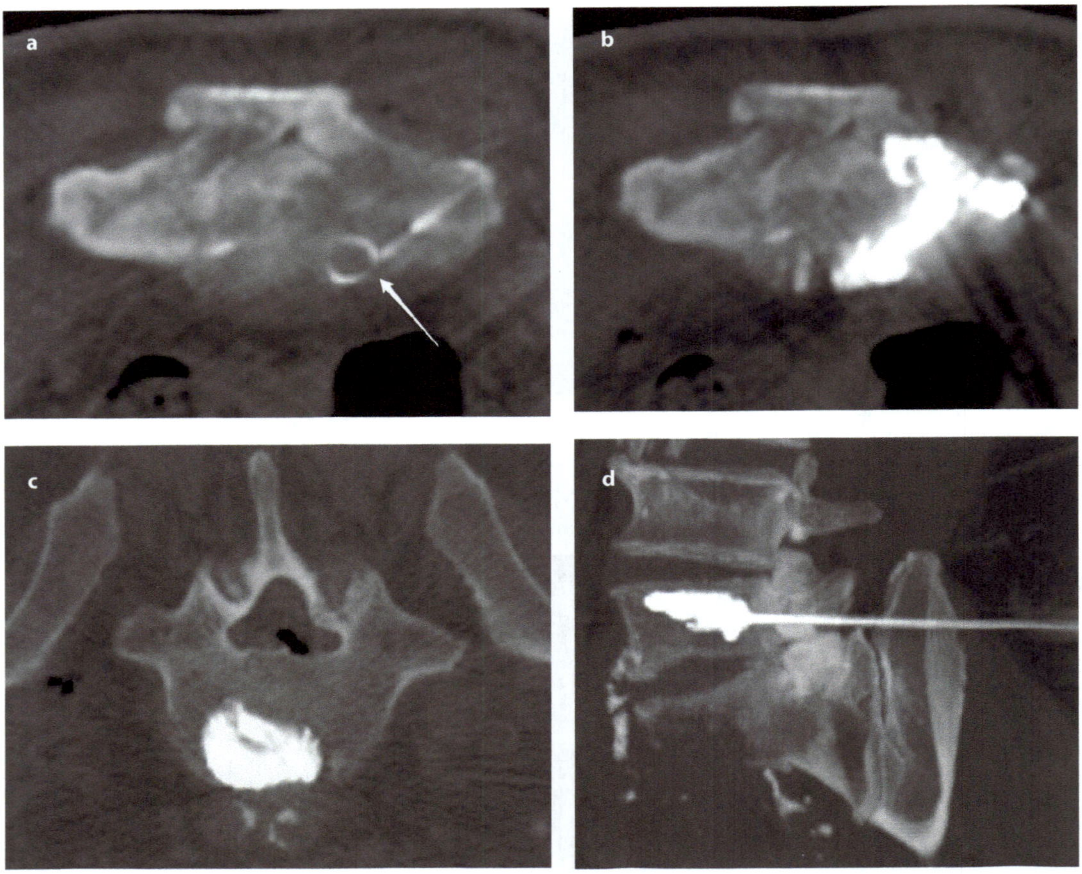

Fig. 15.7 Axial CT slice showing a spring-shaped electrode inside a left sacral wing metastasis (**a**) followed by cement augmentation (**b**). Axial CT slice (**c**) and transparent volume-rendering (**d**) of a L5 somatic metastasis ablated by radiofrequency and then augmented

to surrounding vulnerable tissues (particularly neural structures). Multiplanar reformatting is used intermittently to: monitor extension of the ice ball: confirm appropriate covering of the tumor; ensure the safety of adjacent vulnerable tissues. In addition, cryoablation has intrinsic anesthetic properties that allow carrying out the procedure under mild sedation (or even local anesthetic). Another major benefit of cryoablation in comparison with RFA is the reduction of peri- and post-procedural pain. Furthermore, in contrast to RFA, surgical metallic fixation in contact with the tumor is not contraindicated for cryoablation. Moreover, as with all ablative percutaneous treatments, cryoablation is repeatable in cases of recurrent pain or pain in newly metastatic bone.

The main role of cryoablation in the treatment of bone malignancies lies in the palliative, targeted, minimally invasive ablation of painful metastases secondary to advanced cancer. Patients with metastatic lesions are often in the advanced stages of the disease at the time of diagnosis. Therefore they present with lesions that induce recurrent pain which is often refractory to conventional medical therapy, with consequent significant impairment of QoL. Furthermore, resection is usually contraindicated because these patients often have poor functional status.

Recent studies on small cohorts have reported encouraging results regarding the cryoablation of painful vertebral metastasis. For example, Kurup et al. reported a decrease in the mean score for worst pain from 6.7/10 to 3.8/10 in a 24-h period over 4 weeks. Furthermore, patients reported a reduction in the use of narcotics and pain relief that appeared to be durable, with excellent control of pain in the treated area during the 24-week follow-up period [15]. However the treated lesions are usually osteolytic and, because ablation may further weaken bone, vertebroplasty after ablation may be necessary to reduce the risk of fracture (Fig. 15.6 a–d) [16].

An additional option of cryoablation is tissue displacement with catheter-guided balloons, which is not possible with other heat-based methods due to the thermal limitations of these devices. Finally, although osteoblastic metastases are less commonly treated with cryoablation, the ice ball can penetrate deeply into bone, whereas the use of radiofrequency energy it is less successful. However, in these cases, visual control of the ice ball is reduced and a bone biopsy device or bone drill may be required.

15.5 Conclusions

Cryoablation and RFA are minimally invasive treatments indicated for specific spinal tumors. Treatment strategies vary between conservative options (radiotherapy) to very aggressive surgical interventions. The appropriate indication for each treatment is based on clinical status and the intrinsic characteristics of the tumors. Minimally invasive percutaneous cryogenic and RFA procedures fall between the classifications of aggressive surgery and conservative radiotherapy. With the right indications, these procedures can be used to heal patients who, in most cases, have a short life expectancy and poor QoL.

Cryoablation and RFA may be undertaken as stand-alone treatments or may be followed by cement injections with the aim of bone augmentation. In the latter thermal ablation (RFA or cryoablation) has the double purpose of necrotizing tumor cells and hollowing out the infiltrated osseous segment, thereby increasing cement impregnation through production of a "virtual cavity" (Fig. 15.7a–c). Cement augmentation stabilizes spinal segments in a manner that approaches surgical instrumentation with the huge advantage of being a minimally invasive procedure that is very well tolerated by patients. Moreover, cement injection provides immediate post-procedural relief and, in same cases, prevents future fractures.

References

1. Bailar JC III, Gornik HL (1997) Cancer undefeated. N Eng J Med 336:1569–1574
2. Jacobs WB, Perrin RG (2001) Evaluation and treatment of spinal metastases: an overview. Neurosurg Focus 11:e10
3. Greenlee RT, Murray T, Bolden S et al (2000) Cancer statistics, 2000. CA Cancer J Clin 50:7–33
4. Harrop JS, Schmidt MH, Boriani S et al (2009) Aggressive "benign" primary spine neoplasms: osteoblastoma, aneurysmal bone cyst, and giant cell tumor. Spine (Phila Pa 1976) 34 (22 Suppl.):S39–S47
5. Fisher CG, DiPaola CP, Ryken TC et al (2010) A novel classification system for spinal instability in neoplastic disease: an evidence-based approach and expert consensus from the Spine Oncology Study Group. Spine (Phila Pa 1976) 35:E1221–E1229
6. Fourney DR, Frangou EM, Ryken TC et al (2011) Spinal instability neoplastic score: an analysis of reliability and validity from the Spine Oncology Study Group. J Clin Oncol 29:3072–3077
7. Paton GR, Frangou E, Fourney DR (2011) Contemporary treatment strategy for spinal metastasis: the "LMNOP" system. Can J Neurol Sci 38:396–403
8. Maranzano E, Latini P, Checcaglini F et al (1991) Radiation therapy in metastatic spinal cord compression. A prospective analysis of 105 consecutive patients. Cancer 67:1311–1317
9. Faul CM, Flickinger JC (1995) The use of radiation in the management of spinal metastases. J Neurooncol 23:149–161
10. Ryu SI, Chang SD, Kim DH et al (2001) Image-guided hypo-fractionated stereotactic radiosurgery to spinal lesions. Neurosurgery 49:838–846
11. Leksell L (1983) Stereotactic radiosurgery. J Neurol Neurosurg Psychiatry 46:797–803
12. Gerszten PC, Ozhasoglu C, Burton SA et al (2004) CyberKnife frameless stereotactic radiosurgery for spinal lesions: clinical experience in 125 cases. Neurosurgery 55:89–98 (discussion, 98–99)
13. Ahmed M, Brace CL, Lee FT Jr et al (2011) Principles of and advances in percutaneous ablation. Radiology 258:351–369
14. Marcove RC, Miller TR (1969) The treatment of primary and metastatic localized bone tumors by cryosurgery. Surg Clin North Am 49:421–430
15. Callstrom MR, Kurup AN (2009) Percutaneous ablation for bone and soft tissue metastases – why cryoablation? Skeletal Radiol 38:835–839
16. Masala S, Guglielmi G, Petrella MC et al (2011) Percutaneous ablative treatment of metastatic bone tumours: visual analogue scale scores in a short-term series. Singapore Med J 52:182–189

Indications and Results for Minimally Invasive Spinal Surgery

16

Olga Corriero, Oreste de Divitiis,
Giancarlo Guizzardi and Paolo Cappabianca

16.1 Introduction

For a neurosurgeon, "minimally invasive surgery" is not so much a procedure undertaken with a small incision in the skin with a needle or through a cannula but instead "appropriate surgery" which involves the best possible result with minimal adverse effects for the patient. This means discarding *a priori* all therapies that have been proven to have few or no benefits but which are considered to be minimally invasive for reasons that we do not agree with.

Another concept that needs to be stressed is that the surgeon and the interventional neuroradiologist must make the correct diagnosis and establish the appropriate therapy. That is, they must undertake the procedure on patients themselves (rather than on their radiological images), and the objective is care of patients to heal them of their symptoms, which must be consistent with the imaging tests. Advanced imaging techniques such as magnetic resonance imaging (MRI) and computed tomography (CT) can sometimes detect anomalies that are not connected to specific symptoms, which are called "incidentalomas."

P. Cappabianca (✉)
Department of Neurological Sciences, University of Naples Federico II, Naples, Italy
e-mail: paolo.cappabianca@unina.it

In the case of spinal disease, the neurosurgeon is consulted if the:

- family doctor sends the patient directly to the neurosurgeon;
- disease cannot be treated using interventional neuroradiology;
- interventional neuroradiologist cannot resolve the problem and suggests a neurosurgical examination;
- procedures used by neuroradiologists are also used by neurosurgeons.

16.2 Biomechanics of the Vertebral Column

Appropriate surgical treatment of degenerative spinal disease must respect the biomechanics of the rachis [1]. The vertebral column is a complex system that be analogized to that of a crane with arms of different lengths. The crane is supported by a central pillar upon which two arms rest. The one at the front is very long, whereas the one behind is much shorter, and provided with a counterweight that balances the crane. The spine corresponds to the central supporting pillar. The force of gravity to the long arm would cause the crane to fall forward were it not for the complex musculature of the vertebral column (which corresponds to the rear arm of the crane with its heavy counterweight that maintains balance, which is known as the "crane principle") (Fig. 16.1).

M. Muto (ed.), *Interventional Neuroradiology of the Spine*,
DOI 10.1007/978-88-470-2790-9_16, © Springer-Verlag Italia 2013

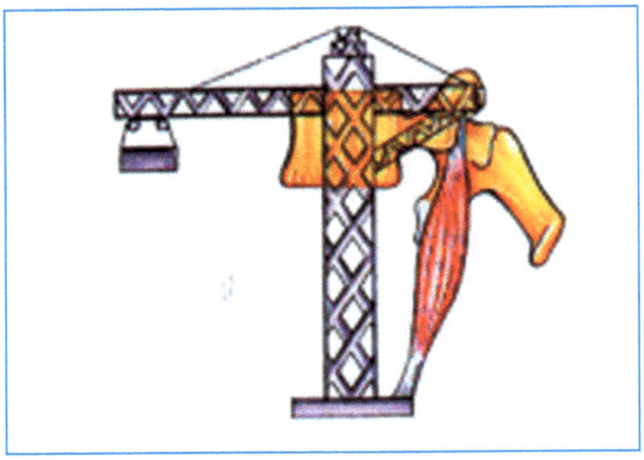

Fig. 16.1 The "crane principle" of understanding the biomechanics of the spinal column (schematic)

Another important biomechanical concept is that of "sagittal balance", a term used to indicate the orientation of the vertebral column and its balance in the sagittal plane (Fig. 16.2). The sagittal plane runs in an anterior-to-posterior direction and divides the body into two parts, which mirror each other. Furthermore, together with the pelvis, the vertebral column can be considered to be an open linear chain connecting the head to the pelvis, in which the form and orientation of each anatomical segment are closely related and influenced by the adjacent segment. The ultimate goal is to maintain stable balance and posture with the lowest possible expenditure of energy. A correct sagittal balance involves a cervical lordosis, a dorsal kyphosis, a lumbar lordosis and correct inclination of the pelvis with respect to the spine. An illness or surgery that alters this system produces an "unbalanced spine" and consequent problems ranging from simple pain to debilitating neurological damage.

From an anatomical viewpoint, vertebrae are different from one individual to another, as are the angles between them and the insertions of the disk. Conventionally, thoracic–lumbar balance is defined by a straight radiographic line that falls between C7 and S1. If the line ends at the terminal portion of the diskal plate S1, sagittal balance is considered to be positive, and if the line ends at the front it is defined as negative. For appropriate assessment of individual balance, morphodynamic studies of the conventional spinal column are very important, such as radiographs under dynamic loading or, preferably, stand-up MRI or the EOS® system. A more or less rapid "degenerative cascade" (see below) corresponds to altered sagittal balance.

Another important parameter is the ratio between the vertebral column and the pelvis, two structures with complex inter-relationships (especially during movement). A fixed anatomical

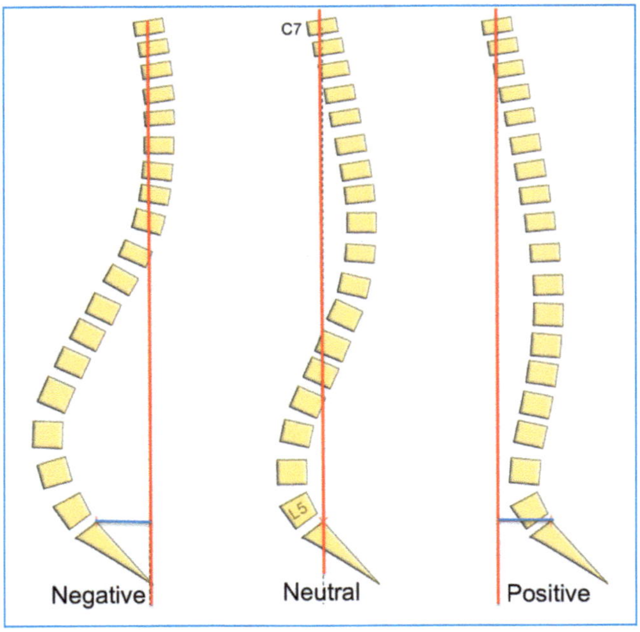

Fig. 16.2 A plumb line can be drawn from the center of the C7 vertebral body to the pelvis. Negative sagittal imbalance: the plumb line falls behind the posterosuperior corner of the S1 vertebral body. Neutral sagittal balance: the plumb line intersects the posterosuperior corner of the S1 vertebral body. Positive sagittal imbalance: the plumb line falls in front of the posterosuperior corner of the S1 vertebral body

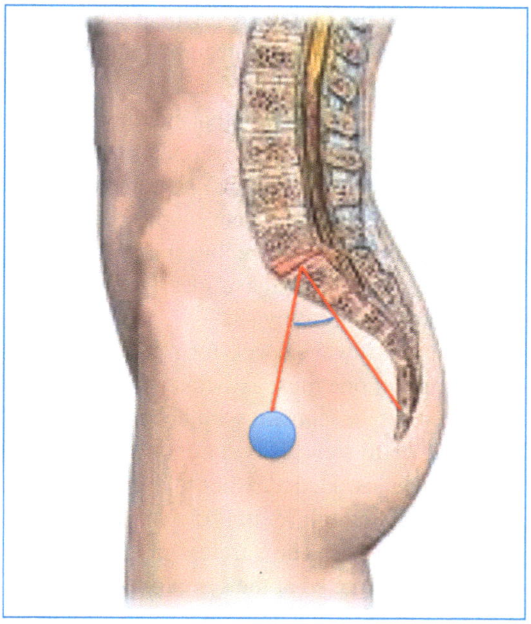

Fig. 16.3 The pelvic incidence is the angle formed between the perpendicular line drawn from the midpoint of a line tangent to the plate of S1 and the perpendicular line drawn from the midpoint of the femoral head

parameter called "pelvic incidence" (PI) correlates the two structures. PI is determined on the basis of the measurement of the pelvic tilt and sacral slope. PI is the angle formed between the perpendicular line drawn from the midpoint of the line tangent to the plate of S1 and the perpendicular line drawn from the midpoint of the head of the femur (Fig. 16.3). A patient with a low PI has limited ability to tilt the pelvis and a lower compensation in the case of disease of the vertebral column. A patient with a high PI has a large capacity of pelvic inclination through a wide range of angles.

Consequently, pelvic orientation is determined directly by the morphology of the pelvis in the sagittal plane in the same way that lumbar lordosis is closely related to pelvic morphology. Therefore, a patient with a high PI will probably need a wide lumbar lordosis. These parameters show that, under physiological conditions, the line of gravity is positioned between the femoral heads and the posterior portion of the upper plate of S1. If the pelvis is rotated backwards, the distance between the posterior edge of S1 and the line of gravity increases, and the patient's posture must change to adapt to this condition.

The vertebral column and the pelvis are mobile segments with multiple muscle attachments. The muscles are of paramount importance for maintaining correct balance, allowing adaptation of the vertebral column to its various physiological and pathological conditions.

Stresses of various types affect the spine and alter its operating conditions, which can lead to the onset of disease. The pathological development of the physiological aging process is called the degenerative cascade and it can lead to biomechanical and functional changes to the vertebral column such as dramatic degenerative scoliosis and overt instability.

16.3 Stenosis of the Spinal Canal

Marginal osteophytosis, fissuring of intervertebral disks and their "bulging" into the spinal canal (with consequent loss of height of the intervertebral disk space and pseudohypertrophy or true hypertrophy of the ligamentum flavum), hypertrophy of the facets, and stenosis of the lateral recess represent the pathophysiological basis of stenosis. They must all be treated by surgical means because they cause stenosis of the spinal canal. Nevertheless, the specific surgical treatment to be adopted varies according to whether the anterior or posterior segment is affected, or if there is a spinal deformity.

Three types of stenosis of the spinal canal can be distinguished:

- "soft stenosis" (in which the stenosis mainly affects the soft parts, with a protrusion of the disk and the ligamentum flavum into the canal);
- "hard stenosis" (in which the bony elements are hypertrophic);
- "dynamic stenosis" (in which the stenosis is the product of an abnormal mobility of the affected vertebral segment or of a deformity of the spine, as in the case of degenerative scoliosis).

In the case of soft stenosis, in which the stenosis is located in the posterior elements, the determinant anatomical basis is the ligamentum flavum. Consequently, the surgical procedure must address this target. In the absence of listhesis or deformity, surgical treatments can consist of flavectomy, stretching of the ligament, or limitation of extension.

Soft stenosis tends to be unstable. Hence, if radiological investigation suggests dynamic instability, decompression must be associated with stabilization of the segment. In young patients, dynamic stabilization is recommended to maintain lumbar mobility. Surgical treatment for this type of stenosis includes the use of dynamic interlaminar spacers. These devices stretch the ligamentum flavum, causing a reduction in pressure on the degenerative disk and thereby reducing stress on the facet joints. At the lumbar level, the main contraindications for the use of such devices are:

- instability at L5–S1 (where the lamina is shorter and therefore less likely to support this type of device);
- spondylolisthesis greater than grade I;
- severe osteoporosis;
- a significant reduction of the disk space;
- degenerative scoliosis.

The use of systems of dynamic transpedicular stabilization is another alternative. These systems reduce the normal physiological range of motion, prevent hypermobility, lead to recalibration of the disk space, and preserve the physiological pump effect of the disk. This results in an interruption of the degenerative cascade. Contraindications to the use of such devices are soft disk herniation, osteoporosis, and overt instability.

In principle, the most appropriate treatment of younger patients is "step by step" treatment starting with an interlaminar spacer, continuing with dynamic stabilization, and ending with laminectomy and fixation of the segment. In the case of elderly patients, aggressive treatment is appropriate from the beginning.

In the case of hard stenosis, the surgical options are:

- bilateral fenestration and enlargement of the foramen;
- a unilateral approach with bilateral decompression;
- laminectomy of the "Christmas tree" type, with laminectomy, facetectomy, and bilateral foraminotomy.

In multilevel cervical stenosis, laminoplasty is associated with greater postoperative pain and a lower quality of life (QoL) as compared with laminectomy. Indeed, recent studies show that, especially in cases where instability is absent, laminoplasty does not have clear benefits compared with laminectomy [2].

One must always check for signs of instability. If present, one must associate stabilization of the hypermobile segment with decompression of the canal. Hard stenosis is commonly a multisegmental stenosis. Hence, when planning surgery, one should not try to improve movement but rather preserve it. The surgical procedure must therefore be targeted at the symptomatic level.

In the case of dynamic stenosis the treatment should be modulated according to its extent. Treatment ranges from simple ligamentoplasty to segment stabilization with transpedicular screws and bars.

16.4 Herniation of Spinal Disks

In industrialized countries, "back pain" affects >80% of the adult population. It is the second most common cause of illness for which people seek a medical consultation and the number-one cause of absence from work. The highest incidence is among people between 30 years and 50 years of age. The social cost of herniated disks is therefore very high. Epidemiological studies have revealed that the health of 30% of patients with herniated disks becomes chronic, whereas 70% of cases resolve in 3–8 weeks and, in the latter group, recurrence occurs in 70% of subjects within 1 year. The pathogenesis of disk herniation is related to mechanical factors which cause fissure in the central area of the disk, with consequent abnormal redistribution of the loads on the disk segment. This redistribution results in the loss of the effect of the diskal pump which, due to its connection with the subchondral venous plexus, causes degeneration of the cartilage plate and adipose involution of the vertebral body, which is defined as the "Modic effect" in radiographic images [3]. With respect to the natural history of disk herniation, the relationship between the hernia and the posterior longitudinal ligament is very important (i.e., whether or not it is intact).

In cases of extruded herniated disks, there is a 75% probability of spontaneous reduction/re-absorption, resulting in clinical improvement and the disappearance of pain. There is no correlation between the initial diameter of the herniated fragment and the degree of reduction/re-absorption of the fragment. The rupture of the posterior longitudinal ligament is associated with production of a large volume of granulation tissue. Most of the inflammatory cells contain interstitial collagenase (matrix metalloproteinase-1 (MMP-1)) and stromelysins (e.g., MMP-3), which deal specifically with the decomposition of type-II collagen and proteoglycans. The presence of these proteinases with direct actions on the components of intervertebral disks explains the high percentage of reduction/re-absorption of the extruded herniated fragment.

In contrast, this cellular response is virtually absent in subligamentous hernias. These kinds of herniated disks are less likely to heal spontaneously and therefore need surgical intervention more often. The first type of treatment for a patient suffering from disk herniation is conservative. It is based on local and/or general pharmacotherapy and on personalized physio-kinesio-therapeutic rehabilitation. Surgeons should be aware that: (i) asymptomatic patients have herniated disks in >75% of cases; (ii) symptomatic disk herniation resolves spontaneously in 6–8 weeks in 80% of cases; and (iii) 95% of patients return to work within 3 months without recourse to invasive treatment. Surgery should be considered:

- in the presence of a severe neurological deficit;
- in the presence of a persistent "disability" that is resistant to the various types of conservative treatment;
- upon request from the patient after he/she has been clearly informed of the advantages and disadvantages of surgery.

The formation of periradicular fibrosis is one of the most important causes of failed back surgery syndrome (FBSS) after surgery for lumbar disk herniation. Numerous materials have been used and studied to reduce the formation of scar tissue. In our department, we tend to respect the periradicular anatomical structures as much as possible [4, 5]. In fact, preservation of the ligamentum flavum, sparing of periradicular fat, and careful hemostasis encourage the preservation of the ecology of the spinal root [3].

Surgery is indicated in cervical hernia if there is radiographic evidence suggesting myelopathy. Cervical diskectomy *via* the anterior route is the prevalent surgical approach for degenerative disease of the cervical rachis.

The introduction of increasingly sophisticated prosthetic implants onto the market has undoubtedly revolutionized treatment. These implants have improved the prevalence of intersomatic fusion and overall cervical alignment, reduced postoperative immobilization and improved clinical outcomes. Mobile implants are being used increasingly frequently, which aids preservation of the mobility of the cervical spine. However, these disk substitutes are used only in selected cases. Long-term data that show conclusively the greater effectiveness of mobile prostheses with regard to fixed prostheses are not available.

16.5 Spinal Tumors

Spinal tumors represent 15% of all primary tumors of the central nervous system (CNS), and most are benign. The most common presenting symptom is pain, followed by clinical signs of myelo-radicular compression. Spinal tumors can be divided into three major classes: extradural; intradural extramedullary; and intradural intramedullary [7, 8, 9].

16.5.1 Extradural Tumors

Extradural tumors account for 55% of all spinal tumors. They originate from vertebral bodies and epidural tissues. They are usually osteolytic metastases (lymphoma, lung cancer, breast cancer, prostate cancer) or osteoblastic (prostate cancer, breast cancer) and primitive spinal tumors (chordomas, osteomas, aneurysmal bone cysts, chondrosarcomas, osteosarcomas, vertebral hemangiomas, plasmacytomas, multiple myelomas, Ewing's sarcoma).

Vertebral metastases occur in 10% of patients with systemic disease. In 80% of cases they are patients with primary tumors of the lung, breast, prostate gland and kidney as well as melanomas and lymphomas. The lesions are usually in the thoracic area because of its greater extension.

Surgery is indicated in the case of:

- unknown primary tumors (for diagnostic purposes);
- instability of the spinal column;
- pathological fracture resulting in vertebral collapse and medullary compression;
- radio-resistant tumors such as renal cell carcinoma and melanoma;
- tumor progression during radiotherapy or if there are rapidly worsening neurologic deficits.

Surgical methods are dependent upon greater or lesser invasion of the vertebra. They can range from simple vertebral plastic repairs to relieve pain and prevent collapse, to posterior decompression, curettage, or partial *excision* of the lesion, to total corpectomy and stabilization. All surgical methods are dependent on physical status, the prognosis, and the cost:benefit ratio for the patient. Radiotherapy may also be indicated. It is the oncologist's duty to guide the team in the various therapeutic strategies.

16.5.2 Intradural Extramedullary Tumors

Meningiomas show peak incidence in subjects aged between 40 years and 70 years with a predominance in females. Eighty-two percent of cases have a thoracic location, 15% are in the cervical area, and 2% are in the lumbar region. In most cases they are completely intradural with a lateral location, but they can also have an intra-extradural localization (5%). The initial symptoms are local or radicular pain, followed by signs of nerve compression with pyramidal syndrome, difficulty in walking, paraplegia and quadriplegia, which can lead to sensorimotor plegia and sensory symptoms as well as sphincter disturbances.

Schwannomas are benign, slow-growing tumors. They are localized mainly in the dorsal area. Initial symptoms are of a radicular type with local pain, and they belatedly develop only neurological deficits. Most of these lesions are completely intradural. However, they can be extradural in 8–30% of cases, and intradural and extradural hourglass-tumors in 6–20% of cases. Only 1% of cases are intramedullary. The treatment of these lesions is primarily surgical, with a posterior approach to intracanalar and intraforaminal lesions and with an anterior or combined approach for lesions with an extended extraforaminal component. The roots from which the lesion originates must be severed. This modest (but necessary) procedure is, in almost all cases, asymptomatic.

16.5.3 Intradural Intramedullary Tumors

Intradural intramedullary tumors account for 5% of all spinal tumors. They are mostly astrocytomas and ependymomas. Thirty percent of intradural intramedullary tumors are malignant gliomas, dermoids, epidermoids, teratomas, hemangioblastomas or lipomas. The most common presenting symptom is pain (which can be local or radicular) with recrudescence that is typically nocturnal, accompanied by paresthesia experienced as a burning sensation and dysesthesia. Other symptoms include: motor disorders with weakness; atrophy; fasciculations and muscle tics; sensory disturbances with loss of thermosensitivity to pain and paresthesia; and sphincter disturbances (which are most commonly urinary). The onset of symptoms is usually insidious and progressive.

Astrocytomas have a peak of incidence around the third-to-fifth decade of life. The ratio between lesions of low degree and high degree is 3 to 1. The localization is mainly in the chest, followed by the neck. Thirty-eight percent of cases have a cystic component and the cerebrospinal fluid may show an increase in protein levels. Surgery is the first-line treatment.

Ependymomas are the most common type of glioma of the distal spinal tract, with localization predominantly at the level of the cone and the filum. The second most common location is cervical. Ependymomas are prevalent in adults. They are slow-growing tumors that may have a cystic component in 46% of cases and, in terms of histology, they are most commonly myxopapillar (World Health Organization grade 1). In most cases, they are encapsulated and poorly vascularized lesions. The only treatment is surgical treatment: complete resection.

Epidermoids are rare after infancy. They have a slight predominance in females and are most commonly located at the cone.

Lipomas occur together with spinal dysraphism. The peak incidence is at around 2, 3 and 5 days of life. The most common symptoms are unilateral or bilateral ascending paraparesis, sphincter disturbances in the more caudal lesions, and the presence of a palpable subcutaneous mass. Surgical treatment is the only option.

All of the surgical procedures for the different types of spinal tumors (particularly in the case of intradural tumours) involve minimally invasive approaches. Such approaches cause little damage to muscle and allow reconstruction of the bone cage (which is particularly important in younger subjects). This is done to prevent future problems such as severe scarring or deformity, which can lead to overt instability. In this type of surgery, the technique, the surgeon's experience and intraoperative neurophysiological monitoring (which provides constant and continuous information to the operator during the procedure) have key roles.

16.6 Spinal Vascular Malformations

There are three types of spinal vascular malformation: arteriovenous fistulas (AVFs), intradural arteriovenous malformations (AVMs) and cavernous angiomas.

Dural AVFs are the most common variant. They are localized in the dura, in the proximal portion of the spinal root, and the corresponding dura. The anatomopathological basis is an abnormal connection between an artery and a dural vein that leads blood to the arterialized coronal venous plexus, which consequently becomes enlarged and tortuous. These lesions begin in adulthood (commonly with pain) and result in symptoms of deficit (more or less rapidly progressive) predominantly in the lower limbs. This condition requires prompt treatment. The damage is always linked to food deprivation, which causes ischemia of nervous tissue. The only treatment is to close the fistula.

In most cases, good endovascular treatment of occlusion of the malformation is sufficient to solve the problem. Rehabilitation of the fistula through other branches is possible after surgery or endovascular treatment, with a success rate that is slightly lower than that for surgical occlusion. Some more complex AVFs may have intradural and extradural drainage, the first in the medullary vein and the second in an epidural vein. In this type of lesion, the nidus of the fistula must be removed together with the dura that contains it, and the dural defect must be repaired with the standard materials available for reconstruction.

Intradural AVMs have a less predictable clinical course. Treatment must thus be determined on a case-by-case basis. Surgery is first-line treatment.

Spinal AVMs can be divided into two groups: juvenile and glomus. They are characterized by the intramedullar location of the nidus, most commonly in the ventral portion. The afferent vessel is the anterior medullary artery. Symptomatology is characterized by myelopathy caused by repeated hemorrhage, venous hypertension, progressive ischemia with seizures, and compression and distortion of the spine.

Juvenile-type AVMs consist of tortuous vessels with interposed nervous tissue, from which they cannot be separated. They become symptomatic in childhood or in young adulthood, and surgery carried considerable risks. Treatment is therefore endovascular, but the results are inconsistent because excluding the nidus from the circle is not possible.

Glomus-type AVMs consist of small vessels with a nidus located in a limited segment of the bone. They commonly have a single afferent vessel. Glomus-type AVMs become symptomatic in adulthood. For posterior lesions and those that are not too extensive, surgical removal is possible and is effectively curative. However, if the lesions are posterior or too extensive, it is preferable to adopt endovascular treatment due to the high risk of postoperative neurological deficits with repeated embolizations.

Spinal cavernous angiomas are basically no different from those observed in the brain. They become symptomatic as a result of micro-intramedullary hemorrhage (isolated or repeated). This results in intermittent and progressive myelopathy. In the presence of progressive myelopathy, the only option is surgery.

Lesions that benefit from surgical treatment can be tackled with surgical microscopes with intravenous injection of indocyanine green. This dye can provide optimal visualization of the direction of flow and, therefore, clear identification of the afferent and efferent vessels as well as of the points of the fistula or anastomosis.

16.7 Summary

The concept of minimally invasive neurosurgery as applied to spinal surgery must involve respect for tissues and neurovascular structures and not be considered surgery of small dimensions or that has better cosmetic results as its primary goal. Spinal surgery has received a major impetus from technological advances such as neuro-navigation, preoperative and intraoperative monitoring, introduction of new hemostatic agents, and better visualization provided by new types of surgical operating microscopes. This allows the surgeon to respect parenchymal structures, in addition to intraoperative neurophysiological monitoring, which can be integrated with preoperative tests and examinations. The crucial phase of the procedure attempts to understand the physiology and pathology of the spinal column. The biomechanics of the spine and respect for the muscles, bones and joints is of great importance, but to deliver the best results, it is equally important to respect neurovascular tissue.

References

1. Simeone R (2006) The spine. Saunders, Philadelphia
2. Nurboja B, Kachramanoglou C, Choi D (2012) Cervical laminectomy vs laminoplasty: is there a difference in outcome and postoperative pain? Neurosurgery 70:965–970 (discussion 970)
3. Modic MT, Ross JS, Masaryk TJ (1989) Imaging of degenerative disease of the cervical spine. Clin Orthop Rel Res (239):109–120
4. Caspar W (1977) A new surgical procedure for lumbar disc herniation causing less tissue damage through a microsurgical approach. In: Wullenweber RBM, Hamer J, Klinger M, Spoerri O (eds) Advances in neurosurgery. Springer-Verlag, Berlin, p 74–77
5. De Divitiis E, Spaziante R, Stella L (1979) Some technical modifications of surgical treatment of lumbar disc lesions. Neurochirurgia 22:95–98
6. de Divitiis E, Spaziante R, Cappabianca P, Donzelli R (1984) Lumbar disk. Surgical tricks for safeguarding the "root's ecology". Surgical Neurol 22:73–75
7. Brotchi J, Bruneau M, Lefranc F, Baleriaux D (2006) Surgery of intraspinal cord tumors. Clin Neurosurg 53:209–216
8. L. Sekhar and R. G. Fessler, Eds (2006) Atlas of neurosurgical techniques: spine and peripheral nerves, vol. 2, Thieme, New York
9. Luis R (1982) Chirurgie du rachis: anatomie chirurgicale et voies d'abord. Springer-Verlag, Berlin

Radiotherapy for the Treatment of Bone Metastases

17

Rossella Di Franco, Sara Falivene,
Vincenzo Ravo and Paolo Muto

17.1 Introduction

Bone metastases are a frequent and severe complication of advanced neoplastic disease. After the lungs and liver, bone is the most frequent site of metastasis. Many advanced cancers, such as lung cancer and prostate cancer in men as well as breast cancer in women, have a strong tropism for the bone. The pain related associated with bone metastases is a major cause of morbidity in cancer patients. Events related to bone metastasis include impaired quality of life (QoL), bone fractures, hypercalcemia, neurological deficits, and movement limitation.

Bone is not an inert body because it undergoes continuous remodeling with phases of resorption and formation [1]. This process is coordinated by osteoclasts (responsible for the resorption phase) and osteoblasts (responsible for formation phase). If the bone has tumor involvement, the normal process of bone turnover is compromized [2]. Bone resorption and the regulation of osteoclastic activity are under the influence of the receptor activator of nuclear factor-kappa B ligand (RANKL)/RANK/osteoprotegerin (OPG) system. RANK-L belongs to the tumor necrosis factor (TNF) superfamily. It is the key mediator of the formation, survival and function of osteoclasts. RANK-L is expressed as a membrane on the surface of stromal cells/osteoblasts. It can be expressed in a soluble form, binding to the RANK receptor on osteoclasts, and stimulating the activation and differentiation of osteoclasts as well as inhibiting apoptosis [3]. OPG can bind to RANK-L and inhibit its function, thereby leading to inhibition of bone resorption [4]. An increase in the RANKL/OPG ratio is associated with an increase in bone resorption. This phenomenon is implicated in the formation of bone metastases and their maintenance [5].

17.2 Clinical and Imaging-based Diagnoses of Bone Metastases

In most cases, subjects with bone metastases present with local or radicular pain with or without limitation in motor control, sensory impairment and poor sphincter control [6, 7]. The pain develops over weeks or months, and becomes increasingly severe. It is usually described as "dull" and "constant", and the intensity is progressive. It is usually localized in a particular area, and often occurs at night or with loadbearing.

The mechanism of pain from bone metastases is incompletely understood. It can be caused by: mechanical instability; irritation of the receptors caused by stretching of the periosteum; osteolysis; nerve injury induced by the tumor; production of nerve growth factor; or the stimulation of cytokine receptors [8–10].

P. Muto (✉)
Radiotherapy Unit, INT IRCCS Fondazione G. Pascale, Naples, Italy
e-mail: p.muto@istitutotumori.na.it

M. Muto (ed.), *Interventional Neuroradiology of the Spine*,
DOI 10.1007/978-88-470-2790-9_17, © Springer-Verlag Italia 2013

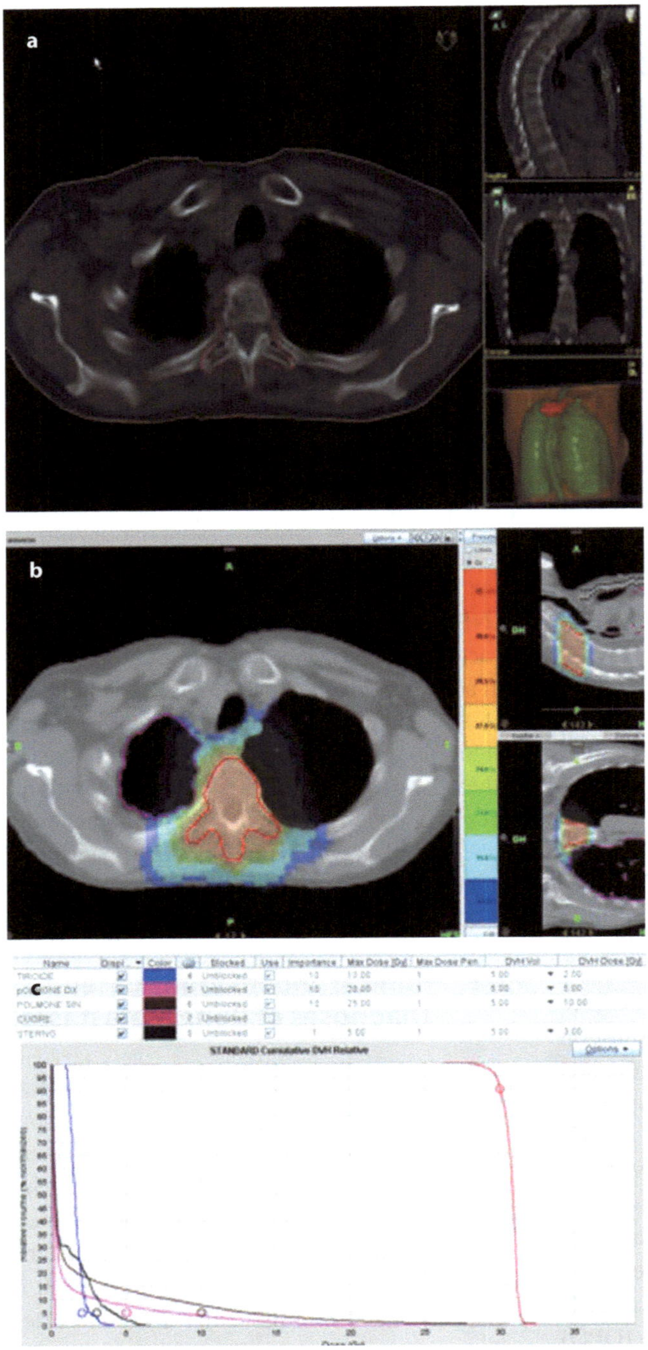

Fig. 17.1 Contouring, treatment plan, and dose-volume histogram to treat tumor of vertebral body (D3). **a** Example of contouring for a treatment with radiotherapy of a metastasis of the vertebra T3. **b** Example of the dose distribution in the planned treatment of the same case. **c** Dose-volume histogram of the irradiated volumes in the same treatment

Bone metastases are often described as "osteolytic" or "osteoblastic". Cancers of the breast and lung usually cause osteolytic-appearing lesions; cancers of the prostate and thyroid glands more often cause an osteoblastic appearance. However, only myeloma is associated with purely osteolytic lesions [11]. Most other tumors have a combination of osteolytic and osteoblastic components. Increased bone resorption occurs even in prostate-cancer metastases with an osteoblastic appearance.

Bone metastases may be diagnosed by vari-

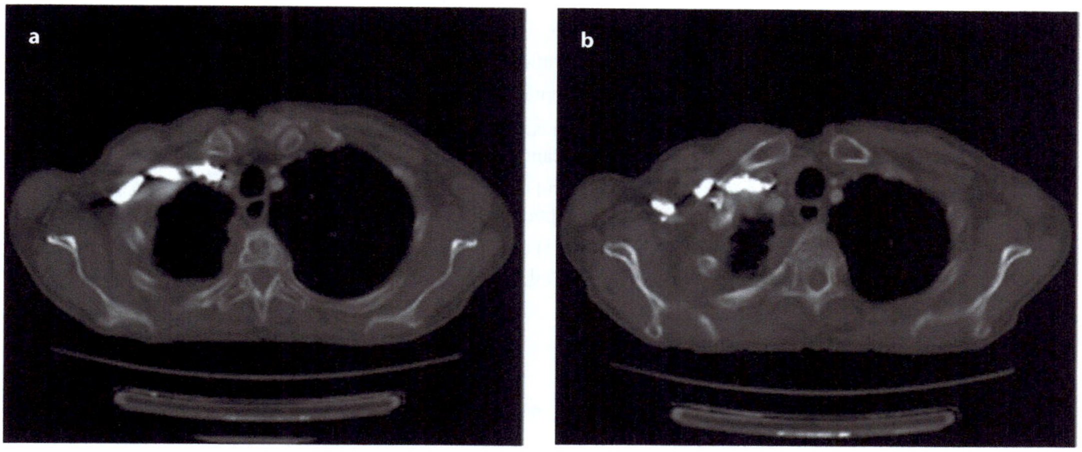

Fig. 17.2 Revaluation with a CT scan of the patient treated with the planned therapy showed in Fig. 17.1 after 6 months from radiotherapy

ous methods: radiography, scintigraphy, computed tomography (CT) and magnetic resonance imaging (MRI). CT allows identification of the type of metastases and is more sensitive than the other methods. MRI is better than plain radiography or bone scintigraphy for assessment of the involvement of trabecular bone ("red marrow"), especially in the vertebral bodies. However, MRI may be more sensitive than bone scintigraphy in the vertebral body region. The sensitivity of MRI has been reported to be 91–100%, compared with 62–85% for bone scintigraphy [12–14]. MRI can be used to distinguish whether a compression fracture of the vertebral body is due to a tumor or osteoporosis. Positron emission tomography (PET) with 2-deoxy-2-[18F] fluoro-D-glucose (18-FDG) can be used to evaluate areas of increased metabolic activity. It shows osteolytic bone metastases, but is less sensitive for osteoblastic metastases. Simultaneous use of CT with PET allows identification of the exact location of the abnormal uptake of lesions that is difficult to achieve with PET alone. PET may be useful as a whole-body screening tool [15, 16]. Comparative studies have shown PET to be more sensitive than technetium-99m (Tc-99m) scintigraphy or whole-body MRI for the detection of bone metastases. However, there may be limitations in the sensitivity of PET in the skull, where the intense physiological uptake from the adjacent brain parenchyma may obscure small metastases in the skull [17, 18].

17.3 Prediction of Survival in Patients with Vertebral Bone Metastases

After the lung and liver, the skeleton is the organ most affected by metastases. Bone metastases can give produce different degrees of disability depending on their location. Bone metastases (especially those localized to the spine) are more frequently observed in tumors of the lung, prostate gland, breast, and hematopoietic organs. The axial skeleton is the most common site of bone metastasis, with metastasis most frequently occurring in the spine, pelvis, and ribs. The lumbar spine is the single most frequent site of bone metastasis [19, 20]. In the appendicular skeleton, the proximal femurs are the most common site of metastatic disease, and humeral lesions also occur frequently. The acral sites (feet and hands) are rarely involved. Certain skeletal sites are associated with specific areas of bone metastases. For example, scapular metastases are seen more frequently from primary tumors of the kidney [21].

Involvement of the skull is more common with breast primaries. The distal appendicular

Table 17.1 Harrington classification of metastases to the spinal column

Class	Criteria
I	No significant neurologic involvement
II	Involvement of bone without collapse or instability
III	Major neurologic impairment (sensory or motor) without significant involvement of bone
IV	Vertebral collapse with pain due to mechanical causes or instability but without significant neurologic compromize
V	Vertebral collapse with pain due to mechanical causes or instability combined with major neurologic impairment

skeleton (tibia, fibula) and acral sites (especially the hands) are more common with lung primaries. Involvement of the toes is seen more commonly with genitourinary primaries.

Pain is the main symptom of bone metastases, but neurological symptoms can occur with compression of the spinal cord or spinal nerves. The therapeutic approach varies according to the type of lesion, bone compression, and involvement of the bone marrow or nerves. Estimation of life expectancy is difficult and warrants a multidisciplinary approach. In 1986, Harrington proposed initial identification of bone metastases during spine loading, from which treatment strategies could be formulated (Table 17.1) [22].With this classification, Harrington provided radiation treatment in patients of classes I–III, whereas primary surgical treatment was recommended for patients of classes IV–V. A secondary surgical approach was planned for these patients, with pain or neurological symptoms, which could not be subjected to radiotherapy.

Various attempts have been made to establish a valid method for predicting survival [23]. A scheme was proposed by Tomita and Tokuhashi to select the most suitable candidates for surgical treatment [24]. Bartles et al. developed a model to predict the survival of patients with vertebral metastases. They evaluated parameters such as: sex; the location of the primary tumor; the intention of curative treatment of the primary tumor; the location of cervical spine metastases; and the Karnofsky Performance Score (KPS) [25]. In 2001, Chow et al. published a review suggesting that the KPS was a suitable predictor [26]. A scoring system was devised by van der Liden et al. that was based on a large randomized trial of radiotherapy for the treatment of pain from bone metastases [27]. The KPS is considered to be one of the strongest predictors of survival, along with the: type of primary tumor; presence of visceral metastases; presence of multiple bone metastases; response to radiotherapy. The Palliative Prognostic Score (PaP Score) can be used to classify cancer patients. The PaP Score is the result of different prognostic factors: the KPS, clinical prediction of survival, anorexia, dyspnea, total number of white blood cells, and the percentage of lymphocytes. The PaP Score can be used to identify three prognostic groups so that the appropriate treatment schedule can be applied, i.e., patients with:

- a median survival of 64 days (which is an indication to a single fraction of radiotherapy);
- limited metastatic disease and good life expectancy (standard or dictated hypofractionated treatments allowing local control of the disease in 2 weeks);
- a poor prognosis and with symptomatic localized areas (monofractionated regimens with rapid improvement in pain and a decrease in the duration of treatment, thereby improving the QoL) [28].

17.4 Treatment

The management of metastatic bone pain must involve a multidisciplinary approach. It includes analgesia, radiotherapy, surgery, chemotherapy, hormone treatment, radioisotopes and bisphosphonates.

17.4.1 Radiotherapy

Radiotherapy is crucial in the treatment of metastatic spinal disease. Radiotherapy is considered to be standard treatment if there is pain, a risk of pathologic fracture, or compression of the spinal cord. It is effective symptomatic treatment of local bone pain [29, 30]. A palliative effect is seen within 4–6 weeks in approximately 80% of patients.

Radiotherapeutic techniques include conventional external beam radiotherapy, intensity-modulated radiation therapy (IMRT), stereotactic radiosurgery and stereotactic radiotherapy. The efficacy of radiotherapy in the treatment of pain and neurological symptoms is dependent upon the sensitivity of tumor cells to ionizing radiation. Primary tumors that are very sensitive to ionizing radiation include lymphomas, myeloma, and seminomatous germ-cell tumors. Most solid tumors such as breast cancer, prostate cancer and lung cancer have intermediate radio-sensitivity. Melanoma, osteosarcoma and renal cell carcinomas are usually radio-resistant [31].

The analgesic effect of radiotherapy on bone-metastases pain is based on the cytocidal effect of ionizing radiation on tumor cells. This can lead to a reduction of mechanical compression and the infiltration of bone tissue. Another important mechanism is reduction of the production of the cytokines that act on the receptors responsible for pain. The precocity of palliation which is observed in around 25% of patients (usually within 48 h of treatment) and which cannot be attributed to the reduction of tumor mass probably involves the action of ionizing radiation on osteoclasts and on the system regulator RANK/RANK-L. Hoskin et al. showed that the reduction of pain after radiotherapy for bone metastases is associated with low concentrations of urinary pyridinoline and deoxypyridinoline, which are markers of bone resorption [32].

In recent years numerous studies have evaluated the most appropriate regimen of fractionation in individual cases. Despite this, a consensus for the choice of a particular fractionation regimen is lacking [33, 34]. The Radiation Therapy Oncology Group (RTOG) 7402 trial showed that the pattern "short-course" in a single fraction of 8 Gy is as effective as a hypofractionated regimen for pain palliation [35]. The Dutch Bone Metastasis Study was a randomized study of 1,171 patients with bone metastases treated with a single fraction of 8 Gy or 24 Gy (4 Gy/fz) in six fractions. The results showed no difference in pain palliation, QoL or side effects between the two regimens. The RTOG 9701 trial compared the efficacy of a single fraction of 8 Gy with a total dose of 30 Gy (3Gy/fz) in 10 fractions. The only difference noted was lower acute toxicity and a higher percentage of reprocessing in patients treated with a single fraction. A review in 2007 and two meta-analyses confirmed the equivalence of a single fraction with multiple fractions in pain management. With the single fraction, an improvement of pain symptoms in 80% of cases and a complete response in 30% of cases were observed. Re-treatment was observed in 10% of multiple-fraction treatments compared with 20% of single-fraction treatments. These studies revealed that there was no difference in efficacy in pain palliation between single-fraction and multiple-fraction treatments. However, there would be a difference in the radiobiological context because only higher doses would activate bone recalcification.

The American Society for Radiation Oncology (ASTRO) convened a Task Force of experts who developed a guideline (published in 2011) regarding the use of palliative radiotherapy. They confirmed that external-beam radiotherapy is the mainstay of treatment for painful, uncomplicated bone metastases, and that various fractionation regimens can provide an equivalent response to pain control (although longer treatment has the advantage of a lower incidence of re-treatment on the same site) [36]. Moreover, radiotherapy techniques may allow conformal dose distribution to reduce the toxicity in normal tissues (Fig. 17.1). These methods (IMRT, stereotactic radiosurgery, stereotactic radiotherapy) permit the safe delivery of higher radiation doses. These methods require a high standard of precision in targeting the beam to the shape and exact location of the tumor [37–41].

New methods have produced promising results for some patients with spinal metastases (Fig. 17.2). Nevertheless, external-beam radiotherapy remains the "gold standard" treatment for spinal metastases. The non-availability and expense prohibit the widespread use of advanced methods for these palliative indications.

17.4.2 Surgical Treatment and Radiotherapy

Pathologic fractures and spinal-cord compression require rapid treatment because they can lead to a worse QoL. A multimodal approach between radiologists, radiotherapists, medical oncologists, surgeons, as well as specialists in pain medicine and palliative care is required. Radiotherapy has a central role because it is effective and is associated with few side effects [42]. The treatment goals are:

- maintenance of good QoL;
- prevention of skeletal events;
- improve mobility;
- improve survival (if possible).

Pathologic fractures in bone metastases occur spontaneously or after minor trauma due to a reduction in bone integrity [43]. Such fractures cause pain and disability. In many cases, they may require a surgical approach, with stabilization techniques and a radiotherapeutic approach [44].

In one study looking at the treatment of metastatic spinal-cord compression, the role of radiotherapy was the removal or reduction of back pain in 89% of patients [45]. Sixty-six percent of patients with urinary dysfunction were shown to respond to radiotherapy. The surgical approach in spinal-cord compression provides circumferential decompression. This is carried out with stabilization of the anterior wall with interposition of methyl methacrylate with or without support by a system applied with a posterior surgical approach. Therefore, laminectomy is reserved for a few rare cases. However, a posterior approach does not exclude access to the vertebral bodies and reconstruction of the anterior column.

Pathologic fractures can have a serious impact not only on QoL but also on outcome. There is no evidence of a significant difference between single- and multiple-fraction radiotherapy in the prevalence of pathological fractures in irradiated regions. This is despite the fact that more fractures occurred after single-fraction radiotherapy than after multiple-fraction radiotherapy in a study by Steenland et al. [46]. Recurrences of metastatic spinal-cord compression in the irradiated region ("in-field recurrences") are more common after single-fraction and short-course multiple-fraction radiotherapy than after long-course radiotherapy [47, 48]. Patients with a favorable prognosis may live long enough to develop recurrences, so these patients should receive long-course radiotherapy and should be considered candidates for decompressive surgery preceding radiotherapy or for high-precision radiotherapy. Selected patients treated with decompressive surgery followed by long-course radiotherapy were shown to have better post-treatment ambulatory status (84% *versus* 57%, $p < 0.001$) than patients treated with radiotherapy alone [49].

The indications for surgery are:

- a radio-resistant tumor;
- progressive neurologic deficit before, during, or after radiotherapy;
- bone fragments in the spinal canal;
- instability of the spine due to a pathologic fracture causing intractable pain or a neurologic deficit [50];
- neurologic deficit ≤24 h;
- a circumscript spinal lesion;
- life expectancy of ≥3 months.

Vertebroplasty involves the injection of polymethyl methacrylate (PMMA) into the involved vertebral body under fluoroscopic guidance. Bone reinforcement and stabilization of the anterior column relieves pain and prevents pathological fractures. PMMA could have anti-tumor activity as a result of cytotoxicity, thermal effects, and ischemia [51]. The indication for this procedure is painful vertebral metastasis without neurological compromise. Partial emptying of the vertebral body and creating a cavity within the body can prevent cement leakage. This can be done using a laser or balloon [52]. The last method is called "kyphoplasty". Both methods can be completed percutaneously or as an open procedure during a standard posterior approach [53, 54].

17.4.3 Bisphosphonates and Radiotherapy

Bisphosphonates have an increasingly important role in oncology, management of bone metastases, and the prevention of skeletal complications [55, 56]. They reduce skeletal morbidity in breast cancer, pain levels, consumption of analgesics, and lead to an improvement in QoL [57]. In addition to inhibiting osteoclast function bisphosphonates also cause apoptosis. However, they seem to have a direct effect on the type of apoptotic tumor cells, as has been demonstrated by *in-vitro* studies on tumor cells of the breast and prostate gland as well as melanoma, osteosarcoma, and myeloma [58–63]. Radiotherapy and bisphosphonates, therefore, through their effects on cellular homeostasis, have a major role in the treatment of bone metastases. The combination of bisphosphonates and radiotherapy can improve the effectiveness of the latter due to the radiosensitizing action of bisphosphonates [64]. Several mechanisms for the interaction of systemic treatment with radiation have been described.

Additive and super-additive effects: Radiotherapy and bisphosphonates have effects upon cellular homeostasis (particularly osteoclast activity) around the bone metastasis. Through their common action on osteoclasts, a positive interaction within an area of bone metastasis may be postulated which is dependent upon the relative extent to which the two are effective. An additive or even super-additive effect may also be seen, with relief of acute pain through the biochemical alteration of osteoclast activity consolidated by additional killing of tumor cells from radiation.

Spatial cooperation: A local treatment such as radiotherapy may deal with the primary site of disease whereas systemic treatment can be added to control microscopic or asymptomatic disease in other areas.

Normal tissue tolerance: Radiotherapy and bisphosphonates used together do not have overlapping toxicity and do not compromise tolerance for either method. Only treatment of large areas of the skeleton with radiotherapy in the setting of widespread metastatic disease may cause significant suppression of the bone marrow. Bisphosphonates have a selective effect upon the mechanisms of bone mineralization and osteoclasts. However, they have no effect upon bone-marrow function and are therefore a safe and predictable "systemic partner" in the management of bone metastasis with radiotherapy [65].

Krempiem et al. investigated the possible benefit of a combination of radiotherapy and bisphosphonates on recalcification and stabilization of osteolytic bone metastases in animal tumor models. They demonstrated that early addition of the bisphosphonate clodronate and radiotherapy significantly improved the density and bone microstructure [66]. In a clinical trial of 33 patients with bone metastases from breast cancer, Kouloulias et al. showed that a combination of radiotherapy and treatment with bisphosphonates induced clinical improvement after 6 months of therapy compared with the control baseline in terms of bone density, pain control, performance status, biochemical markers of bone resorption, and QoL. They also showed better clinical benefit with respect to bone recalcification with a combination of radiotherapy and bisphosphonates compared with that obtained by radiotherapy alone [67]. Many patients receive bisphosphonates in combination with radiotherapy, as documented by a study by Rosen et al. [68] and a review by Hoskin [69].

17.4.4 Morphine Immediate-Release (MIR) and Radiotherapy

Chronic pain due to cancer represents a major medical challenge [70]. Good compliance with treatment is necessary if radiotherapy is to be successful. Indeed, even if these patients are treated with analgesics they do not always achieve adequate control of pain. Positioning during radiotherapeutic procedures often leads to the exacerbation of pain. Different categories of drugs are used for the treatment of chronic pain, but opioids are pivotal in advanced treatment [70, 75]. Therefore, the radiotherapist must often care for patients who are undergoing analgesic therapy but who are suffering from intense pain when they are positioned for radiotherapy. This pain may often be so severe that the patient interrupts the therapy session (or even the therapy cycle).

Recent experience has highlighted the role of MIR. MIR appears to be the ideal agent for the treatment of predictable pain due to its pharmacological features [76, 77]. Prevention of pain onset and resource optimization can be achieved with an opioid with a short half-life that can be administered readily *via* the oral route, such as MIR. Radiotherapy combined with opioid medical therapy is effective treatment for the management of metastatic bone pain. The identification of the features of pain as well as knowledge of how pain changes in terms of intensity and time can improve pain management in cancer patients and, therefore, the effectiveness of the treatments delivered due to improved patient compliance. Consequently, the radiotherapist also has a crucial role with regard to the administration of analgesic treatments by helping to achieve increasingly personalized and effective therapeutic management [78].

References

1. Mundy GR (1987) Bone resorption and turnover in health and disease. Bone 8 (Suppl. 1):S9–S16
2. Mercadante S (1997) Malignant bone pain: pathophysiology and treatment. Pain, 69:1–18
3. Hsu H, Lacey DL, Dunstan CR et al (1999) Tumour necrosis factor receptor family member RANK mediates osteoclast differentiation and activation induced by osteoprotegerin ligand. Proc Natl Acad Sci U.S.A. 96:3540–3545
4. Simonet WS, Lacey DL, Dunstan CR et al (1997) Osteoprotegerin: a novel secreted protein involved in the regulation of bone density. Cell 89:309–319
5. Guise TA, Yin JJ, Thomas RJ, Dallas M, Cui Y, Gillespie MT (2002) Parathyroid hormone-related protein (PTHrP)(1–139) isoform is efficiently secreted in vitro and enhances breast cancer metastasis to bone in vivo. Bone 30(5):670–676
6. Perrin R G, Laxton AW (2004) Metastatic spine disease: epidemiology, pathophysiology, and evaluation of patients. Neurosurg Clin N Am 15:365–373
7. Coleman RE (2006) Clinical features of metastatic bone disease and risk of skeletal morbidity. Clin Cancer Res 12:6243s–6249s
8. Coleman RE (1997) Skeletal complications of malignancy. Cancer 80 (Suppl. 8):1588–1594
9. Goblirsch MJ, Zwolak PP, Clohisy DR (2006) Biology of bone cancer pain. Clin Cancer Res 12:6231–6235s
10. Hoskin PJ, Stratford MRL, Folkes LK, Regan J, Yarnold JR (2000) Effect of local radiotherapy for bone pain on urinary markers of osteoclast activity *Lancet* 355:1428–1429
11. Roodman GD (2004) Mechanisms of bone metastases. N Engl J Med 350:1655-1664
12. Smoker WRK, Godersky JC, Knutzon RK et al (1987) The role of MR imaging in evaluating metastatic spinal disease. AJR Am J Roentgenol 149:1241-8
13. Flickinger FW, Sanal SM (1994) Bone marrow MRI: techniques and accuracy for detecting breast cancer metastases. Magn Reson Imaging 12:829-835
14. 1Hamaoka T, Madewell JE, Podoloff DA et al (2204) Bone imaging in metastatic breast cancer. J ClinOncol 22:2942-2953
15. Evan-Sapr E, Mester U, Mishani E et al (2006) The detection of bone metastases in patients with high-risk prostate cancer: 99mTc-MDP Planar bone scintigraphy, single- and multi-field-of-view SPECT, 18F-fluoride PET, and 18F-fluoride PET/CT. J Nucl Med 47:287-297
16. Fujimoto R, Higashi T, Nakamoto Y et al (2006) Diagnostic accuracy of bone metastases detection in cancer patients: comparison between bone scintigraphy and whole-body FDG-PET. Ann Nucl Med 20:399-408
17. Daldrup-Link HE, Franzius C, Link TM (2001) Whole-body MR imaging for detection of bone metastases in children and young adults: comparison with skeletal scintigraphy and FDG PET. Am J Roentgenol 177:229-236
18. Ohta M, Tokuda Y, Suzuki Y et al (2001) Whole body PET for the evaluation of bony metastases in patients with breast cancer: comparison with 99Tcm-MDP bone scintigraphy. Nucl Med Commun 22:875-879
19. Asdourian PL, Weidenbaum M, DeWald RL, Hammerberg KW, Ramsey RG (1990) The pattern of vertebral involvement in metastatic vertebral breast cancer. Clin Orthop Relat Res 250:164–170
20. Steinmetz MP, Mekhail A, Benzel EC (2001) Management of metastatic tumors of the spine: strategies and operative indications. Neurosurg Focus 11:e2
21. Gurney H, Larcos G, McKay M, Kefford R, Langlands A (1989) Bone metastases in hypernephroma. Frequency of scapular involvement. Cancer 64:1429–1431
22. Harrington KD (1986) Metastatic disease of the spine. J Bone Joint Surg Am 68:1110–1115
23. Harrington KD (1997) Orthopedic surgical management of skeletal complications of malignancy. Cancer 80 (8 Suppl.):1614–1627
24. Tomita K, Kawahara N, Kobayashi T, Yoshida A, Murakami H, Akamaru T (2001) Surgical strategy for spinal metastases. Spine 26:298–306
25. Bartles RH, Feuth T, van der Maazen R (2007) Development of a model with which to predict the life

expectancy of patients with spinal epidural metastasis. Cancer 110:2042–2049
26. Chow E, Harris K, Fung K (2006) Successful validation of a survival prediction model in patients with metastases in the spinal column. Int J Radiat Oncol Biol Phys 65:1522–1527
27. Aglietta M, Mandoliti G, Marangolo M, Maranzano E (2007) La palliazione in radioterapia oncologica. Argomenti Oncologici Quaderni di Oncologia. Medical Communication, Torino, pp 41-47
28. van der Linden YM, Dijkstra SPDS, Vonk EJA, Marijnen CAM, Leer JWH (2005) Prediction of survival in patients with metastases in the spinal column. Cancer 103:320–328
29. Poulson HS, Nielsen OS, Klee M, Rorth M (1989) Palliative irradiation of bone metastases. Cancer Treat Rev 16:41–48
30. Hoskin PJ (1995b) Radiotherapy in the management of bone pain. Clin Orthopaed Res 312:105–119
31. Peters LJ (1990) The EstroRegaud Lecture. Inherent radiosensitivity of tumor and normal tissue cells as a predictor of human tumor response. Radiother Oncol 17:177–190
32. Hoskin PJ, Stratford MR, Folkes LK, Regan J, Yarnold JR (2000) Effect of local radiotherapy for bone pain on urinary markers of osteoclast activity. Lancet 355:1428–1429
33. Hoskin PJ, Yarnold JR, Roos DR, Bentzen S (2001) Radiotherapy for bone metastases. Clin Oncol (R Coll Radiol) 13:88–90
34. Wu JS, Wong RK, Lloyd NS, Johnoston M, Bezjak A, Whelan T (2004) Radiotherapy fractionation for the palliation of uncomplicated painful bone metastases – an evidence-based practice guideline. BMC Cancer 4:71
35. Tong D, Gillik L, Hendrickson FR (1982) The palliation of symptomatic osseous metastases. Final results of the study by the Radiation Therapy Oncology Group. Cancer 50:893–899
36. Lutz S, Berk L, Chang E et al (2011) Palliative radiotherapy for bone metastases. An ASTRO evidence-based guideline. Int J Radiat Oncol 4: 965–976
37. Gibbs IC, Kamnerdsupaphon P, Ryu MR et al (2007) Image-guided robotic radiosurgery for spinal matastases. Radiother Oncol 82:185–190
38. Gerszten PC, Burton SA, Ozhasoglu C, Welch WC (2007) Radiosurgery for spinal metastases: clinical experience in 500 cases from a single institution. Spine 32:193–199
39. Jin JY, Chen Q, Jin R et al (2007) Technical and clinical experience with spine radiosurgery : a new technology for management of localized spine metastases. Technol Cancer Res Treat 6:127–133
40. Ryu S, Fang Y, Rock J et al (2003) Image-guided and intensity-modulated radiosurgery for patients with spinal metastasis. Cancer 97:2013–2018
41. Nieder C, Grosu AL, Andratschke NH, Molls M (2006) Update of human spinal cord reirradiation tolerance based on additional data from 38 patients. Int J Radiat Oncol Biol Phys 66:1446–1449
42. Trodella L, Ramella S, D'Angelilla RM, Orecchia R, Muto P (2011) Radiation therapy for bone metastases. Tumori 12 (suppl. 1):S12–S17
43. Janian N (2001) Bone metastases: approaches to management. Semin Oncol 28:28–34
44. Roos D, Turner S, O'Brien P et al; TROG 96.05 (2005) Randomized trial of 8 Gy in 1 versus 20 Gy in 5 fractions of radiotherapy for neuropathic pain due to bone matastases. Radiother Oncol 75:54–63
45. Maranzano E, Latini P, Checcaglini F et al (1992) Radiation therapy of spinal cord compression caused by breast cancer: report of a prospective trial. Int J Radiat Oncol Biol Phys 24:301–306
46. Steenland E, Leer J, van Houwelingen et al (1999) The effect of a single fraction compared to multiple fractions on painful bone metastases: a global analysis of the Dutch Bone Metastasis Study. Radiother Oncol 52:101–109
47. Rades D, Fehlauer F, Schulte R et al (2006) Prognostic factors for local control and survival after radiotherapy of metastatic spinal cord compression. J Clin Oncol 24:3388–3393
48. Maranzano E, Trippa F, Casale M, Anselmo P, Rossi R (2011) Reirradiation of metastatic spinal cord compression: definitive results of two randomized trials. Radiother Oncol 98:234–237
49. Patchell RA, Tibbs PA, Regine WF et al (2005) Direct decompressive surgical resection in the treatment of spinal cord compression caused by metastatic cancer: a randomised trial. Lancet 366:643–648
50. Hirabayashi H, Ebara S, Kinoshita T (2003) Clinical outcome and survival after palliative surgery for spinal metastases: palliative surgery in spinal metastases. Cancer 97:476–484
51. Pilitsis JG, Rengachary SS (2001) The role of vertebroplasty in metastatic spinal disease. Neurosurg Focus11:e1
52. De Negri P, Tirri T, Paternoster G, Modano P (2007) Treatment of painful osteoporotic or traumatic vertebral compression fractures by percutaneous vertebral augmentation procedures: a nonrandomized comparison between vertebroplasty and kyphoplasty. Clin J Pain 23:425–430
53. Wenger M (2003) Vertebroplasty for metastasis. Med Oncol 20:203–209
54. Fuentes S, Metellus P, Pech-Gourg G (2007) Traitement par Kyphoplastieafoyer ouvert des metastases rachidiennes. Neurochirurgie 53:49–53
55. Poulson HS, Nielsen OS, Klee M, Rorth M (1989) Palliative irradiation of bone metastases. Cancer Treat Rev 16: 41–48
56. Hoskin PJ (1995) Radiotherapy in the management of bone pain. Clin Orthop Rel Res 312:105–119
57. Coleman-Robert E (2000) Management of bone metastases. Oncologist 5:465–466
58. Colston KW (2000) Bisphosphonates induce apoptosis in human breast cancer cell lines. Brit J Cancer 82:366–371
59. Jagdev SP, Coleman RE, Shipman CM, Ro-stami HA, Croucher PI (2001) The bisphosphonates zole-

dronic acid induces apoptosis of breast cancer cells: evidence for synergy with paclitaxel. Brit J Cancer 84:1126–1134
60. Lee MV, Fong EM, Singer FR, Guenette RS (2001) Bisphosphonate treatment inhibits the growth of prostate cancer cells. Cancer Res 61:2602–2608
61. Riebeling C, Forsea AM, Raisova M, Orfanos CE, Geilen CC (2002) The bisphosphonate pamidronate induces apoptosis in human melanoma cells in vitro. Brit J Cancer 87:366–371
62. Mackie PS, Fisher JL, Zhou H, Choong PF (2001) Bisphosphonates regulate cell growth and gene expression in the UMR 106-101 clonal rat osteosarcoma cell line. Brit J Cancer 84:951–958
63. Shipman CM, Croucher PI, Russell RG, Hel-frich MH, Rogers MJ (1998) The bisphosphonate incadronate (YM175) causes apoptosis of human myeloma cells in vitro by inhibiting the mevalonate pathway. Cancer Res 58:5294–5297
64. Ugur-Ural A, Avcuand F, Baran Y (2008) bisphosphonate treatment and radiotherapy in metastatic breast cancer. Med Oncol 25:350–355
65. Mandoliti G, Ramella S, Muto P et al (2011) Integrating radiation therapy and bisphosphonates. I supplementi di Tumori 12:S7-S11
66. Krempiem R, Huber PE, Harms W, Treiber M, Wannenmacher M, Krempiem B (2003) Combination of early bisphosphonates administration and irradiation leads to improved remineralization and restabilization of oste-olytic bone metastases in an animal tumor model. Cancer 98:1318–1324
67. Kouloulias V, Matsopoulos G, Kouvaris J et al (2003) Radiotherapy in conjunction with intravenous infusion of 180 mg sodium pamidronate in the management of oste-olytic metastases from breast cancer: clinical evaluation, biochemical markers, quality of life, and monitoring of recalcification using assessments of gray level histogram in plain radiographs. Int J Radiat Oncol Biol Phys 57:143–157
68. Rosen LS, Gordon D, Tchekmedyian S et al; Zoledronic Acid Lung Cancer and other Solid Tumors Study Group (2003) Zoledronic acid versus placebo in the treatment of skeletal metastases in patients with lung cancer and other solid tumors: a phase III, double-blind, randomized trial. J Clin Oncol 21:3150–3157
69. Hoskin PJ (2003) Bisphosphonates and radiation therapy for palliation of metastatic bone disease. Cancer Treat Rev 29: 321–327
70. Hemming L, Maher D (2005) Cancer pain in palliative care: why is management so difficult? Br J Community Nurs 10:362–367
71. World Health Organization (1986) Cancer pain relief. World Health Organization, Geneva
72. Takeda F (1985) Japanese field-testing of WHO guidelines. PRN Forum 4:4–5
73. Walker VA, Hoskin PJ, Hanks GW, White ID (1988) Evaluation of WHO analgesic guidelines for cancer pain in a hospital based palliative care unit. J Pain Symptom Manage 3:145–149
74. Hanks GW, Conno F, Cherny N et al; Expert Working Group of the Research Network of the European Association for Palliative Care (2001) Morphine and alternative opioids in cancer pain: the EAPC recommendations. Brit J Cancer 2001 84:587–593
75. Ripamonti C, Dickerson ED (2001) Strategies for the treatment of cancer pain in the new millennium. Drugs 61:955–977
76. Lo Presti C, Roscetti A, Muriess D, Mammucari M (2010) Time to pain relief after immediate-release morphine in episodic pain. The TIME Study. Clin Drug Invest 30 (Suppl. 2):49–55
77. Mammucari M, Mediati RD, Vellucci R. (2010) L'uso degli oppiacei nella pratica clinica 2010. Wolters Kluwer Health Italy Ltd, Milan
78. Murino P, Mammucari M, Borrelli D et al (2011) Role of immediate-release morphine (MIR) in the treatment of predictable pain in radiotherapy. J Pain Palliat Care Pharmacother 25:121–124

Classification and Treatment of Vascular Malformations of the Spinal Cord

18

Francesco Causin, Joseph Gabrielli
and Emanuele Orrù

18.1 Introduction

Vascular malformations of the spinal cord (arterial and venous) represent a heterogeneous group of vessel disorders that affect the tissue of the spinal cord either directly or indirectly. This group comprises spinal arteriovenous malformations (AVMs), dural arteriovenous fistulas (DAVFs), spinal hemangiomas, cavernous hemangiomas, aneurysms and vascular tumors.

This chapter is focused on high-flow lesions of the spinal cord such as arteriovenous malformations and arteriovenous fistulas (AVFs). Low-flow vascular malformations without arteriovenous shunts such as capillary telangiectasias and cavernous hemangiomas are not considered. Other lesions, such as highly vascularized tumors (e.g., hemangioblastomas, angiosarcomas, hemangiopericytomas, angiofibromas, angiolipomas, hemangioendotheliomas) are also not discussed.

18.2 Anatomy of the Spinal Cord

The spinal cord is constituted by neural tissue (gray matter, neural pathways, glial cells) and interwoven vasculature that supply the spinal parenchyma. The spinal cord does not extend the entire length of the vertebral column: it extends from the foramen magnum to the conus medullaris at the level of L1–L2 vertebrae. The spinal cord continues with the cauda equina, and terminates with a fibrous extension known as the filum terminalis that anchors the spinal cord to the coccyx. It is ovoid-shaped, around 45 cm in length and has a varying width: it ranges from 15-mm thick in the cervical and lumbar regions to 10-mm thick in the thoracic area.

The spinal cord is protected by the spinal meninges, which continue the three cranial layers. The dura mater is the outermost layer. Between the dura mater and the bone of the vertebrae is the epidural space, which is filled with adipose tissue and contains a network of blood vessels. The arachnoid is the middle protective layer. The interface between the dura mater and the arachnoid is the subdural space. The subdural space of the spinal cord was historically defined as a potential cavity or a "virtual space" between the dura and arachnoid. More recently, authors have stopped identifying this space and instead describe a compartment filled with neurothelial cells termed the "dura–arachnoid interface". The space between the arachnoid and the underlying pia mater is the subarachnoid space. The subarachnoid space contains the cerebrospinal fluid (CSF), the three longitudinal arteries that supply the spinal cord (anterior spinal artery and the right and left posterior spinal arteries), and the medullary veins.

F. Causin (✉)
Neuroradiology Unit, Padua University Hospital,
Padua, Italy
francesco.causin@sanita.padova.it

M. Muto (ed.), *Interventional Neuroradiology of the Spine*,
DOI 10.1007/978-88-470-2790-9_18, © Springer-Verlag Italia 2013

18.3 Vasculature of the Spinal Cord

The complex and extremely delicate vascular system of the spinal cord must be understood to fully appreciate the types of vascular malformations of the spinal cord. A detailed description of the normal and malformed arterial supply and venous drainage should be provided in subjects by using computed tomography (CT) and magnetic resonance imaging (MRI) as well as catheter angiography.

Segmental arteries coming from the aorta and their divisional branches support the spinal radicular and medullary arteries that provide circulation to the vertebral bodies, dural sleeves of the nerve roots, and spinal cord.

The cervical segment and upper thoracic segment are fed by arteries coming from the vertebral arteries (posterior inferior cerebellar arteries, anterolateral spinal arteries, segmental arteries) and from the ascending and deep cervical arteries. Below the cervical region, the blood supply comes from the pair of intercostal and lumbar radicular arteries that provide major anastomoses and which run into the spinal cord alongside the dorsal and ventral nerve roots. The largest of the anterior radicular arteries is the artery of Adamkiewicz (also known as the "artery of the lumbar enlargement"), which usually arises between L1 and L2, but which can arise anywhere from T8 to L4. In 75% of the population, the artery of Adamkiewicz originates on the left side of the aorta between the T8 and L1 vertebral segments [1].

The anterior spinal artery (ASA) descends in front of the medulla oblongata and along the anterior medial fissure of the spinal cord (medulla spinalis) to supply the anterior two-thirds of the spinal cord. It is reinforced by a succession of radicular branches which enter the vertebral canal through the intervertebral foramina and which pierce the dura following the nerve roots. During the embryonic period, 31 pairs of segmental arteries at each level reach the anterior spinal artery. The progressive spontaneous regression of these branches during development leaves 4–8 ventral arteries supplying the anterior spinal artery [1, 2]. A dominant feeding branch in the cervical region is commonly present ("artery of the cervical enlargement") as well as sparse small feeders in the thoracic region. At the lumbar enlargement, as stated above, is the largest supplying artery: the artery of Adamkiewicz. All of these feeding arteries to the anterior spinal artery are termed the "radiculomedullary arteries".

The right and left posterior spinal arteries together supply the posterior third of the cord. They are classically shown as two paired vessels running along the back surface of the cord on each side, but this depiction is not true. They should be shown as a discontinuous longitudinal system on the dorsal aspect of the spinal cord supplied *via* radiculopial branches that run along the pial surface to supply a posterior segment of the spinal artery, which usually involves no more than a few levels. Inferiorly, the anterior and posterior systems are anastomized around the conus medullaris in the arterial "basket".

Thus, the blood supply to the spinal cord is dependent upon two systems: (i) medullary perforating arteries from the anterior spinal artery (sulcocommisural artery) supplying the anterior and central portions and the gray matter, and (ii) pial circumferential arteries (coronary arteries or vasocorona) from the posterior spinal arteries system supplying the periphery [2, 3].

At any cross-sectional level the two sulcocommisural arteries supply the anterior two-thirds of the spinal cord. Sulcocommisual penetrating arteries have few anastomoses, and are in effect end-arteries. The posterior pial network has many feeders and extensive anastomoses.

The blood flow within the spinal cord has two opposite directions [4]: a centrifugal system (supplied by the central sulcocommisural artery) and a centripetal system (supplied by the coronary arteries), which supply distinct territories. There is an intermediate zone which may be supplied by either system.

18.3.1 Centrifugal System

The centrifugal system is also known as the "sulcocommisural system". The ventral spinal axis (anterior spinal artery) gives rise to 200–400 sulcocommissural arteries within the ventral sulcus of the spinal cord. These arteries penetrate the sulcus and enter the central gray matter, where they give off branches radiating outward toward the peripheral white matter. Each sulcocommissural artery usually supplies one-half (right or left) of the cord. The sulcocommissural system supplies most of the gray matter and the ventral half of the cord. Before entering cord tissue, each sulcocommissural artery gives off cranial and caudal anastomotic branches to other sulcocommissural arteries. Craniocaudal anastomoses are also seen within the substance of the cord. The sulcal arteries have a completely horizontal course early in human development. They assume an ascending course with growth due to disproportionate elongation of the spinal column in relation to the spinal cord.

18.3.2 Centripetal System

The centripetal system is also known as the "dorsolateral pial supply" (from posterior spinal arteries). This network covers the dorsal and dorsolateral surface of the spinal cord, and has two dominant craniocaudal channels known as the "posterior spinal arteries". At the craniocervical junction, supply to this system comes directly from the transdural vertebral arteries (or from the posterior inferior cerebellar arteries if their origin is below the dura). Below this level, arterial supply is granted by radiculopial arteries. This system has a dorsal component and a lateral component (located between the dorsal and ventral nerve roots), which are interconnected. This network gives rise to radial arteries (vasa corona), which extend around the circumference of the cord and have anastomoses to the ventral spinal axis. The radial arteries give off perforating branches to the spinal cord all along their course. These short perforating branches extend axially, into the white matter and into the gray matter of the dorsal horns. The perforating arteries have intramedullary anastomoses with branches of the sulcocommissural arteries dorsolaterally, ventrolaterally, and ventrally. There are also short, extramedullary longitudinal (craniocaudal) anastomoses between the radial arteries. These anastomoses are relatively small, however, and cannot provide adequate craniocaudal supply in the case of arterial occlusion. The dorsolateral pial network must therefore be regarded primarily as an axial system of the arterial supply.

The venous drainage of the spinal cord [3, 5, 6] is guaranteed through radially symmetric intrinsic spinal cord veins and small superficial pial veins that open into the superficial longitudinal median spinal cord veins. These veins follow more or less the arteries but have many anastomoses, including transmedullary anastomoses that create a network with more than one anterior and posterior vein. They follow the nerve roots and reach the epidural plexus as well as the extraspinal veins and plexus, with a reflux-impeding mechanism within the dura mater. In the superior cervical region, these veins can run through the occipital foramen to connect the vertebral plexus to the inferior dural sinuses. Blood drainage from the spine occurs through the internal and external venous vertebral plexus, which is connected to the azygos and hemiazygos venous systems.

18.4 Clinical Features of Spinal Lesions

Spinal arteriovenous lesions may be associated with myelopathy (sensory and motor deficits, bowel dysfunction, bladder dysfunction), radicular pain or radicular deficit, back pain [7] or deformities in the spinal column. Damage to the spinal cord can occur *via* hemorrhage, venous hypertension, arterial steal and mass effect.

Hemorrhage can occur in the parenchyma and subarachnoid space of the spinal cord, leading to the acute onset or sudden worsening of neurological deficits. The risk of hemorrhage is greater in spinal cord AVMs than in other types of lesions. Less prevalent is bleeding due to large and giant AVFs in the spinal cord as well as cervical or intracranial DAVFs with perimedullary venous drainage. Small AVFs in the spinal cord as well as thoracic and lumbar DAVFs are less likely to bleed [8, 9]. Spinal artery and intranidal aneurysms are associated with a higher risk of hemorrhage. Venous hypertension is typically associated with arteriovenous lesions with perimedullary venous drainage. This phenomenon is associated with spinal DAVF, but can be seen with any lesion that has perimedullary venous drainage (e.g., pial AVFs of the spinal cord or intracranial dural AVFs).

High-flow arteriovenous shunts may lead to the steal of arterial blood from adjacent normal spinal cord tissue [10]. Lesions in the dorsal aspect of the spinal cord fed by the ASA are also prone to arterial steal because of the low efficacy of collateral supply to normal cord tissue. Mass effect is a rare mechanism in myelopathy. Large aneurysms and large dilated varices (such as the ones seen with giant AVFs in the spinal cord) may compress the spinal cord or nerve roots, leading to myelopathy, radicular pain, radicular deficit and back pain.

18.5 Epidemiology and Classification of Spinal Lesions

The ability to examine the angioarchitecture of these lesions provided by the evolution of selective angiography and MRI has led to accurate classification systems based on topographic and anatomic criteria. However, there remains an element of subjective judgment, and some lesions will defy classification.

The Bicetre group [11, 12] classified spinal cord AVMs into three main groups:

- genetic hereditary lesions that are caused by a genetic disorder affecting vascular germinal cells, such as malformations associated with hereditary hemorrhagic telangiectasia;
- genetic non-hereditary lesions such as the Cobb syndrome (or spinal arteriovenous metameric syndrome), Klippel–Trenaunay and Parkes–Weber syndromes. These patients typically present with multiple shunts of the spinal cord and nerve root, bone, paraspinal, subcutaneous and skin tissue;
- single lesions that may reflect the incomplete expression of one of the situations mentioned above. These include spinal cord, nerve root, and filum terminale arteriovenous lesions. Most of the spinal vascular malformations with pial and dural arteriovenous shunts are included in this group.

Patsalides et al. [13] described a classification based on vascular anatomy and hemodynamic criteria as well as an overview on the anatomy and the pathophysiology of each spinal arteriovenous shunt. This classification was proposed with particular reference to the indications, contraindications, and techniques of endovascular treatment to achieve a safe, effective, multidisciplinary and tailored approach for each lesion. Two distinct categories were proposed.

The first category was an AVM with a nidus between the artery and vein. This could be classified into: (i) intramedullary (also known as type-II or glomus-type AVM); (ii) pial; (iii) epidural; or (iv) intramedullary and extramedullary (also known as type-III, intradural–extradural, juvenile AVM, or metameric AVM).

The second category was AVF with a direct shunt between the artery and vein. This could be classified into: (i) pial AVF (also known as type-IV, spinal cord AVF, ventral intradural AVF, or perimedullary AVF), which could be subdivided into small, large or giant; (ii) dural AVF (also known as type-I or dorsal intradural AVF); and (iii) epidural AVF (also known as extradural AVF).

Despite advancements in imaging modalities and continuous efforts for systematization of these lesions, the classification created between 1991 and 1998 by cooperation between authors [15, 16, 17] is the most widely used.

18.5.1 Type I: DAVFs

DAVFs are the most common type of spinal cord AVMs, comprising 70% of all spinal AVMs. These lesions show a male predominance (80%) and, in general, present in late adulthood (age, 40–60 years) [18]. In cerebral dural fistulas, a strong association with thrombosis in the cerebral vein [19] as well as levels of factor V Leiden and protein C has been demonstrated [20, 21]. These conditions or other causes such as infection [22] or trauma have been proposed as factors, but none of these seem to play a major part [23, 24, 25].

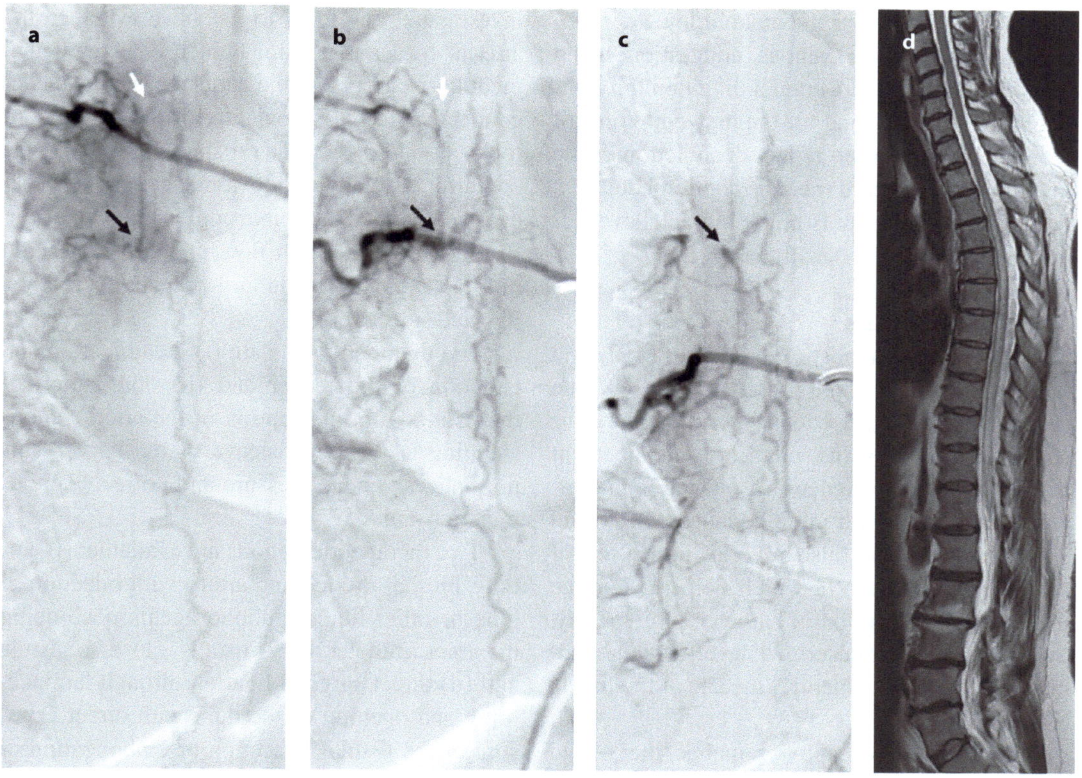

Fig. 18.1 Dural arteriovenous fistula (type I) with multiple feeders. The fistula is fed by left T6 (**a**) T7 (**b**) and T8 (**c**) thoracic radiculomedullary arteries. The main arteriovenous shunt is in T7 (*black arrow*) and is supported by adjacent levels. An additional small feeding vessel (*white arrow*) penetrates the dura at the T6 level and contributes to the venous outflow. T2 sagittal MRI (**d**) shows congestive myelopathy with spinal cord edema from T4 to the conus medullaris

18.5.1.1 Presentation

The typical presentation is radiculomyelopathy followed by progressive neurological deterioration. Subarachnoid hemorrhage is very uncommon, and acute deterioration in neurological function is unlikely. Most fistulas are solitary lesions and are found in the thoraco-lumbar region. Additional small feeding vessels from adjacent levels may also penetrate the dura and contribute to venous outflow (Fig. 18.1). In 2% of patients, double spinal DAVFs or an association of a spinal dural shunt with a spinal pial arteriovenous shunt may be present. The fistula is located inside the dura, where a radiculomeningeal artery enters the corresponding radicular vein, close to the spinal nerve root.

18.5.1.2 Clinical Course

The progressive clinical course is due to increased pressure in the spinal venous system that leads to venous congestion and consequent decreased drainage of normal spinal veins. The increased venous pressure yields chronic ischemia in the spinal cord, cell loss, and atrophy of the spinal cord. The impaired autoregulation yields direct transmission of changes in systemic arterial pressure to the spinal cord without the normal dampening effect of the venous plexus. Apart from the increased pressure caused by the shunt, in patients with AV fistulas, venous outflow may be less efficient to start with than is the case in healthy individuals [26, 27].

There are some differences in anatomic distribution of spinal venous outflow that justify the clinical presentation and clinical course. In general, the lower thoracic region has relatively fewer venous outflow channels at a segmental level than the cervical or lumbosacral regions [28].

These differences in segmental outflow are probably responsible for venous congestion being transmitted in a caudo–cranial direction throughout the spinal cord, and for the first symptoms of myelopathy tending to reflect dysfunction of the lowest part of the cord (i.e., the conus medullaris) even though the shunt is at the thoracic level (or in some cases near the skull base) [29].

18.5.1.3 Diagnosis

The essential diagnostic tools are MRI and selective catheter angiography. On MRI, the combination of cord edema, perimedullary arterialized dilated veins, and cord enhancement is characteristic. Magnetic resonance angiography (undertaken with more advanced 1.5-T and 3-T machines) may also give an indication of the level of the DAVF, which helps to confine the extent and duration of catheter angiography. Some authors have described the effectiveness of multidetector CT to identify the site of the fistula [30, 31, 32, 33].

Catheter angiography remains the "gold standard" in the diagnosis of DAVFs. The examination should be undertaken *via* femoral access using a 5-F catheter carefully studying bilaterally not only the intercostal and lumbar arteries, but also the median sacral artery as well as the hypogastric and lateral sacral arteries. In the upper part, the deep cervical and ascending cervical arteries should be injected selectively. If a dural arteriovenous shunt is not found, then intracranial vessels should be studied selectively, including vertebral arteries, internal carotid arteries (meningohypophyseal trunk) and external carotid branches, such as the ascending pharyngeal artery, middle meningeal artery and occipital artery (Fig. 18.2). An essential part of the examination is to identify the artery of Adamkiewicz. If needed, because of clinical status or excessive administration of the contrast medium, selective angiography should be divided into different sessions. If the fistula is not detected, the examination should be repeated few weeks later.

18.5.1.4 Treatment

The angio-architecture of the fistula should be investigated carefully to establish whether the arterial feeder is a dural branch or a segmental medullary artery. In the latter case, the feeder contributes to the vasculature of the spinal cord (anterior and posterolateral spinal arteries). This condition excludes endovascular treatment because damage to the spinal cord is likely to occur. In rare cases, the high flow of the fistula could hide a segmental medullary branch, even when injected selectively.

The treatment goals are (i) identification and isolation of the feeder and (ii) obliteration of the fistula with interruption of the arteriovenous shunting at the dural sleeve of the nerve. This normalizes venous pressure and corrects venous hypertension.

Two therapeutic options are available: (i) embolization of the feeding artery with injection of glue or other liquid embolic agents positioning the microcatheter very distally close to fistula and (ii) direct surgical ligation through laminectomy and opening of the dura with direct exposure of the fistula. Resection or embolization of arterialized veins should be avoided. Embolization in well chosen cases is a safe and effective therapy for DAVFs. Direct surgical exposure is preferred if glue migration in the draining veins can be predicted or if the feeder is a segmental medullary artery.

18.5.2 Type II: Intramedullary Glomus AVMs

Intramedullary glomus AVMs are "true" intramedullary AVMs of the spinal cord. They are distributed along the entire spinal cord axis, and may be located inside the parenchyma (intramedullary AVMs), at the surface of the spinal cord (pial AVMs), in the epidural space (epidural AVMs), or may have a more complex anatomy with intramedullary and extramedullary components without tissue boundaries. AVMs located in the conus medullaris represent a distinct type, and can extend to the cauda equina and along the filum terminale.

The glomus type is the most commonly encountered intramedullary vascular malformation,

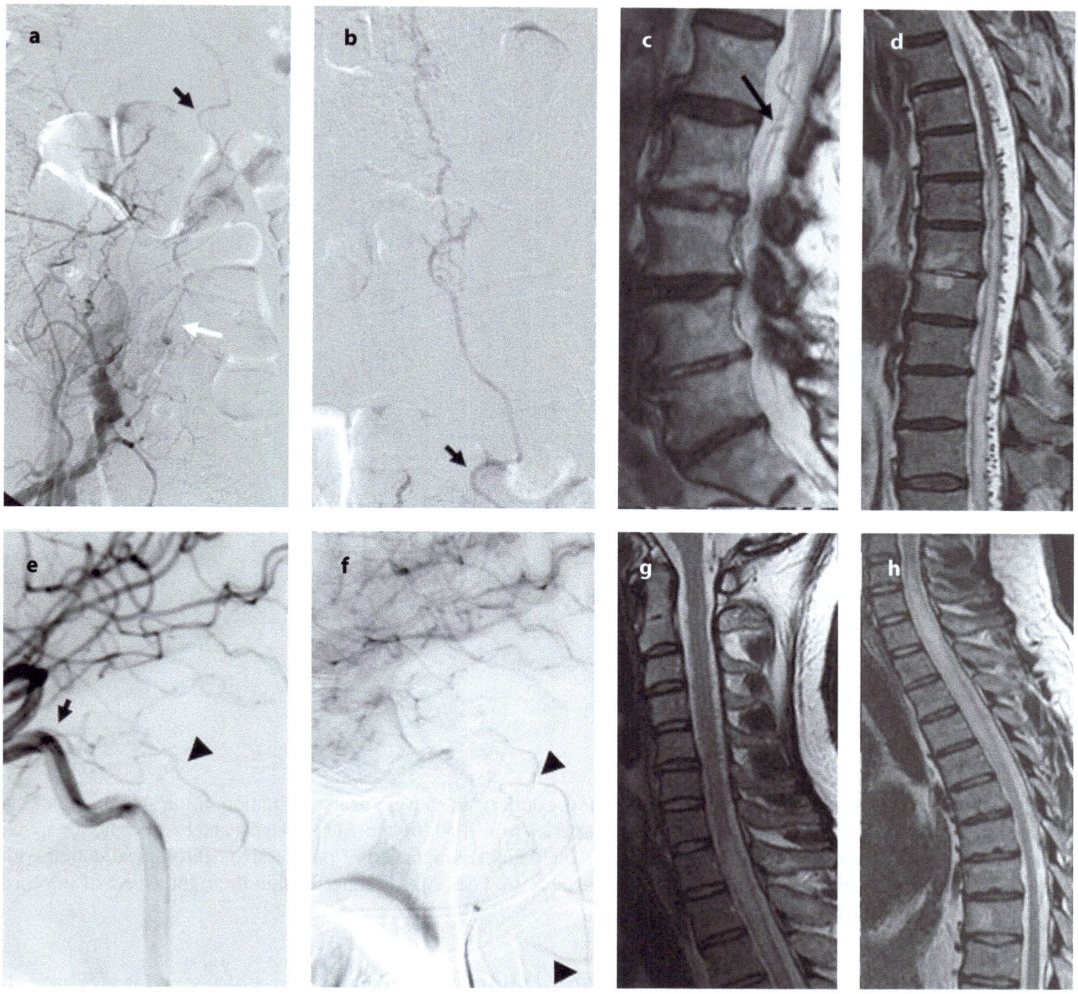

Fig. 18.2 Atypical dural arteriovenous fistulas. These cases highlight the importance of complete angiographic evaluation that should be done from the cranium to the sacrum. **a–d**: A 73-year-old patient. Dural arteriovenous fistula (type I) supported by tiny arteries arising from the left hypogastric artery. The feeder pierces the dura at the S2 level and communicates with the sacral epidural veins (*white arrow*). The spinal venous drainage (black arrow) runs along the cauda and reaches the conus medullaris at the L1 level. MRI shows congestive myelopathy of the conus medulalris with perimedullary dilated veins. **e–h**: A 42-year-old patient with progressive neurological impairment. Selective angiography shows a type-V Cognard intracranial dural arteriovenous fistula fed by the meningohypophyseal trunk of the left internal carotid artery (*black arrow*). The fistula drains into the petrous and spinal perimedullary veins (*black arrowheads*). There are no feeders from the external carotid and vertebral branches or from the radiculomedullary arteries. MRI shows congestive myelopathy of the upper thoracic segment (from C7 to T6) with perimedullary dilated veins

representing 20% of all spinal vascular malformations. These lesions are characterized by a compact intramedullary nidus that occupies a short segment of the spinal cord, with multiple feeding vessels arising from the anterior or posterior spinal arteries (or both) and drainage into an arterialized coronal venous plexus [10, 34]. Analogous to brain AVMs, they represent a focal network of arteriovenous shunts that drain into the spinal veins (Fig. 18.3). Associated aneurysms of the feeding arteries and the nidus are common [35].

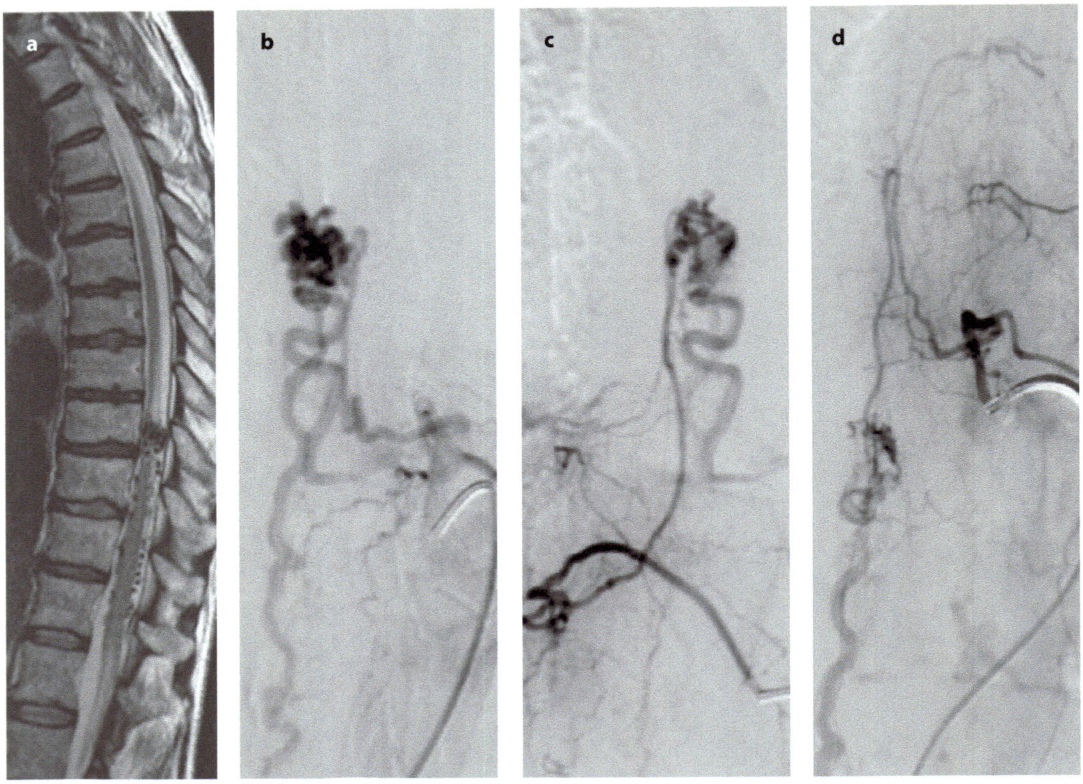

Fig. 18.3 Glomus-type spinal cord AVM (type II). Intramedullary arteriovenous malformation of the spinal cord at the T9 level (**a**). The AVM is fed by posterolateral spinal arteries from T10 (**b**) and T11 (**c**) levels and by the anterior spinal artery from the left T8 radiculo-medullary artery (**d**). The patient complained of progressive neurological deficit with painful paraplegia (as well as sensory and sphincter disorders). The AVM is superficial in the right aspect of the cord and drains downwards in the epidural plexus

18.5.2.1 Presentation and Clinical Course

Intramedullary AVMs show an equal distribution between men and women and, in general, present at an early age. The clinical course of these lesions is marked by progressive and fluctuating myelopathy, paraplegia and pain, overlaid by periods of acute neurological deterioration secondary to hemorrhage within the AVM. Sudden-onset presentation (often with profound neurological impairment and possible transverse myelopathy) is common. Subarachnoid and intramedullary hemorrhage often occurs in these lesions. The mortality related to type-II malformations has been reported to be 17.6%. After initial hemorrhage, the prevalence of re-bleed is 10% within the first month and 40% within the first year.

18.5.2.2 Diagnosis

Despite advances in CT and MRI, selective angiography remains the gold standard. Through femoral access, all feeders must be selectively catheterized (using a 5-F catheter) and evaluated. Undertaking the examination with the patient under general anesthesia improves the quality of the study. In this condition, the patient remains comfortable during a potentially long study and apnea can be carried out to reduce motion artefacts. In patients complaining of pain and sensimotor disturbances, selective injection could be even more painful.

18.5.2.3 Treatment

There is a general consensus among physicians/surgeons dealing with spinal lesions regarding the need to treat intramedullary AVMs or to modify the natural history and decrease the risk of future hemorrhage.

The prognosis for untreated spinal cord

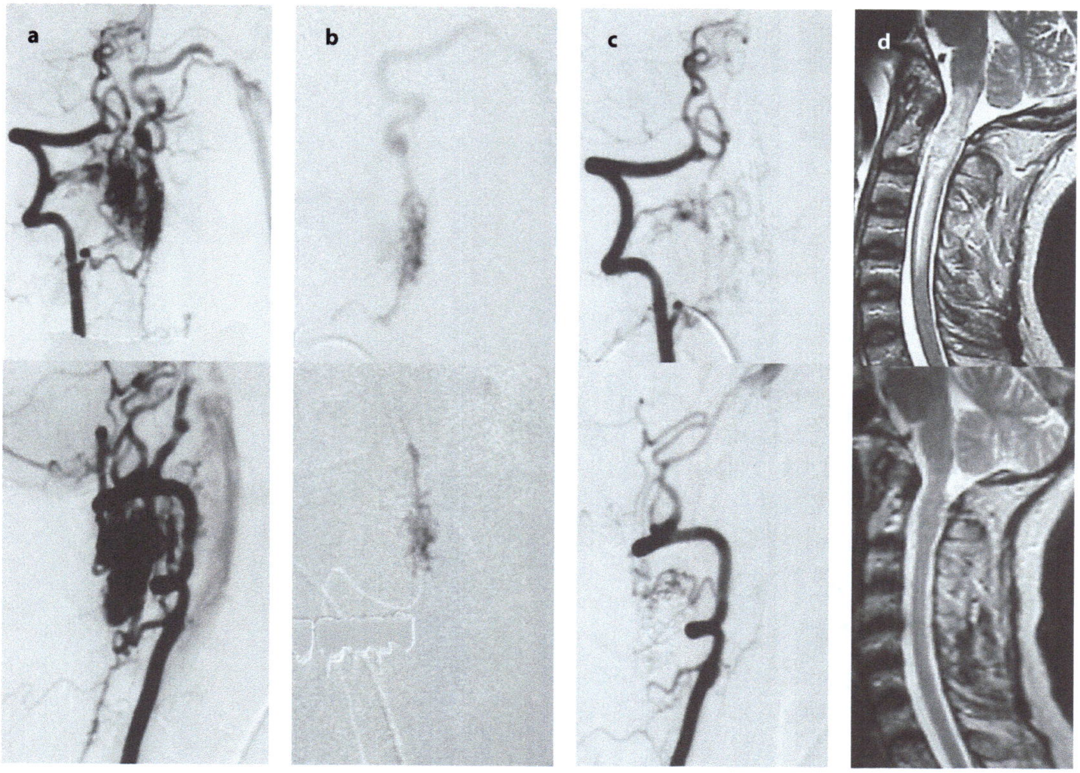

Fig. 18.4 Glomus-type spinal cord AVM (type II). (**a**) Anteroposterior and lateral view of a C1–C2 intramedullary diffuse arteriovenous malformation fed by segmental branches of the right and left vertebral arteries. (**b, c**) Super-selective angiography of a right segmental feeder and NBCA-selective injection. (**d**) T2 sagittal MRI undertaken the following day shows diffuse myelopathy that recovered at 6-months. The patient showed good recovery with residual neurological deficits

AVMs is poor, with 36% of patients younger than 40 years of age developing severe impairment after 3 years of evolution [36, 37, 38].

Therapeutic options are available: embolization, surgery, or both. Surgical obliteration can be associated with a high intraoperative risk of neurological injury (especially for lesions in the anterior cord). Posterior superficial location makes a lesion more amenable to safe surgical resection [39]. In selected cases, resection of the residual nidus after embolization can be considered.

Embolization plays an important part in the management of intramedullary AVMs as primary treatment or as an adjunct to surgery. Even partial embolization can improve the prognosis. Endovascular treatment can be undertaken using particulate material or liquid embolic agents (Fig. 18.4). As primary treatment, through reduction in arterial steal and improved perfusion in the spinal cord, immediate clinical improvement has been noted in >50% of patients after embolization. Recanalization, however, occurs over time, with the continued risk of hemorrhage. Liquid agents such as n-butyl-cyanoacrylate (NBCA) glue and Onyx can achieve a permanent occlusion with a very low prevalence of recanalization [10, 40] but carry the concurrent risk of inadvertent embolization of normal perforating arteries that may not be visible on angiography. Hence, a liquid agent should be used when feasible, especially if embolization is the primary or sole treatment. In addition, treatment of selected intramedullary AVMs with the CyberKnife Robotic Radiosurgery System™ has been reported [41].

Conus medullaris AVMs are a particular category of type-II malformations characterized

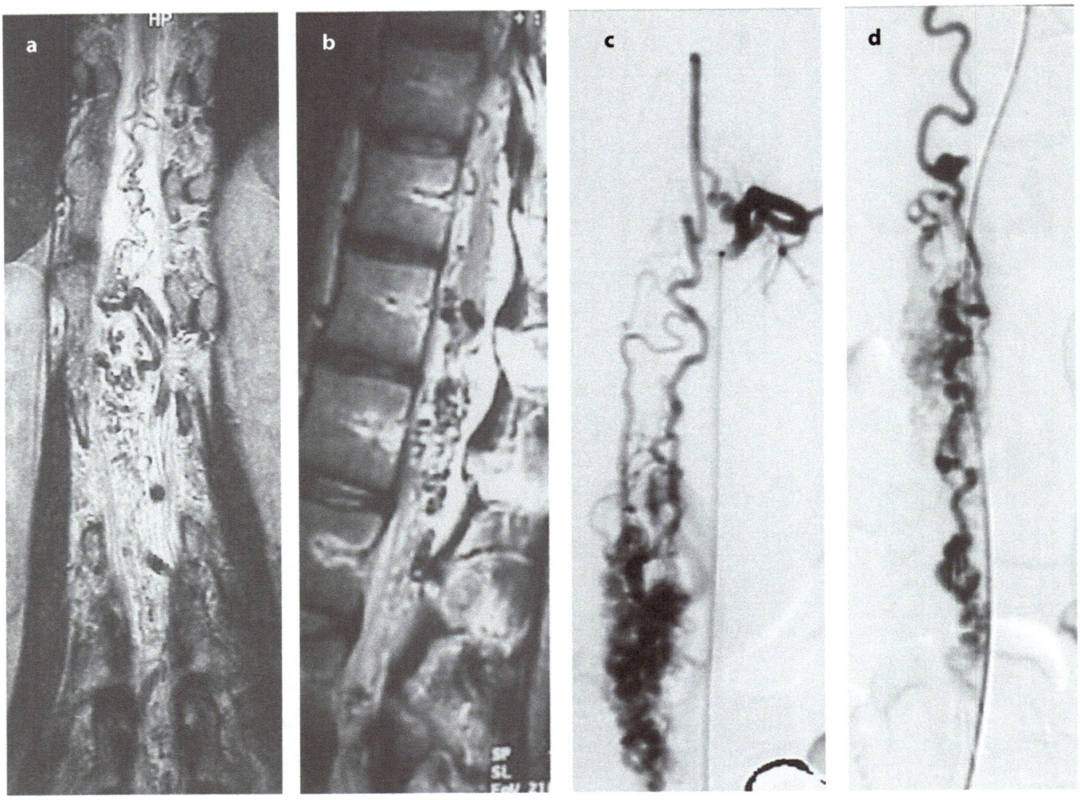

Fig. 18.5 **a-d** Juvenile diffuse-type AVM (type III). Large and complex high-flow AVM of the conus medullaris fed by posterolateral spinal arteries and by the anterior spinal artery. An associated aneurysm of the anterior spinal artery is present

by the simultaneous presence of an anterior and dorsal intradural arteriovenous shunt with multiple feeders and an intramedullary AVM. The association with a tethered cord has been reported. Presentation is usually with myelopathy, radicular symptoms and early bowel/bladder deficits. Their extensive nature and multiple arterial feeders make them difficult to treat by embolization alone. Initial embolization followed by resection might be the optimal treatment.

18.5.3 Type III: Juvenile AVMs (Diffuse-type AVMs)

Juvenile spinal AVMs are extremely rare. These lesions are true AVMs with an intramedullary nidus that may occupy the entire spinal canal at the involved level. Cord tissue is present within the AVM interspaces. They are extensive lesions with abnormal vessels that can be intramedullary and extramedullary in location. Extension of extraspinal paraspinous structures is possible. Juvenile AVMs are large and complex lesions, with multiple arterial feeding arteries often arising from different cord levels [10, 13]. Associated aneurysms of the feeding arteries and within the nidus are common (Fig. 18.5). With regard to hemodynamics, they are very high-flow lesions. Cardiac output requirements may be significantly increased and a bruit is commonly noted. They occur most commonly in childhood and young adults with various clinical scenarios.

18.5.3.1 Presentation

Presentation is similar to that seen with type-II AVMs. Acute onset of symptoms can occur secondary to subarachnoid hemorrhage (SAH), whereas progressive motor and sensory deterioration as well as sphincter disturbance usually result from vascular steal, venous hypertension, or mass effect on the spinal cord and/or nerve roots from the dilated veins. SAH usually occurs from venous rupture or aneurysm rupture. Hematomyelia has also been observed after rupture of subpial spinal veins. The mass effect caused by dilated veins on the cord or nerve roots explains the sometimes asymmetric nature of deficits.

18.5.3.2 Diagnosis

Selective spinal angiography reveals scattered vessels in the spinal cord matter, direct AVM feeders passing from the ventral or dorsal spinal arteries (and sometimes from the radiculopial arteries). The AVM is drained by dilated perimedullary veins. Intramedullary AVMs are typically limited by the spinal cord or the conglomeration of vessels spread on the surface of the spinal cord.

18.5.3.3 Treatment

Considering their size and vascular complexity, the natural history and prognosis after any type of treatment for these lesions should be considered very poor. A multidisciplinary approach is tailored on the extension, location and angioarchitectural features of these lesions. Surgery and embolization may be used alone or in combination. Achieving complete cure in these types of AVMs is extremely difficult and probably associated with increased morbidity. Palliative treatment could be considered, and targeted endovascular or surgical approaches could be done to relieve symptoms that may be caused by a hematoma, arterial steal, venous hypertension, or direct mass effect.

18.5.4 Type IV: Perimedullary AVFs

These lesions are not true AVMs but AVFs. The fistulous connection is intradural but extramedullary, located on the ventral or dorsal surface of the spinal cord (Fig. 18.6). They result from a direct communication between one or more feeding arteries arising from the anterior spinal artery and an enlarged draining vein without an interposed vascular network. Presentation occurs in the third-to-sixth decade [10]. SAH is possible, with subsequent acute neurological deterioration. A gradual but progressive neurological deterioration is common. Three subcategories of intradural spinal AVFs have been recognized.

Type-IVa AVFs feature a single feeding artery (often the artery of Adamkiewicz) with low flow through the arteriovenous shunt and moderate venous enlargement. Endovascular techniques are difficult due to the small size of feeding vessels. Surgical excision is therefore often preferred.

Type-IVb AVFs are intermediate in size, often with multiple feeding arteries, and more marked venous enlargement. Venous ectasia may develop at the shunting site. Embolization in these lesions is possible due to the increased size of feeding arteries. In cases of incomplete obliteration of the shunt, direct surgical excision may be needed.

Type-IVc AVFs are the largest one of these types of fistulas. They are multipediculated, with high blood flow, and enlarged, tortuous draining veins. Spinal ischemia may develop in these lesions secondary to vascular steal. Surgery is technically difficult due to the size of these lesions. Treatment is through a combination of endovascular reduction followed by surgical excision of residual elements.

18.5.5 Other Types: Spinal Aneurysms

Spinal aneurysms not related to a vascular malformation are extremely rare. They seldom occur at branching points, instead they develop along the course of an artery [47]. Spinal aneurysms lack a clear neck and usually appear as fusiform dilations. The fusiform nature of these lesions makes clipping difficult and favors sacrifice of the parent artery. Endovascular techniques can also be considered.

18.5.6 New Classifications

Vascular malformations represent rare and insufficiently studied pathological entities characterized by considerable variability. As mentioned

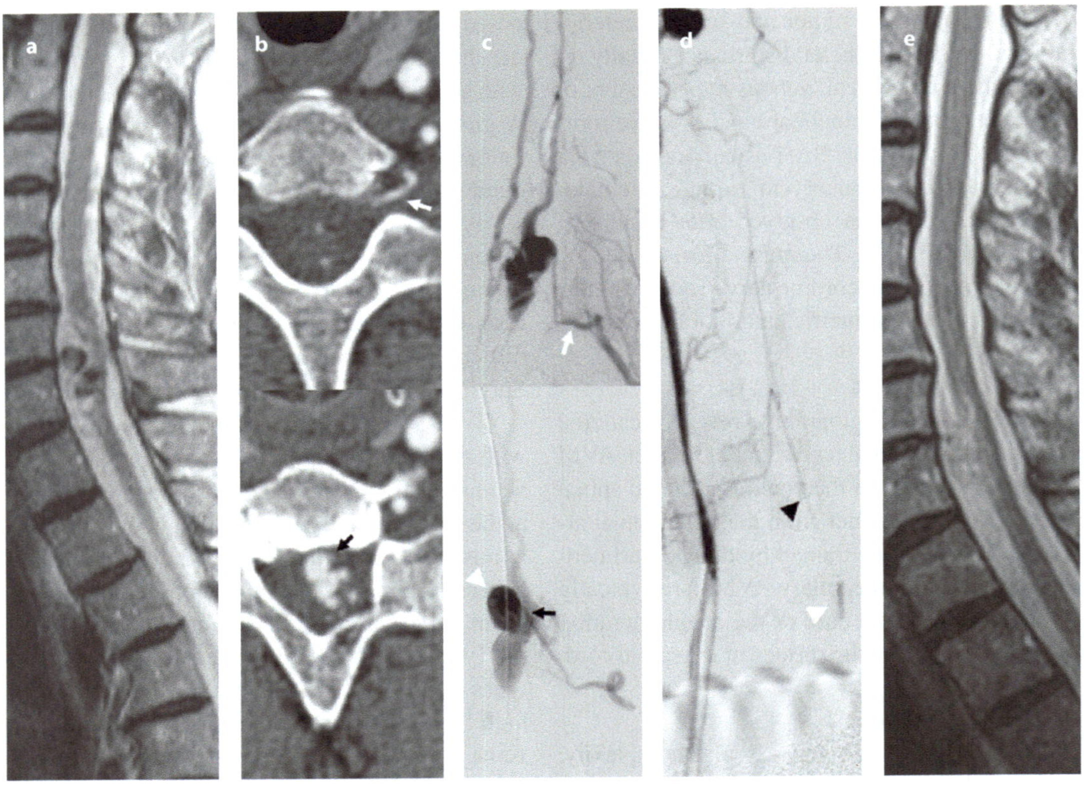

Fig. 18.6 Perimedullary arteriovenous fistula (type IV). 64-year-old patient with paresthesia in the right arm and upper trunk with a C6 type-IVb arteriovenous fistula. The arteriovenous fistula is fed by the left anterior radiculomedullary artery arising from the deep cervical artery. There is direct communication between the C6 main feeder and ventral enlarged venous pouch. An aneurysm is seen in the course of the radiculomedullary artery (*white arrowhead*). The fistula receives a low-flow feeder from the anterior spinal artery. There is marked venous enlargement with ascending drainage in the perimedullary veins.
a T2 sagittal MRI shows venous dilatations that compress and displace the cervical spinal cord with anterior myelopathy. **b** Axial CT images and left C6 selective angiography show a hypertrophic left ventral radiculomedullary artery at the C6 level (*white arrow*). An aneurysm (*black arrow*) is seen just before the entrance of the ventral radiculomedullary artery in the hypertrophic venous drainage (**c**). **d** Right vertebral selective angiography shows the anterior spinal artery supported by upper-level segmental arteries (*black arrowhead*). Very low-flow communication between the anterior spinal artery and the aneurysm (*white arrowhead*) is shown. **e** Sagittal T2 MRI obtained 1 week after endovascular occlusion shows disappearance of the venous enlargements with persistent edema of the anterior aspect of the cord

above, advancement in MRI and CT technology, improved definition of angiography and a more dedicated super-selective catheterization armamentarium have extended our knowledge significantly and led to new classification systems based on hemodynamic, topographic and anatomical criteria. Until now, a detailed and widely accepted systematization of spinal vascular malformations has not been proposed. Such a scheme should facilitate treatment planning and different tactics for endovascular and surgical interventions [44, 48]. Treatment options should be differentiated with regard to the localization, angio-architectural type and hemodynamic peculiarities of malformations: this would allow optimization of the results of treatment.

Different authors have tried to find a clear systematization of spinal vascular lesions. Spetzler et al. [48, 49] and Zozulya et al. [44] offered new classifications of spinal vascular pathological entities (Tables 18.1 and 18.2) based on anatomical, pathophysiological or angio-architectural features. Patsalides et al. [10] offered a classification based on hemodynamic criteria.

A new classification system has been proposed recently by Geibprasert et al. [50] for dural AVFs (cranial and spinal). This classification system describes not only the topographies, arterial feeders and drainage patterns, but also considers the different parts played by each epidural area involved, as revealed during the development and embryology of the venous system. They redefined AVFs in three groups on the basis of the embryologic development of the venous drainage of the surrounding structures: the ventral, dorsal, and lateral epidural groups.

The ventral epidural group consists of shunts into those veins that normally drain structures developed from the notochord (i.e., the vertebral body at the spinal level). These veins are known as the "basivertebral venous plexus", which subsequently drain into the anterior internal vertebral venous plexus, located at the ventral epidural space of the spinal canal, which joins the basilar venous plexus and cavernous sinus cranially. The previously called "epidural," "osteodural," or "paravertebral" arteriovenous shunts can be categorized into this group. Because the draining veins of these shunts do not drain the spine but instead the bone, these shunts will not become symptomatic due to venous congestion of the cord. They may become symptomatic due to compression of the spinal cord or of the nerve roots by the enlarged epidural venous pouches. Only a few case reports have described the associated perimedullary reflux causing congestive myelopathy. A hypothesis about a possible defective valve-like mechanism impeding retrograde flow from the epidural plexus to perimedullary veins has been put forward to explain this finding. However, it could also be argued that the reflux is due to an extensive thrombosis of the normal epidural outlets that leads to secondary retrograde drainage into the perimedullary veins [8].

The dorsal epidural group of arteriovenous shunts is related to veins that normally drain the spinous process and lamina at the spinal level. Although they are related to the major dural venous sinuses (superior sagittal sinus as well as torcular and transverse sinuses) at the cranial level, the corresponding veins at the spinal level are poorly developed and comprise a pair of longitudinal channels (i.e., the posterior internal venous plexus). Patients with dural arteriovenous shunts within this space typically present with spontaneous epidural hematomas. These shunts are extremely rare.

Table 18.1 Classification of vascular lesions in the spinal cord proposed by Spetzler et al. in 2002 based on anatomical and pathophysiological features. Authors identified three primary or broad categories: neoplasms, aneurysms, and arteriovenous lesions. Arteriovenous lesions are further subdivided based on their neuroanatomy [49]

Mechanism
Neoplastic vascular lesions
hemangioblastoma
cavernous malformation
Spinal aneurysms
Arteriovenous fistulas
extradural
intradural
ventral (A, small shunt; B, medium shunt; C, large shunt)
dorsal (A, single feeder; B, multiple feeders)
Arteriovenous malformations
extradural–intradural
intradural
intramedullary
compact
diffuse
conus medullaris

The most common "classic" types of spinal DAVFs are lateral epidural DAVFs. These arteriovenous shunts develop in the lateral epidural space at the junction of the bridging (or radicular) veins that connects the spinal cord drainage to the epidural venous system. Outflow obstruction of its adjacent venous outlet due to thrombosis or fibrosis related to aging leads to immediate drainage into the perimedullary veins. As a result, subjects present with aggressive symptoms and at an older age. A strong male predominance is also observed, which is similar to that observed in the cranially located lateral epidural DAVFs, such as in the foramen magnum (medulla bridging vein) and tentorial (petrosal bridging vein) locations [8].

Table 18.2 Classification of vascular malformations in the spinal cord proposed by Zozulya et al in 2006 based on anatomical characteristics as well as angio-architectural and hemodynamic features. Reproduced with permission from [44]

Axial	Lengthwise	Feeding Vessels	Structural Features	Drainage	Hemodynamic Features
I. Intramedullary	1. Cervical 2. Thoracic 3. Conus medullaris	1. Ant. spinal art. 2. Post. spinal art. 3. Radiculopial art. 4. Combined	1. Glomus or compact 2. Diffuse	1. Perimedullary veins	A. Low flow B. Mod. flow C. high flow
II. Intradural or Perimedullary	1. Cervical 2. Thoracic 3. Conus medullaris	1. Ant. spinal art. 2. Ant. radiculomed. art. 3. Post. spinal art. 4. Ant. radiculomed. art. 5. Combined	1. Glomus AVM 2. AVF	1. Ant. perimedullary veins 2. Post. perimedullary veins	A. Low flow B. Mod. flow C. High flow
III. Dural	1. Cervical 2. Thoracic 3. Lumbar	1. Radiculo-meningeal artery	1. Microglomus AVM 2. AVF	1. Retrograde into ant. perimedullary veins 2. Retrograde into post. perimedullary veins 3. Anterograde into epidural veins	A. Low flow
IV. Epidural	1. Cervical 2. Thoracic 3. Lumbar	1. VAs 2. Spinal branch of segmental arteries 3. Post-central branches 4. Pre-laminar branches 5. Combined	1. Glomus AVM 2. AVF	1. Epidural veins 2. Paravertebral veins	A. Low flow B. Mod. flow C. High flow
V. Intravertebral	1. Cervical 2. Thoracic 3. Lumbar	1. Ventrolateral branches of segmental arteries 2. Post-central branches 3. Pre-laminar branches 4. Combined 4.1 One side 4.2 Both sides	1. Glomus AVM limited by vertebra 2. Glomus AVM w/ paravertebral spreading	1. Epidural veins 2. Paravertebral veins 3. Combined	A. Low flow B. Mod. flow C. High flow
VI. Combined	1. Cervical 2. Thoracic 3. Lumbar	1. Mainly from spinal branches 2. Mainly from radiculo-medullary arteries	1. Mainly intradural glomus AVM 2. Mainly intradural glomus AVM	1. Mainly perimedullary veins 2. Mainly epidural veins 3. Mainly paravertebral veins 4. Combined	A. Low flow B. Mod. flow C. High flow

Ant, anterior; *AVF*, arteriovenous fistula; *AVM*, arteriovenous malformation; *mod*, moderate; *post*, posterior; *radiculo-med. art.*, radiculomedullary artery; *radiculopial art*, radiculopial artery.

18.6 Therapeutic Options

The decision to undertake treatment on any individual with an AVM requires careful consideration of possible benefits *versus* risks. The natural history of an individual AVM is difficult to predict. However, left untreated, they can cause significant damage and hemorrhage, which may result in severe neurological deficits or death. Conversely, embolization, surgery or radiosurgery on any part of the central nervous system (and particularly in the spinal cord) carry risks. There is no easy "formula" that can allow physicians and patients to reach a decision on optimal therapy. all therapeutic decisions must be made on a case-by-case basis (especially for AVMs in the spinal cord).

All treatment options exist for AVMs and AVFs: microsurgery, endovascular embolization, and radiosurgery. The choice of treatment is dependent largely on the symptoms, location and angio-architectural features (size, arterial supply, venous drainage) of the malformation [51].

In type-I AVFs, symptoms increase over an extended period of months-to-years, and include progressive weakness of the legs and concurrent difficulties in the bowel or bladder. In these patients, surgical or endovascular treatment is essential, and it is imperative to occlude the shunt as soon as possible to interrupt and revert damage to the spinal cord [52]. In 2008, Narvid et al. [53] described a 20-year experience with surgical and endovascular approaches. Thirty-nine patients underwent an initial endovascular embolization, and 69% required only the first procedure for complete obliteration compared with 83% of the 24 patients that were treated successfully with a single surgical procedure. The ability to treat spinal AVFs definitively using endovascular embolization has significantly improved over the last years. Overall rates of definitive embolization have ranged between 25% and 100% and are dependent upon the embolic agent used and partially on the use of variable-stiffness microcatheters. Most of the recent studies in which *N*-butyl cyanoacrylate or other liquid embolic agents were used have reported success rates of 70–90%. Surgery remains the definitive option in cases of failed embolization and recanalization or in lesions not amenable to embolization. Clinical outcomes have been comparable with surgical treatment if the fistula and draining vein remain persistently occluded. Improvements in gait and motor function are more likely after successful treatment, whereas urinary disorders are less likely to improve.

In subjects with intradural AVMs/AVFs (types 2 and 4), an important consideration before intervention is preoperative neurological status. Typically, these patients present acutely after intraparenchymal hemorrhage or SAH. Rarely, patients present because of vascular steal or chronic myelopathy, in which oxygenated arterial blood shunted through the AVM causes the surrounding normal parenchyma to become hypoperfused or high-flow fistulas cause venous engorgement. Lastly, patients with intradural lesions can present with the mass effect caused by the growth of feeders and draining veins of the AVM. Enlargement of the vascular malformation compresses the surrounding neural tissue, impairing neurological function. Treatment planning is based on the hemodynamics of the lesion, on its location in the axial and longitudinal plane, and on the angio-architecture.

Embolization is the first-line treatment for many arteriovenous anomalies. However, surgery continues to have a key role, and a multidisciplinary approach is essential. Maximum functional results can be obtained in patients treated early before advanced deterioration. In patients with severe neurological impairment, partial results can be obtained. Particular consideration is necessary in hemorrhagic patients. In 2004, Rodesch et al. [12] described their experience with 155 patients with high-flow spinal cord arteriovenous shunts. Although bleeding can have severe consequences, the short-term prognosis after the hemorrhage seems less serious than initially thought. In their series, improvement was seen in >70% of patients, and therefore emergency treatment (surgical or endovascular) should not be considered as primary management. Early acute rebleedings were mostly due to re-rupture of an associated false aneurysm. In such cases, early target embolization should be considered [54].

Embolization plays an important part in the management of dural and intramedullary spinal AVMs as primary treatment or as an adjunct to surgery. A few basic considerations should always be taken into account. The migration of embolic agents distally with occlusion of the venous drainage of a large arteriovenous shunt carries increased risks. In an AVM, this might lead to increased pressure in the nidus and subsequent hemorrhage whereas, in an AVF, this may lead to increased venous engorgement due to occlusion of the normal drainage of the spinal cord. A too-proximal occlusion of a feeding artery to an arteriovenous shunt is usually ineffective because other arterial anastomoses may subsequently be recruited to supply the shunt. This may also lead to increased arterial steal because blood will now be diverted to the shunt. Simultaneously, the ability to access the shunt for further embolization is diminished or definitely compromised. Occlusion of high-flow feeding arteries of a lesion with arterial steal leads to diminution of the arterial steal and to the possible appearance of normal spinal arteries which are not opacified in the pre-embolization angiogram. This event should be considered to avoid or limit inadvertent embolization of normal territories.

Microcatheters allow selective catheterization of tiny arteries feeding the AVM/AVF. As a rule, coils are not used in these lesions. They can achieve only proximal embolization, which may lead to the development of collateral flow to the shunts. The use of particles has the advantage of stepwise embolization and the ability to follow the results *via* clinical and angiographic means during the procedure, but has the serious disadvantage of recanalization. Treatment with particle embolization requires annual angiographic control and additional embolizations [10, 56]. Liquid agents have the advantage of achieving more permanent occlusion with a very low rate of recanalization. In general, a liquid agent (e.g., NBCA or Onyx) should be used if embolization is the primary or sole treatment [10, 40]. The liquid agent should be delivered within (or as close as possible to) the shunt to better control the injection and to ensure complete occlusion.

References

1. Lasjaunias PL, Berenstein A, Ter Brugge KG (2001) Surgical neuroangiography, vol 1: clinical vascular anatomy and variations. Springer Verlag, Heidelberg
2. Lazorthes G, Gouaze A, Zadeh O (1971) Arterial vascularisation of the spinal cord: recent studies of the arterial substitution pathways. J Neurosurg 35, 253–262
3. Santillan A, Nacarino V, Greenberg E, Riina HA, Gobin YP, Patsalides A (2011) Vascular anatomy of the spinal cord. J NeuroIntervent Surg 4:67–74
4. Krings T, Geibprasert S, Thron A (2009) Spinal vascular anatomy. In: Naidich T (ed) Neuroradiology of the brain and spine. Elsevier, New York
5. Thron AK (1988) Vascular anatomy of the spinal cord: Neuroradiological anatomy and clinical syndromes. Springer Verlag, Vienna
6. Gillilan LA (1970). Veins of the spinal cord. Anatomic details; suggested clinical applications. Neurology 20:860–868
7. Jellema K, Tijssen CC, van Gijn J (2006) Spinal dural arteriovenous fistulas: a congestive myelopathy that initially mimics a peripheral nerve disorder. Brain 129:3150–3164
8. Krings T, Geibprasert S (2009) Spinal dural arteriovenous fistulas. Am J Neuroradiol 30:639–648
9. Hurth M, Houdart R, Djindjian R et al (1978) Arteriovenous malformations of the spinal cord: clinical, anatomical and therapeutic consideration: a series of 150 cases. Progr Neurol Surg 9:238–266
10. Patsalides A, Knopman J, A. Santillan A, Tsiouris AJ, Riina H, Gobin YP (2011) Endovascular treatment of spinal arteriovenous. Lesions: beyond the dural fistula. Am J Neuroradiol 32:798–808
11. Rodesch G, Hurth M, Alvarez H et al (2002) Classification of spinal cord arteriovenous shunts: proposal for a reappraisal – the Bicetre experience with 155 consecutive patients treated between 1981 and 1999. Neurosurgery 51:374–379
12. Rodesch G, Hurth M, Alvarez H et al (2004) Angioarchitecture of spinal cord arteriovenous shunts at presentation: clinical correlations in adults and children – the Bicetre experience on 155 consecutive patients seen between 1981–1999. Acta Neurochir (Wien)146:217–226
13. Krings T, Mull M, Gilsbach JM et al (2005) Spinal vascular malformations. Eur Radiol 15:267–278
14. Jellema K, Canta LR, Tijssen CC et al (2003) Spinal dural arteriovenous fistulas: clinical features in 80 patients. J Neurol Neurosurg Psychiatry 74:1438–1440
15. Bao YH, Ling F (1997) Classification and therapeutic modalities of spinal vascular malformations in 80 patients. Neurosurgery 40:75–81
16. Barrow DL, Awad IA (eds) (1999) Conceptual overview and management strategies in spinal vascular malformations. American Association of Neurological Surgeons, Park Ridge, p 169–180
17. Berenstein A, Lasjaunias P (1992) Spinal dural arteriovenous fistulas. In: Surgical neuroangiography: en-

dovascular treatment of spine and spinal cord lesions. Springer, Berlin
18. Koch C (2006) Spinal dural arteriovenous fistula. Curr Opin Neurol 19:69–75.
19. *Tsai LK, Jeng JS, Liu HM, Wang HJ, Yip PK (2004).* Intracranial dural arteriovenous fistulas with or without cerebral sinus thrombosis: analysis of 69 patients. *Neurol Neurosurg Psychiatry* 75: 1639–1641
20. Kraus JA, Stuper BK, Berlit P (1998) Association of resistance to activated protein C and dural arteriovenous fistulas. J Neurol 245:731–733
21. Kraus JA, Stuper BK, Nahser HC, Klockgether T, Berlit P (2000) Significantly increased prevalence of factor V Leiden in patients with dural arteriovenous fistulas. J Neurol 247:521–523
22. Foix CH, Alajouanine T (1926) La myelite necrotique subaigue. Rev Neurol 46:1–42
23. Jellema K, Tijssen CC, Fijnheer R, de Groot PG, Koudstaal PJ, van Gijk J (2004) Spinal dural arteriovenous fistulas are not associated with prothrombotic factors. Stroke 35:2069–2071
24. Gerlach R, Boehm-Weigert M, Berkefeld J et al (2008) Thrombophilic risk factors in patients with cranial and spinal dural arteriovenous fistulae. Neurosurgery 63:693–698
25. Jellema K, Tijssen CC, Sluzewski M, van Asbeck FW, Koudstaal PJ, van Gijn J (2006) Spinal dural arteriovenous fistulas – an underdiagnosed disease. A review of patients admitted to the spinal unit of a rehabilitation center. J Neurol 253:159–162.
26. Merland JJ, Riche MC, Chiras J (1980) Intraspinal extramedullary arteriovenous fistulae draining into the medullary veins. J Neuroradiol 7:271–320.
27. Thron A (2001) Spinal dural arteriovenous fistulas. Radiologe 41:955–960
28. Tadié M, Hemet J, Freger P, Clavier E, Creissard P (1985) Morphological and functional anatomy of spinal cord veins. J Neuroradiol 12:3–20
29. Asakawa H, Yanaka K, Fujita K, Marushima A, Anno I, Nose T (2002) Intracranial dural arteriovenous fistula showing diffuse MR enhancement of the spinal cord: case report and review of the literature. Surg Neurol 58:251–257
30. Mull M, Nijenhuis RJ, Backes WH et al (2007) Value and limitations of contrast-enhanced MR angiography in spinal arteriovenous malformations and dural arteriovenous fistulas. Am J Neuroradiol 28:1249–1258
31. Yamaguchi S, Eguchi K, Kiura Y et al (2007) Multidetector-row CT angiography as a preoperative evaluation for spinal arteriovenous fistulae. Neurosurg Rev 30:321–326
32. Hetts SW, Moftakhar P, English JD et al (2012) Spinal dural arteriovenous fistulas and intrathecal venous drainage: correlation between digital subtraction angiography, magnetic resonance imaging, and clinical findings. J Neurosurg Spine 16:433–440
33. Yamaguchi S, Eguchi K, Kiura Y et al (2007) Multidetector-row CT angiography as a preoperative evaluation for spinal arteriovenous fistulae. Neurosurg Rev 30:321–326
34. Berenstein A, Ter Brugge K, Lasjaunias P (2004) Surgical neuroangiography vol. 2: clinical and endovascular treatment aspects in adults. Springer, Berlin
35. Biondi A, Merland JJ, Hodes JE, Pruvo JP, Reizine D (1992) Aneurysms of spinal arteries associated with intramedullary arteriovenous malformations. I. Angiographic and clinical aspects. Am J Neuroradiol 13:913–922
36. Aminoff MJ, Logue V (1974) The prognosis of patients with spinal vascular malformations. Brain 97:211–218
37. Hurth M, Houdart R, Djindjian R et al (1978) Arteriovenous malformations of the spinal cord: clinical, anatomical and therapeutic consideration: a series of 150 cases. Progr Neurol Surg 9:238–266
38. Bostrom A, Krings T, Hans FJ, et al (2009) Spinal glomus-type arteriovenous malformations: microsurgical treatment in 20 cases. J Neurosurg Spine 10:423–429
39. Connolly ES Jr, Zubay GP, McCormick PC et al (1998) The posterior approach to a series of glomus (type II) intramedullary spinal cord arteriovenous malformations. Neurosurgery 42:774–785
40. Corkill RA, Mitsos AP, Molyneux AJ (2007) Embolization of spinal intramedullary arteriovenous malformations using the liquid embolic agent, Onyx: a single center experience in a series of 17 patients. J Neurosurg Spine 7:478–485
41. Sinclair J, Chang SD, Gibbs IC, Adler JR Jr (2006) Multisession CyberKnife radiosurgery for intramedullary spinal cord arteriovenous malformations. Neurosurgery 58:1081–1089
42. Tai PA, Tu YK, Liu HM (2001) Surgical treatment of spinal arteriovenous malformations: vascular anatomy and surgical outcome. J Formos Med Assoc 100:389–396
43. Hida K, Iwasaki Y, Goto K, Miyasaka K, Abe H (1999) Results of the surgical treatment of perimedullary arteriovenous fistulas with special reference to embolization. J Neurosurg 90:198–205
44. Zozulya YP, Slin'ko EI, Al-Qashqish II (2006) Spinal arteriovenous malformations: new classification and surgical treatment. Neurosurg Focus 20:E7
45. Rodesch G, Hurth M, Alvarez H et al (2003) Embolization of spinal cord arteriovenous shunts: morphological and clinical follow-up and results – review of 69 consecutive cases. Neurosurgery 53:40–49
46. McDougall CG, Deshmukh VR, Fiorella DJ et al (2005) Endovascular techniques for vascular malformations of the spinal axis. Neurosurg Clin N Am 16:395–410
47. Gonzalez LF, Zabramski JM, Tabrizi P, Wallace RC, Massand MG, Spetzler RF (2005) Spontaneous spinal subarachnoid hemorrhage secondary to spinal aneurysms: diagnosis and treatment paradigm. Neurosurgery 57:1127–1131
48. Kim LJ, Spetzler RF (2006) Classification and surgical management of spinal arteriovenous lesions: arteriovenous fistulae and arteriovenous malformations. Neurosurgery 59:S195–S201
49. Spetzler RF, Detwiler PW, Riina HA, Porter RW

(2002) Modified classification of spinal cord vascular lesions. J Neurosurg 96:145–156
50. Geibprasert S, Pereira V, Krings T et al (2008) Dural arteriovenous shunts: a new classification of craniospinal epidural venous anatomical bases and clinical correlations. Stroke 39:2783–2794
51. Krings T, Thron AK, Geibprasert S et al (2010) Endovascular management of spinal vascular malformations. Neurosurg Rev 33:1–9
52. Cenzato M, Versari P, Righi C et al (2004) Spinal dural arteriovenous fistulae: analysis of outcome in relation to pretreatment indicators. Neurosurgery 55:815–822
53. Narvid J, Hetts SW, Larsen D, et al (2008) Spinal dural arteriovenous fistulae: clinical features and long-term results. Neurosurgery 62:159–166
54. Konan AV, Raymond J, Roy D (1999) Transarterial embolization of aneurysms associated with spinal cord arteriovenous malformations: report of four cases. J Neurosurg 90:148–154.
55. Biondi A, Merland JJ, Hodes JE, Aymard A, Reizine D (1992) Aneurysms of spinal arteries associated with intramedullary arteriovenous malformations. II. Results of AVM endovascular treatment and hemodynamic considerations. Am J Neuroradiol 13:923–931.

Practical Guidelines for Percutaneous Vertebral Cementoplasty

19

Pedro Nunnes, Vitor Mendes Pereira and Mario Muto

19.1 Introduction

Minimally invasive percutaneous vertebral cementoplasty (PVC) is an interventional neuroradiological procedure. It comprises percutaneous injection of bone cement (usually polymethyl methacrylate (PMMA)) [1–8] in a weakened vertebral body under imaging guidance (computed tomography (CT) or digital subtraction angiography (DSA)). PVC provides mechanical reinforcement and stabilization with or without plastic restoration of the height of the vertebral body, thereby reducing or eliminating pain. There is appreciable scientific consensus (supported by a consensus document published in 2007 [9] that PVC is a successful, safe and effective minimally invasive procedure in selected patients with painful vertebral compressive fractures (VCFs) or microfractures [5–29]. Several case series and retrospective studies have shown statistically significant pain relief and improvement of mobility and function with a consistently high success rate.

Galibert and Deramond were the first to carry out PVC in 1984; it was for treatment of an aggressive cervical vertebral body hemangioma [1–2]. In 1991, Debussche-Depriester reported a series of cases with substantial pain relief in osteoporotic VCFs [3]. Since then, as PVC has grown in popularity worldwide, the importance of restoring vertebral-body height (VBH) and minimizing the associated kyphotic deformity with intrasomatic expandable devices has been recognized. Research has led to several technical improvements.

Restoration of VBH can be achieved with cement injection or by using intrasomatic expandable devices while creating a cavity to be filled with bone cement [31–38]. Both methods have been shown to produce substantial immediate and long-term pain relief and early-improved mobilization with a major positive effect on quality of life (QoL) all with acceptable levels of safety. They are not mutually exclusive procedures, and one may be preferable to the other depending on medical history, etiology of the painful VCFs, age at fracture, vertebral level, and degree of kyphotic deformity. The outcome data for PVC with expandable intrasomatic devices are not as extensive as for PVC without expandable devices. The potential cost-effective benefits and advantages of both procedures are controversial [31–38]. The best long-term outcome of PVC in appropriately selected patients is reliant on the procedure being carried out by physicians experienced in percutaneous interventions with optimal neuroradiological evaluation under the best fluoroscopy guidance available.

M. Muto (✉)
Neuroradiology Department, A. Cardarelli Hospital, Naples, Italy
e-mail: mutomar2@gmail.com

M. Muto (ed.), *Interventional Neuroradiology of the Spine*,
DOI 10.1007/978-88-470-2790-9_19, © Springer-Verlag Italia 2013

19.2 Patient Selection

The major indications for PVC are painful VCFs or microfractures secondary to osteoporosis, trauma, primary bone tumors (e.g., symptomatic hemangioma), secondary bone tumors or hematologic malignancies (e.g., multiple myeloma and lymphoma).

PVC should be proposed in porotic cases to patients with subacute or chronic back pain refractory to a long period (usually 4–8 weeks) of conservative medical therapy. There is no optimal waiting time between onset and the procedure. Most patients would benefit most immediately after the symptomatic fracture, thereby preventing height loss and enabling a prompt return to function with minimal short-term complications.

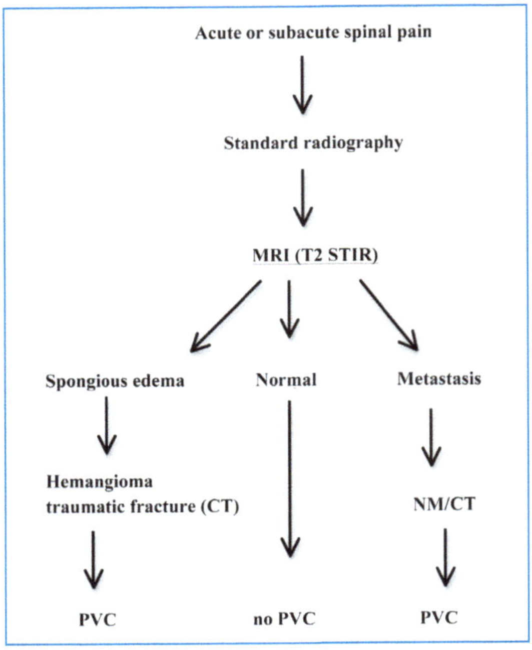

Fig. 19.1 Diagnostic flow-chart for percutaneous vertebral cementoplasty. *CT* computed tomography, *MRI* magnetic resonance imaging, *NM* nuclear medicine, *PVC* percutaneous vertebral cementoplasty, *STIR* short-term inversion recovery

19.3 Clinical Evaluation and General Pre-procedure Considerations

Written informed written consent must be obtained before PVC with a description and discussion of the procedure, expected outcome, and possible complications. Recent hematologic screening with coagulation tests, platelet counts and white blood counts are necessary before the procedure. Osteomyelitis or systemic infections are absolute contraindications for PVC.

Upon physical examination, the anatomical location of the VCF considered for treatment should be consistent with the location of pain. Percussion of the spine usually elicits pain within 1–2 vertebral levels contiguous to the weakened vertebral body. Patients may also complain of referred pain (e.g., referred hip pain due to a lower lumbar fracture) and that should not be considered a contraindication.

The etiology of the disease underlying the painful VCFs (e.g., osteoporosis, trauma, tumoral or hematologic malignancies) must be documented because the fracture characteristics are different, as is the disposition to complications. The degree of kyphotic deformity as determined by imaging should also be documented.

Various standardized questionnaires are available to report patient evaluation, procedure, outcome and complications. Such questionnaires provide standard reporting and archiving of interventional procedures. The visual analog scale (VAS) is a well-established method of documenting pain levels [39–44]. The VAS should be used before and after the procedure. The Oswestry Disability Index (ODI) [40] and Roland Morris Disability Questionnaire [39] are well-established condition-specific outcome measures in the management of low back pain. Short Form-36 (SF36) comprises 36 questions with an eight-scale profile of scores as well as summary measures of physical and mental health [45–46].

19.4 Diagnostic Imaging

Neuroradiological evaluation of painful VFCs with or without kyphotic deformity includes conventional radiographs, magnetic resonance imaging (MRI), CT, or bone scintigraphy (Fig. 19.1).

MRI is the "gold standard" imaging for patient selection. MRI has high sensitivity and specificity for bone-marrow edema (BME) of the affected vertebral body. BME is defined as increased signal intensity on T2 short-term inversion recovery (STIR) sequence and decreased signal intensity on T1-weighted images. BME is presumably the result of microfractures within the medullar bone and the resultant hemorrhage. After 1–3 months, most osteoporotic VCFs become isointense to normal bone on all sequences, which is considered a sign of fracture healing [66]. Decrease in pain intensity after PVC is more frequently observed if BME is fully present [66]. Bone scintigraphy may help in the selection of symptomatic vertebrae amenable to PVC, especially in patients with contraindications to MRI. In such patients, CT evaluation is also important.

19.5 PVC Procedure

19.5.1 Image Guidance

PVC should be carried out under guidance by CT or high-quality fluoroscopy (preferably in DSA units) with real-time control of cement injection. The patient is placed in the prone position for lumbar and thoracic levels and in the supine position for the cervical segment.

19.5.2 Sedation

PVC is a painful procedure. The sedation required is usually dependent upon the overall health and comorbidity of the patient. Most patients can tolerate the procedure under conscious sedation and local anesthesia. However, patients undergoing PVC of the cervical vertebrae, or those with multilevel vertebral disease or poor cardiopulmonary status may require general anesthesia. Antibiotics can be administered intravenously on the day of the procedure to prevent infection according to local protocols.

19.5.3 Needles

A wide spectrum of trocar-cannula systems with multiple shapes, diameters and lengths is available. The choice of needle size may be influenced by the planned approach to the vertebral body. The size of the needle may also affect extravasation along the needle tract (as well as the complications associated with needle placement). A beveled or diamond-shaped tip needle with smaller gauge (10–15 G) is usually preferred. Mono- or bipedicular introductory routes can be used by transpedicular, parapedicular, anterolateral (e.g., in the cervical region) and transoral (C2 vertebral body) approaches.

19.5.4 Cement

PMMA is the most commonly used cement. Many PMMA compositions and other cements are available for PVC. Each type is reliant on its own physical, chemical, and mechanical properties, as well as its viscosity. These properties affect mainly the distribution and handling of cement, which are adjustable at each disease process and for each operator. However, PMMA is not biodegradable and cannot induce the formation of new bone. It becomes a permanent implant that may interfere with the natural remodeling process of bone. Some recently developed bone cements containing calcium phosphate, calcium sulfate hydroxyapatite, as well as composite resins have shown promise not only in terms of bone growth but have also revealed improved physical and biomechanical (osteoconductive and osteoinductive) properties.

The "ideal" cement characteristics should be matched as closely as possible to the biomechanical properties of the bone according to resistance as well as axial and torsion stress capacity, with long working time and good opacification. The mechanism for pain relief is based upon mechanical stabilization of vertebral body fractures or microfractures *via* direct structural reinforcement. Cement polymerization is accompanied by a transient exothermic reaction that may induce tumor necrosis and thermal neurolysis to small peripheral sensory nerve endings.

The amount of cement to be injected has not been established. There is general consensus that there is no clinical advantage in overfilling the vertebral body. Cement diffusion over the fracture and the vertebral body without vascular or extra-body leaks is necessary to provide fracture stabilization with pain relief [47–50].

19.5.5 Osteoporotic Compression Fractures

Osteoporotic VCFs represent a common cause of severe back pain among the elderly. It is estimated that ≤50% of post-menopausal Caucasians will experience an osteoporosis-related fracture in their lifetime [11, 51]. Other subgroups with a significant incidence of fractures include patients receiving long-term corticosteroid therapy, patients with chronic kidney disease, or who are immobilized for a long time. Chronic pain in these individuals typically lasts from 2 weeks to 3 months with secondary physical debilitation, increased susceptibility of short-term complications (e.g., lung atelectasis with a predilection for pneumonia, cardiac failure, deep-vein thrombosis and pulmonary embolism) associated with an overall higher incidence of mortality [9].

In a recent randomized, controlled clinical trial, PVC was shown to be more effective than continued conservative medical therapy (CMT), with superior pain relief, and prompt return of mobility and function to normal activities [30, 31]. CMT is neither benign nor risk-free and, in some cases, may lead to adverse outcomes related to low mobility, immobilization with bed rest, and narcotic anesthesia (particularly in older patients) [9]. In a similarly designed study, patients who received PVC with intrasomatic expandable devices experienced superior improvements in QoL *versus* CMT at one-year follow-up [32]. PVC should be undertaken according to patient status as soon as possible to avoid exacerbation of the kyphotic deformity due to progression of collapse of the vertebral body.

19.5.6 Vertebral Hemangioma

Vertebral hemangiomas are benign lesions typically confined to the vertebral body. They are a common incidental and asymptomatic finding upon imaging. Symptomatic destructive vertebral hemangiomas are rare [52, 53]. The presentation of a painful hemangioma differs between patients. It can include referred pain to progressive neurological deficits related to a fracture, mass effect with compression of the thecal sac or compromise in the neural foraminal space. PVC is the gold-standard therapeutic option for symptomatic hemangiomas without neurologic deficits [1, 54–56]. The best long-term results are achieved if there is complete cement filling of the angiomatous venous network and mechanical stabilization. A decompressive laminectomy can be done afterwards if needed [56].

19.5.7 Metastatic Fractures and Hematologic Malignancies

Metastatic vertebral disease is the most common tumoral disorder of the spine. Patients usually have severe pain secondary to osseous involvement with or without vertebral collapse, mimicking osteoporotic fractures. Therefore, biopsy should always be undertaken in cases of unknown primary tumor, multiple primary neoplasms, or if there is doubt of a secondary localization of the known primary neoplasm. Multidisciplinary discussion is necessary for careful evaluation of the benefits and risks before therapeutic or palliative approaches. Adjunctive PVC can be done in association with radiotherapy or chemotherapy. Some European Oncology Centers advocate PVC as the first-line treatment of painful VCFs related to spinal metastases due to breast cancer before radiotherapy based on an apparent "carcinolytic" effect associated with the exothermal polymerization reaction of PMMA cement.

PVC is a good indication for osteolytic neoplastic vertebral lesions (e.g., metastasis, multiple myeloma, lymphoma), including considerable destruction of the posterior vertebral wall [15, 16]. Some studies have shown that PVC can be used for pure osteoblastic or mixed spinal metastases with satisfactory analgesic efficacy. In these lesions, the cement fills first the lytic zones in the heterogeneous vertebra, including the microfractures that are present in the periphery and sometimes inside pure osteoblastic lesions [45].

Radiofrequency ablation is an adjunctive therapeutic option for selected patients with tumors extending beyond the vertebral wall (infiltrating the surrounding soft tissues and foramina or compressing the spinal cord) without neurologic deficits [57–61]. In these cases, the goal is first to destroy the tumor and secondly provide mechanical reinforcement stabilization with cement injection.

Patients with multiple myeloma are at high risk for VCFs due to osteoporosis, which results simultaneously from the molecular pathophysiology of the disease and frequent use of associated corticosteroid therapy. Most myeloma patients have diffuse and focal bone involvement due to direct invasion by myeloma cells. Specifically, PVC appears to offer rapid and long-lasting treatment of pain in multilevel osteolytic vertebral lesions due to multiple myeloma.

19.5.8 Traumatic Fractures

The use of cementoplasty in patients with traumatic vertebral fractures is complicated by the complexity of the injuries and the multifaceted demographics of the patient population. PVC indication must be evaluated carefully and discussed in a multidisciplinary team depending on clinical status, type of fracture, and comorbidities. Recent traumatic lesions are technically challenging to treat because of the higher risk of cement leakage through compressive or burst fractures and potential vertebral dislodgement.

According to the Magerl classification, PVC should not be used in patients with type-B or type-C fractures. Patients with acute VCFs (Magerl type A1) in the earliest onset of the traumatic event could be proposed for vertebral cementoplasty with intrasomatic expandable devices followed by cement injection [52, 53]. The goal is to restore VBH while creating a cavity in which the cement remains without excessive leakage. In these cases a bilateral approach and preferably high-viscosity cement is recommended. Alternatively, this procedure can be done simultaneously with posterior surgical fixation, reducing the need for second anterior stabilization surgery [52, 53].

19.6 Complications

The prevalence of complications of PVC with or without expandable devices is 1–10% [9]. Some studies report a higher risk of complications in patients with malignant disease (including myeloma and osteolytic metastasis). The major cause is related to leakage of cement (PMMA) beyond the confines of the collapsed vertebral body, through areas of cortical destruction, needle tracks, paravertebral venous complexes, or into the epidural space [9, 47, 48]. Cement leakage is usually asymptomatic without short or long-term consequences and does not require therapy. Other rare complications include: fracture of the pedicle; epidural abscess; paravertebral hematoma; symptomatic pulmonary embolism; cerebrospinal fluid (CSF) leak; increased pain; paraplegia; and death [9, 47, 48]. Symptomatic complications are most likely to occur during or immediately after treatment. An increased risk of vertebral fracture at an adjacent level is contentious [62]. There are presumed differences in leakage rates between PVC with or without expandable intrasomatic devices. There is less leakage in the latter and it is attributed to the cavity creation approach. This is believed to help contain the cement within the vertebral body by sealing osseous defects and venous pathways [63]. Other authors, however, have demonstrated that cement viscosity and injection volume are the critical factors for controlling cement leakage [64].

19.7 Follow-up

Patients must be followed up after PVC at ≥1–2 years. Methodical reporting of patient evaluation, outcome and complications in standardized questionnaires is available. This provides standard data and enables archiving of minimally invasive PVC procedures. The standardized data and experience accumulated over the years are important to improve the quality and relevance of the research reporting of PVC.

Medical treatment in the years after PVC includes the addition of vitamin D and calcium in the diet and using bisphosphonates or new drugs such as parathormone derivatives. The continuous development of new materials and techniques may extend and improve indications and outcomes while maintaining a low prevalence of complications.

19.8 Conclusions

PVC is a safe and useful technique in the treatment of spinal pain. Cement injection can be extended also to extravertebral locations in selected patients. The correct diagnostic clinical and neuroradiological approach is essential to understand which patients will benefit from treatment. Radiological guidance with high-quality fluoroscopy or CT is strongly recommended to avoid complications. Cooperation with endocrinologists, physical therapists, pain therapists, oncologists and neurosurgeons is required to obtain the best results.

References

1. Galibert P, Deramond H, Rosat P et al (1987) Note préliminaire sur le traitement des angiomes vertébraux par vertebroplastie percutanée. Neurochirurgie 33:166–168
2. Deramond H, Darrason R, Galibert P (1989) Percutaneous vertebroplasty with acrylic cement in the treatment of aggressive spinal angiomas. Rachis 1:143–153
3. Debussche-Depriester C, Deramond H, Fardellone P et al (1991) Percutaneous vertebroplasty with acrylic cement in the treatment of osteoporotic vertebral crush fracture syndrome. Neuroradiology 33 (Suppl):149–152
4. Jensen ME, Evans AE, Mathis JM et al (1997) Percutaneous polymethylmethacrylate vertebroplasty in the treatment of osteoporotic vertebral body compression fractures: technical aspects. Am J Neuroradiol 18:1897–1904
5. Deramond H, Depriester C, Galibert P et al (1989) Percutaneous vertebroplasty with polymethylmethacrylate: technique, indications and results. Radiol Clin North Am 36:533–546
6. Cotten A, Boutry N, Cortet B et al (1998) Percutaneous vertebroplasty: state of the art. Radiographics 18:311–320
7. Barr JD, Mathis JM, Barr MS et al (2001) Standard for the performance of percutaneous vertebroplasty. American College of Radiology Standards 2000–2001. American College of Radiology, Reston, pp 441–448
8. McGraw JK, Cardella JC, Barr JD et al (2003) Quality improvement guidelines for percutaneous vertebroplasty. J Vasc Interv Radiol 14:827831
9. Jensen ME, McGraw JK, Cardella JF, Hirsch JA (2007) Position statement on percutaneous vertebral augmentation: a consensus statement developed by the American Society of Interventional and Therapeutic Neuroradiology, Society of Interventional Radiology, American Association of Neurological Surgeons/Congress of Neurological Surgeons, and American Society of Spine Radiology. Am J Neuroradiol 28:1439–1443
10. American College of Radiology (2009) Practice guideline for the performance of percutaneous vertebroplasty. ACR Practice Guidelines revised 2009 (resolution 25). American College of Radiology, Reston
11. Radvany MG, Murphy KJ, Millward SF et al (2009) Research reporting standards for percutaneous vertebral augmentation. J Vasc Interv Radiol 20:1279–1286
12. Kaemmerlen P, Thiesse P, Bouvard H et al (1989) Vertébroplastie percutanée dans le traitement des métastases: technique et résultats. J Radiol 70:557–562
13. Nguyen JP, Djindjian M, Pavlovitch JM et al (1989) Vertebral hemangioma with neurologic signs: therapeutic results—survey of the French Society of Neurosurgery. Neurochirurgie 35:299–303 and 305–308
14. Gangi A, Kastler BA, Dietemann JL (1994) Percutaneous vertebroplasty guided by a combination of CT and fluoroscopy. Am J Neuroradiol 15:83–86
15. Cotten A, Dewatre F, Cortet B et al (1996) Percutaneous vertebroplasty for osteolytic metastases and myeloma: effects of the percentage of lesion filling and the leakage of methyl methacrylate at clinical follow-up. Radiology 200:525–530
16. Weill A, Chiras J, Simon J et al (1996) Spinal metastases: indications for and results of percutaneous injection of acrylic cement. Radiology 199:241–247
17. Barr JD, Barr MS, Lemley TJ et al (2000) Percutaneous vertebroplasty for pain relief and spinal stabilization. Spine 25:923–928
18. Martin JB, Jean B, Sugiu K et al (1999) Vertebroplasty: clinical experience and follow- up results. Bone 25:11S–15S
19. Kaufmann TJ, Jensen ME, Schweickert PA et al (2001) Age of fracture and clinical outcomes of percutaneous vertebroplasty. *Am J Neuroradiol* 22:1860–1863
20. Evans AJ, Jensen ME, Kip KE et al (2003) Vertebral

compression fractures: pain reduction and improvement in functional mobility after percutaneous polymethylmethacrylate vertebroplasty—retrospective report of 245 cases. Radiology 226:366–372

21. Muto M, Muto E, Izzo R, Diano AA, Lavanga A, Di Furia U (2005) Vertebroplasty in the treatment of back pain. Radiol Med109:208–219
22. Heini PF, Walchli B, Berlemann U (2000) Percutaneous transpedicular vertebroplasty with PMMA: operative technique and early results—a prospective study for the treatment of osteoporotic compression fractures. Eur Spine J 9:445–450
23. McGraw JK, Lippert JA, Minkus KD et al (2002) Prospective evaluation of pain relief in 100 patients undergoing percutaneous vertebroplasty: results and follow-up. J Vasc Interv Radiol 13:883–886
24. Zoarski GH, Snow P, Olan WJ et al (2002) Percutaneous vertebroplasty for osteoporotic compression fractures: quantitative prospective evaluation of long-term outcomes. J Vasc Interv Radiol 13:139–148
25. Diamond TH, Champion B, Clark WA (2003) Management of acute osteoporotic vertebral fractures: a non-randomized trial comparing percutaneous vertebroplasty with conservative therapy. Am J Med 114:257–265
26. Do HM, Marcellus ML, Weir RU et al (2002) Percutaneous vertebroplasty versus medical therapy for treatment of acute vertebral body compression fractures: a prospective randomized study. Proceedings of the Annual Meeting of the American Society of Neuroradiology, Vancouver
27. Kallmes DF, Comstock BA, Heagerty PJ et al (2009) A randomized trial of vertebroplasty for osteoporotic spinal fractures. N Engl J Med 361:569–579
28. Buchbinder R, Osborne RH, Ebeling PR et al (2009) A randomized trial of vertebroplasty for painful osteoporotic vertebral fractures. N Engl J Med 361:557–568
29. Rousing R, Andersen MO, Jespersen SM (2009) Percutaneous vertebroplasty compared to conservative treatment in patients with painful acute or subacute osteoporotic vertebral fractures: three-months follow-up in a clinical randomized study. Spine 34:1349–1354
30. Voormolen MH, Mali WP, Lohle PN (2007) Percutaneous vertebroplasty compared with optimal pain medication treatment: short-term clinical outcome of patients with subacute or chronic painful osteoporotic vertebral compression fractures. The VERTOS study. Am J Neuroradiol 28:555–560
31. Venmans A, Klazen CA, Lohle PN, Mali WP, van Rooij WJ (2012) Natural history of pain in patients with conservatively treated osteoporotic vertebral compression fractures: Results from VERTOS II. *Am J Neuroradiol* 33:519–521
32. Wardlaw D, Cummings SR, Van Meirhaeghe J et al (2009) Efficacy and safety of balloon kyphoplasty compared with non-surgical care for vertebral compression fracture (FREE): a randomised controlled trial. *Lancet* 373:1016–1024
33. Feltes C, Fountas KN, Machinis T et al (2005) Immediate and early postoperative pain relief after kyphoplasty without significant restoration of vertebral body height in acute osteoporotic vertebral fractures. Neurosurg Focus 18:e5
34. Kasperk C, Hillmeier J, Noldge G et al (2005) Treatment of painful vertebral fractures by kyphoplasty in patients with primary osteoporosis: a prospective nonrandomized controlled study. J Bone Miner Res 20:604–612
35. Gaitanis IN, Hadjipavlou AG, Katonis PG et al (2005) Balloon kyphoplasty for the treatment of pathological vertebral compressive fractures. Eur Spine J 14:250–260
36. Berlemann U, Franz T, Orler R et al (2004) Kyphoplasty for treatment of osteoporotic vertebral fractures: a prospective non-randomized study. Eur Spine J 13:496–501
37. Fribourg D, Tang C, Sra P et al (2004) Incidence of subsequent vertebral fracture after kyphoplasty. Spine 29:2270–2276 (discussion 2277)
38. Majd ME, Farley S, Holt RT (2005) Preliminary outcomes and efficacy of the first 360 consecutive kyphoplasties for the treatment of painful osteoporotic vertebral compression fractures. Spine J 5:244–255
39. Fairbank JC, Pynsent PB (2000) The Oswestry Disability Index. Spine 15:25:2940–2952 (discussion 2952)
40. Bombardier C. (2000) Outcome assessments in the evaluation of treatment of spinal disorders: summary and general recommendations. Spine 25:3100–3103
41. Mousavi SJ, Parnianpour M, Mehdian H, Montazeri A, Mobini B (2006) The Oswestry Disability Index, the Roland–Morris Disability Questionnaire, and the Quebec Back Pain Disability Scale: translation and validation studies of the Iranian versions. Spine 31:E454–E459
42. Calmels P, Béthoux F, Condemine A, Fayolle-Minon I (2005) Low back pain disability assessment tools. Ann Readapt Med Phys 48:288–297
43. DeLoach LJ, Higgins MS, Caplan AB, Stiff JL (1998) The visual analog scale in the immediate postoperative period: intrasubject variability and correlation with a numeric scale. Anesth Analg 86:102–106
44. Bodian CA, Freedman G, Hossain S, Eisenkraft JB, Beilin Y (2001) The visual analog scale for pain: clinical significance in postoperative patients. Anesthesiology 95:1356–1361
45. Calmels V, Vallée JN Rose M, Chiras J (2007) Osteoblastic and mixed spinal metastases: evaluation of the analgesic efficacy of percutaneous vertebroplasty. Am J Neuroradiol 28:570–574
46. Shiely JC, Bayliss MS, Keller SD et al (1996) SF-36 health survey annotated bibliography: first edition (1988–1995). New England Medical Center, Boston
47. Nussbaum DA, Gailloud P, Murphy K (2004) A review of complications associated with vertebroplasty and kyphoplasty as reported to the food and drug administration medical device related website. J Vasc Interv Radiol 15:1185–1192

48. Choe DH, Marom EM, Ahrar K et al (2004) Pulmonary embolism of polymethyl methacrylate during percutaneous vertebroplasty and kyphoplasty. Am J Roentgenol 183:1097–1102
49. Lim TH, Breback GT, Renner SM et al (2002) Biomechanical evaluation of an injectable calcium phosphate cement for vertebroplasty. Spine 27:1297–1302
50. Lieberman IH, Togawa D, Kayanja MM (2005) Vertebroplasty and kyphoplasty: filler materials. Spine J 5 (Suppl):S305–S316
51. Siris ES, Brenneman SK, Barrett-Connor E et al (2006) The effect of age and bone mineral density on the absolute, excess, and relative risk of fracture in postmenopausal women aged 50-99: results from the National Osteoporosis Risk Assessment (NORA). Osteoporos Int 17:565–574
52. Anselmetti GC, Bonaldi G, Carpeggiani P, Manfré L, Masala S, Muto M (2010) Vertebral augmentation: 7 years experience. ACTA Neurochirurgica Supplementum 108:147–161
53. Muto M, Perrotta V, Guarnieri G et al (2008) Vertebroplasty and kyphoplasty: friends or foes? Radiol Med 113:1171–1184
54. Callstrom MR, Charboneau JW (2007) Image-guided palliation of painful metastases using percutaneous ablation. Tech Vasc Interv Radiol 10:120–131
55. Simon CJ, Dupuy DE (2006) Percutaneous minimally invasive therapies in the treatment of bone tumours: thermal ablation. Semin Musculoskelet Radiol 10:137–144
56. Schaefer O, Lohrmann C, Markmiller M, Uhrmeister P, Langer M (2003) Technical innovation. Combined treatment of a spinal metastasis with radiofrequency heat ablation and vertebroplasty. Am J Roentgenol 180:1075–1077
57. Callstrom MR, Atwell TD, Charboneau JW et al (2006) Painful metastases involving bone: percutaneous image-guided cryoablation–prospective trial interim analysis. Radiology 241:572–580
58. Geogy BA, Wong W (2007) Plasma-mediated radiofrequency ablation assisted percutaneous cement injection for treating advanced malignant vertebral compression fractures. Am J Neuroradiol 28:700–705
59. Fox M, Onofrio B (1993) The natural history and management of symptomatic and asymptomatic vertebral hemangiomas. J Neurosurg 78:36–45
60. Acosta FL, Christopher FD (2006) Current strategies and outcomes in management of symptomatic vertebral hemangiomas. Neurosurgery 58:287–295
61. Guarnieri G, Ambrosanio G, Vassallo P et al (2009) Vertebroplasty as treatment of aggressive and symptomatic vertebral hemangiomas: up to 4 years of follow-up. Neuroradiology 51:471–476
62. Guarnieri G, Ambrosanio G, Pezzullo MG et al (2009) Management of vertebral re-fractures after vertebroplasty in osteoporotic patients. Interv Neuroradiol 29:153–157
63. Pateder DB, Khanna AJ, Lieberman IH (2007) Vertebroplasty and kyphoplasty for the management of osteoporotic vertebral compression fractures. Orthop Clin North Am 38:409–418; Abstract vii
64. Gregory BA (2010) Clinical experience with high viscosity cements for percutaneous vertebral body augmentation: occurrence, degree, and location of cement leakage compared with kyphoplasty. Am J Neuroradiol 31:504–508

Index

M. Muto (ed.), *Interventional Neuroradiology of the Spine*,
DOI 10.1007/978-88-470-2790-9, © Springer-Verlag Italia 2013

MIX
Papier aus verantwortungsvollen Quellen
Paper from responsible sources
FSC® C105338

If you have any concerns about our products,
you can contact us on
ProductSafety@springernature.com

In case Publisher is established outside the EU,
the EU authorized representative is:
Springer Nature Customer Service Center GmbH
Europaplatz 3, 69115 Heidelberg, Germany

Printed by Libri Plureos GmbH
in Hamburg, Germany